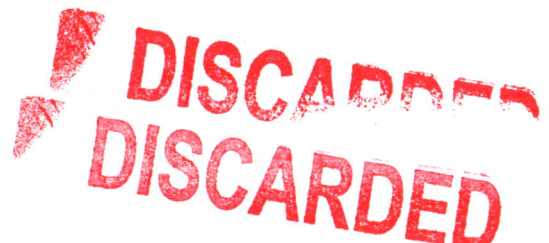

# Filling-In

# Filling-In

## From Perceptual Completion to Cortical Reorganization

*Edited by*

LUIZ PESSOA
PETER DE WEERD

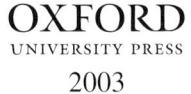

UNIVERSITY PRESS
2003

# OXFORD
UNIVERSITY PRESS

Oxford   New York
Auckland   Bangkok   Buenos Aires   Cape Town   Chennai
Dar es Salaam   Delhi   Hong Kong   Istanbul   Karachi   Kolkata
Kuala Lumpur   Madrid   Melbourne   Mexico City   Mumbai
Nairobi   São Paulo   Shanghai   Taipei   Tokyo   Toronto

Copyright © 2003 by Oxford University Press, Inc.

Published by Oxford University Press, Inc.
198 Madison Avenue, New York, New York, 10016
http://www.oup-usa.org

Oxford is a registered trademark of Oxford University Press

All rights reserved. No part of this publication may be reproduced,
stored in a retrieval system, or transmitted, in any form or by any means,
electronic, mechanical, photocopying, recording, or otherwise,
without the prior permission of Oxford University Press.

Library of Congress Cataloging-in-Publication Data
Filling-in : from perceptual completion to cortical reorganization /
edited by Luiz Pessoa, Peter De Weerd.
p. ; cm.   Includes bibliographical references and index.
ISBN 0-19-514013-3
1. Visual cortex.   2. Visual perception.
3. Senses and sensation.
I. Pessoa, Luiz.   II. De Weerd, Peter.
[DNLM:   1. Perceptual Closure.   2. Form Perception.
3. Perception—physiology.
WW 105 F486 2003]   QP383.15.F55 2003   612.8'4—dc21   2002074922

2 4 6 8 9 7 5 3 1

Printed in the United States of America
on acid-free paper

*To my family,
Djalma, Mariluce, Cristiana,
and Maria Clara
and Arezou
(L.P.)*


*To my family,
especially my parents,
my brother Wim,
and my sister Veerle
and Scotia
(P.D.W.)*

# Preface

There is a long tradition in perceptual psychology in which investigators study perceptual illusions with the goal of gaining insight into normal mechanisms of perception. To a certain extent, the present book adheres to that tradition, and applies it to the topic of "perceptual filling-in," an illusion resulting from the filling-in of information that is not directly given in the sensory input. In this book, however, we suggest that studying the neural mechanisms underlying perceptual filling-in can provide us with insights that have implications beyond the domain of perception.

A well-known example of perceptual filling-in is the visual filling-in of edges, contours and surfaces across the retinal blind spot. However, there are a variety of other types of filling-in in different sensory systems, and in addition to types of filling-in that reflect the normal functioning of the sensory system, others follow peripheral or central damage. Are there common principles underlying these filling-in phenomena? How are they related to each other? One of us approached these questions from a sensory, perceptual, and computational point of view (LP). The other considered that the neuronal processes underlying filling-in could provide a new perspective on plasticity in the brain (PDW). The balance between both viewpoints resulted in a book with insights from a number of research traditions in different sensory systems and the motor system, which have been combined to yield, we believe, a well-integrated and unique volume on the topic of filling-in. A central, integrative thesis is that the neural processes that underlie filling-in under some circumstances can contribute to significant, long-term reorganization in the adult brain.

This book targets a number of audiences. In Part I, readers with an interest in mechanisms of filling-in in the more classical (perceptual) sense will find an up-to-date overview of current neurophysiological and psychophysical data, as well as computational approaches. Readers with an interest in the reorganization of the brain after injury, and in the effects of skill learning and behavioral therapy on such reorganization, may choose to focus their attention on Parts II and III. Readers with a theoretical interest in the principles that bridge the seemingly disparate topics of perceptual filling-in, reorganization after injury, skill learning, and attention will enjoy reading the entire book. Although the volume has been structured to maximize integration between its different chapters, each chapter is a self-contained unit that can be read separately. The chapters contain up-to-date materials and new viewpoints that will be enjoyed by investigators in the different research fields covered in this book. At the same time, there is sufficient background information in the Introduction and in each chapter to make most of this volume accessible to beginning graduate students and advanced undergraduate students with a minimal background in cognitive neuroscience. Hence, *Filling-In* can provide exciting material for a number of courses in cognitive neuroscience on the topics of perceptual illusions, skill learning, recovery after injury to sensory and motor systems, and principles of neural plasticity.

Our desire to produce a streamlined book has led to intense and prolonged exchanges with many of our contributors. We thoroughly enjoyed these enriching and stimulating interactions, and we appreciate the thought and care that has been invested in each of the chapters. We hope that the result of our collective efforts will be enjoyed by many in the field of cognitive neuroscience! In addition, we would like to thank Fiona Stevens from Oxford University Press for being enthusiastic about this project from the beginning and for keeping our schedule not too far from target. We would also like to acknowledge Nancy Wolitzer, also from Oxford University Press, for her expert assistance in the final production stages of the book. Finally, we are grateful to Professor V.S. Ramachandran for a stimulating Foreword to our book.

| | |
|---|---:|
| *Tucson, Arizona* | P.D.W. |
| *Bethesda, Maryland* | L.P. |

# Contents

Foreword, xi
*V.S. Ramachandran*

Contributors, xxiii

Chapter 1. Introduction: Filling-In: More Than Meets the Eye, 1
*Peter De Weerd and Luiz Pessoa*

Part I  Fast-Acting Filling-In in Normal Vision

Chapter 2. Filling-In the Forms: Surface and Boundary Interactions in Visual Cortex, 13
*Stephen Grossberg*

Chapter 3. Contextual Shape Processing in Human Visual Cortex: Beginning to Fill-In the Blanks, 38
*Janine Mendola*

Chapter 4. Surface Completion: Psychophysical and Neurophysiological Studies of Brightness, 59
*Andrew F. Rossi and Michael A. Paradiso*

Chapter 5. Mechanisms of Surface Completion: Perceptual Filling-In of Texture, 81
*Lothar Spillman and Peter De Weerd*

Chapter 6. Searching for the Neural Mechanism for Color Filling-In, 106
*Rüdiger von der Heydt, Howard S. Friedman, and Hong Zhou*

Chapter 7. Effects of Modal versus Amodal Completion Upon Visual Attention: A Function for Filling-In? 128
*Greg Davis and Jon Driver*

Chapter 8. Completion Phenomena in Vision: A Computational Approach, 151
*Heiko Neumann*

## Part II  From Permanent Scotomas to Cortical Reorganization

Chapter 9. Completion Through a Permanent Scotoma: Fast Interpolation Across the Blind Spot and the Processing of Occulsion, 177
*Mario Fiorani, Jr., Leticia de Oliveira, Eliane Volchan, Luiz Pessoa, Ricardo Gattass, and Carlos Eduardo Rocha-Miranda*

Chapter 10. The Reactivation and Reorganization of Retinotopic Maps in Visual Cortex of Adult Mammals After Retinal and Cortical Lesions, 187
*Jon H. Kaas, Christine E. Collins, and Yuzo M. Chino*

Chapter 11. The Blind Leading the Mind: Pathological Visual Completion in Hemianopia and Spatial Neglect, 207
*Jason B. Mattingley and Robin Walker*

## Part III  Long-Term Cortical Remapping

Chapter 12. Plasticity of the Human Auditory Cortex, 231
*Christo Pantev, Nathan Weisz, Michael Schulte, and Thomas Elbert*

Chapter 13. Plasticity in Adult M1 Cortex During Motor Skill Learning, 252
*Julien Doyon and Leslie G. Ungerleider*

Chapter 14. Cortical Reorganization and the Rehabilitation of Movement by CI Therapy After Neurological Injury, 281
*Victor W. Mark and Edward Taub*

Chapter 15. Conclusion: Contributions of Inhibitory Mechanisms to Perceptual Completion and Cortical Reorganization, 295
*Liisa A. Tremere, Raphael Pinaud, and Peter De Weerd*

Index, 323

# Foreword

## V.S. RAMACHANDRAN

The manner in which the brain deals with undersampled regions of the visual field—for example, the blind spot—is potentially of great interest to perceptual psychologists, neurophysiologists, artificial intelligence researchers, and even philosophers. The phenomenon of *filling in* was first noticed by Sir David Brewster in the nineteenth century but was largely ignored as being little more than a curiosity. During the past 10 years, however, there has been a revival of interest in the topic, mainly because of a convergence of ideas from visual psychophysics (*artificial scotomas*), single-unit neurophysiology (demonstrating dynamic changes in receptive fields) and computational modeling. This resurgence of interest was also fueled partly by a fruitful exchange of ideas between philosophers and neuroscientists, something that happens very rarely (e.g., see Dennett, 1991; Churchland and Ramachandran, 1993). This book, compiled and edited by Pessoa and De Weerd, represents a culmination of the interactions between these various research disciplines and fills in a much needed gap in the field.

## Scotomas: Finding Out About Filling-In

My own interest in scotomas began over two decades ago when, as a student of neurology, I encountered patients with focal lesions in the visual cortex. Such patients usually have a scotoma—a region in the visual field within which nothing can be consciously perceived (Weiskrantz et al., 1974). Remarkably, the patients themselves are often unaware of this gaping hole in the visual field. When they look at a colored wall or a regular pattern of any kind (e.g., a carpet or a tile floor), the scotoma gets *filled in* by the surrounding color or pattern. Or if they gaze at a companion seen against a background of wallpaper, the companion's head may vanish and be *replaced* by the wallpaper pattern. According to folklore, King Charles II used to decapitate his ladies-in-waiting using this benign procedure, although he used his natural blind spot rather than a scotoma. Of the natural blind spot (corresponding to the optic nerve head), Sir David Brewster (1832) has written: "We should expect, whether we use one or both eyes, to see a black or dark spot upon every landscape within 10 degrees of the point which most particularly attracts our notice. The Divine Artificer, however, has not left his work thus imperfect . . . the spot, in place of being black has always the same color as the ground." Curiously, Sir David was apparently not troubled by the question of why the "Divine Artificer" should have created an imperfect eye to begin with!

Does the filling in of scotomas involve *referring* a sensory representation of the surrounding pattern to the region of the scotoma in a manner loosely analogous to what we have seen for phantom limbs (Ramachandran and Hirstein, 1998)? Or is there simply a failure to notice the absence of signals from this region of the visual field? Indeed, is the phenomenon any more mysterious than the fact that we do not ordinarily notice the gap behind our heads? This distinction comes perilously close to being a philosophical one, but it isn't. It is one of the many issues dealt with in this stimulating and wide-ranging book.

## *Artificial Scotomas*

To investigate filling-in, Richard Gregory and I (1991) created what we called an *artificial scotoma*, using a twinkling pattern of dots that resembles the "snow" seen on a detuned television set. You can repeat our experiment by using your own television set at home. Pick a channel on which you can see only snow. In the middle of the screen, stick a small circular gummed label with a tiny black dot in its center. The purpose of the black dot is to ensure steady fixation. About 7 or 8 cm from this dot, stick a 1 cm square piece of gray paper (pick a shade of gray that has roughly the same mean luminance as the twinkle on the television screen). If you view the display from a distance of about 1 m and fixate the central dot very steadily for 5 to 10 seconds, you will find that the square vanishes completely and is replaced by the twinkle invading from the surround. Most people are astonished the first time they see the square vanish. The filling-in with the twinkle is obviously analogous to the filling-in of scotomas and blind spots and may be based, in part, on similar neural mechanisms.

But what causes the square to fade in the first place? The effect is vaguely reminiscent of Troxler fading, the tendency for small stationary objects in the peripheral visual field to disappear completely on steady, prolonged fixation. However, unlike Troxler fading, the effect that we have observed cannot be due to local adaptation to the luminance edges that define the square because these edges are being refreshed constantly on the screen. Indeed, the fading is actually enhanced if a dynamic noise background, that is, two-dimensional noise, is used.

De Weerd et al. (1995) and Gilbert and Wiesel (1992) have carried out ingenious experiments in which they investigated the neurophysiological mechanisms contributing to perceptual filling-in. In essence, they found that neurons with their classical receptive field confined inside an artificial scotoma, and surrounded by dynamic texture, become responsive to the texture outside their receptive field within minutes or even seconds. These observations are important for two reasons. First, they imply that the classical receptive field is just the tip of the iceberg and that ongoing visual stimulation can change even the basic structure of the receptive field by disinhibiting silent surrounds (I suggest that receptive fields henceforth be called *deceptive fields*). Second, this observation provides a neat explanation for perceptual filling-in. Since these cells were originally responding to stimuli inside the scotoma, perhaps higher brain centers are "fooled" into "thinking" that stimuli immediately outside the scotoma are now inside it (see Kapadia et al., 1994, for a stimulating discussion). This idea points out that filling-in can be considered a (temporary) remapping of the visual field on the cortex. This has surprising implications, which are explored in the second and third parts of this book.

## *Scotomas of Cortical Origin*

So far, I have considered the filling of artificial scotomas, but do similar principles hold also for scotomas caused by cortical damage? The resulting filling-in phenomenon is usually taken for granted by clinical neurologists, even though in one of the few systematic studies on this topic, the very existence of the phenomenon has been questioned. Sergent (1988), for example, presented semicircles and other geometric figures to patients with hemianopia (blindness in an entire half of the visual field) and commissurotomy (*split brain*). Common knowledge predicted that partial figures presented in the seeing hemifield might be completed in the blind hemifield, but Sergent (1988) found no evidence that this actually occurred. More recently, Dennett and Kinsbourne (1992) have argued, on philosophical grounds, that filling-in does not really occur, and may merely amount to an inappropriate metaphor that requires the assumption of an audience in a Cartesian theater. To resolve these issues empirically, Diane Rogers-Ramachandran, Hanna Damasio, and I examined two patients who had damage to the right occipital pole (visual cortex) producing a small 6 degree diameter scotoma to the immediate left of the center of gaze. The scotoma was of relatively recent onset (about 8 months) in both patients and was caused by lesions in the posterior poles of the right occipital lobe (Ramachandran, 1992a, 1992b, 1993; Ramachandran and Blakeslee, 1998). To begin with, we presented the two halves of a vertical white line on either side of the scotoma and found that the line was completed but, intriguingly, the process took 4 or 5 seconds to occur. (A time delay of this kind is never seen for bridging lines across the natural blind spot.) Furthermore, when the lines were switched off after completion had occurred, one of the two patients reported that he could clearly see a persisting white phantom of the completed part of the line lingering inside the scotoma for several seconds. Instead of using a continuous vertical line, what would happen if one used a more complex pattern, such as a vertical column of X's? Would the subject then actually see X's inside the scotoma? To our surprise, both subjects reported that this was indeed the case—especially when the X's were sufficiently small (0.3 degree). If the X's were large (>1 degree), however, they were clearly reported to be missing from the region of the scotoma. This failure to complete the large X's is important, for it implies that the other completion effects observed in these patients are probably not confabulatory in origin (and that even though you can guess that there is a large X inside the scotoma, you don't fill in large X's in the way you do small ones). We then presented an illusory vertical strip (defined by a gap in a set of parallel horizontal lines) to patient R.J. so that it passed through the region corresponding to his scotoma. Interestingly, he reported completion of the illusory strip rather than completion of the horizontal lines (Ramachandran, 1992b, 1993), which we also observed for the natural blind spot (Ramachandran, 1992a). When we used a field of flickering red dots, the red color seemed to bleed into the scotoma and fill it completely first, so that it looked homogeneously red for several seconds before it became filled-in with the pattern as well. These remarkable effects suggest that mechanisms for the filling-in of colors, motion, and texture can be dissociated, and may correspond to processes in higher-order areas that are specialized for these attributes. Finally, we presented a square or a circle to one of the patients (B.M.) so that a portion of the figure fell inside the scotoma. When one corner of the square was inside the scotoma, he initially reported that the corner was missing, but he claimed that it emerged gradually over a period of 6 or 7 seconds. Similar gradual completion occurred when an arc of a circle fell on the scotoma. The effect occurred whether or not the relevant part of the figure (corner of the square or arc of the circle) was deleted physically from the display. These effects contrast sharply with observations on the natural blind spot. When the corner of a square or an arc of a small circle falls on the blind spot, no perceptual completion occurs (Ramachandran, 1992b, 1993; see below). Why is there a difference? One possibility is that there is a normal patch of visual cortical cells in area 17 in the region corresponding to the blind-spot cells that receive input from the other eye. These cells could signal the absence of a corner or arc, thereby preventing perceptual completion by higher extrastriate visual areas. (This argument holds whether or not the other eye is closed.) In patient B.M., however, the relevant part of area 17 is simply missing, and in the absence of conflicting signals, higher visual areas are allowed to complete the figure without interference. Taken collectively, these findings suggest that the visual system uses information from the region surrounding the scotoma to interpolate perceptually across the gap, and the process seems very different from (say) your failure to notice the gap behind your head. Can the same be said for filling-in of the natural blind spot?

## *Filling-In the Blind Spot*

What types of patterns can be completed across the blind spot? How sophisticated is the process? What are the spatial and temporal constraints on the process? And what does it have in common with other types of perceptual interpolation, such as the filling-in of artificial scotomas and scotomas of cortical origin, and amodal completion? With some simple experimentation (which the reader can carry out using a felt pen and a piece of paper), it can be shown that straight lines are completed readily across the blind spot but that there are clear limits to this filling-in process (Ramachandran, 1992a, 1992b, 1993). For example, if you aim the blind spot on the corner of a square or the arc of a small circle, these figures do not appear complete. They are clearly chopped off by the blind spot (Ramachandran, 1992, 1993). This means that the filling-in of the blind spot is a primitive process that occurs at a relatively early stage in visual processing. What if there are two separate orthogonal lines running through the blind spot, one black and the other white? Would you see a grayish smear at the center of the cross? If you try this experiment, you will find that the two lines compete for completion. Typically, the line you are paying attention to seems to be complete and seems to partially occlude the other line. If the two lines are of unequal length, however, the longer line seems to be completed more readily than the shorter one. These observations are important, for they imply that the filling-in mechanism uses information from an extended distance, rather than just from the area immediately surrounding the blind spot, and that filling-in can be influenced by attention. These topics are explored further in quite original ways in several chapters in the first part of this book.

## What Exactly Does "Filling-In" Mean?

As I have emphasized in previous papers (e.g., Churchland and Ramachandran, 1993; Ramachandran, 1993), I use the term *filling-in* in a strictly metaphorical sense. I certainly do not wish to imply that there is a pixel-by-pixel rendering of the visual image or some internal neural screen (or Cartesian theater) and am in complete agreement with Dennett's views on this issue (Dennett, 1992). I disagree, however, with his specific claim that there is no *neural machinery* corresponding to the blind spot. (There is, in fact, a patch of cortex corresponding to each eye's blind spot that receives input from the other eye as well as from the region surrounding the blind spot in the same eye; see Fiorani et al., 1992; Churchland and Ramachandran, 1993; Ramachandran, 1993.) There is, however, so much confusion associated with the exact meaning of *filling-in* that I would like to take this opportunity to clarify the term. What I mean by *filling-in* is simply this: that one quite literally sees visual stimuli (e.g., patterns or colors) as arising from a region of the visual field where there is actually no visual input. This statement applies to both blind spot filling-in and filling-in of artificial scotomas (an analogous definition can be provided for cortical scotomas). In neural terms, this means that a set of neurons is being activated in such a way that a visual stimulus is perceived as arising from a location in the visual field where there is, in fact, no visual stimulus. This is a purely descriptive theory-neutral definition of filling-in, and one does not have to invoke—or debunk—little homunculi watching screens or Cartesian theaters, or whatever, to accept this definition.

## Blind Spot Filling-In: Similarities with Amodal Completion

Obviously, it is very unlikely that the visual system has evolved dedicated neural machinery for the specific purpose of filling-in the blind spot. What we are seeing here, instead, may be a manifestation of a very general visual process—one that we call *surface interpolation* (Ramachandran, 1992a, 1992b, 1993). Hence the process may have much in common with—and may show some of the same neural machinery as—certain other types of perceptual filling-in such as the perceptual continuity of occluded objects (amodal completion, Kanizsa, 1979). If this conjecture is correct, then it would be instructive to look for similarities and differences between blind spot completion and a variety of other perceptual completion effects that have been reported in the literature (e.g., cortical scotomas, artificial scotomas, illusory contours, amodal completion). There are clearly similarities between amodal completion (i.e., completion behind occluders) and blind spot filling-in. For example, one can readily see continuity of lines behind occluders and perhaps continuity of some types of visual textures as well. Even the "lining up" of noncollinear line segments seems to occur behind occluders in peripheral vision (Durgin et al., 1995), just as it does across the blind spot and scotomas (Lettvin, 1976; Ramachandran, 1992a, 1992b, 1993). There are, however, important differences between completion across the blind spot and amodal completion, which implies that although the two processes are similar, they are not identical, contrary to the views of Durgin et al. (1995). For example, pigs and lizards are similar—they are both vertebrates—but we certainly wouldn't say that therefore they must be identical. The most important difference, of course, is that filling-in across the blind spot is modal, whereas filling-in behind occluders is, by definition, amodal (to use Kanizsa's terminology). What this means is simply that in one case you literally see the filled-in section; in the other case, you don't. This is not a distinction that will appeal to behaviorists, but it should be obvious to anyone who has looked at these displays and is not wholly devoid of common sense. Another important difference is that the corner of a square or the arc of a circle will be completed amodally behind an occluder, but it will not be completed modally across the blind spot (Ramachandran, 1992, 1993). Some evidence for common aspects of a neural mechanism underlying modal and amodal completion comes from the work of Fiorani et al. (1992), reviewed in Chapter 9 of this book. They found that a neuron in the patch of area 17 corresponding to (say) the left eye's blind spot responds not only to the right eye (as expected) but also to two collinear line segments lying on either side of the left eye's blind spot—as though it was filling-in this segment. Remarkably, this neural correlate of filling-in could sometimes be seen in the rest of the normal visual field if an occluder was used instead of the blind spot. The implication is that, at least in the early stages of processing, both modal completion across the blind spot and amodal completion behind occluders may be based on similar neural mechanisms. But if so, why is there such a compelling phenomenological difference between the two? One possibility is that the presence of the occluder itself (as indicated by T-junctions, for example) might be signaled by a different set of neurons that vetoes the modal completion. The net result may be a total pattern of neural activity that is different from modal completion, although there may be a shared subset of neurons that is active in both cases (Ramachandran, 1993). The results of Driver and colleagues (Chapter 7 of this book) are consistent with this idea.

## Filling-In: A Solution to the Riddle of Qualia

The filling-in phenomenon may give us clues to understanding the functional significance of what philosophers call *qualia*—the raw feel of sensations (e.g., the painfulness of pain, the yellowness of yellow). With the term *qualia*, I am referring exclusively to sensory qualia; philosophers often use the word more loosely to refer to any fleeting mental impression, but in my view, this confuses rather than clarifies issues. There are at least three questions to be asked about qualia (see also Crick and Koch, 2002): First, which subset of neurons need to be active for you to experience qualia? Second, why do only these neurons have qualia associated with them, whereas others do not (e.g., your pupil will contract in response to a light even when you are asleep)? Third, what are the functional characteristics that distinguish qualia-laden events from unconsciously processed ones? Elsewhere I suggested that four functional characteristics need to be present for the emergence of qualia (Ramachandran and Hirstein, 1997; Ramachandran and Blakeslee, 1998). I refer to these as the *four laws of qualia*. The first law is that qualia are irrevocable and beyond dispute (i.e., "this is yellow"—not "maybe this is yellow, but I can also choose to perceive it as blue"). The second law is that qualia are linked to short-term memory; they are held in a short term *buffer* to provide enough time for subsequent decisions about processing (i.e., to allow the luxury of choice). Third, whereas for a spinal reflex arc only one output is possible, qualia have potentially unlimited implications, or *meanings* (i.e., yellow flowers, yellow teeth, yellow egg yolk). The key idea is that you cannot change your mind about what it *is* (law 1), but you can change your mind about what you can *do* with it. This choice is achieved most parsimoniously, perhaps, by the information being "sent" to a central executive system that also has access to and can manipulate memories. This may not be carried out in a specific place in the brain (although the temporo-parieto-occipital junction and the anterior cingulate, by virtue of their anatomical connections, might be important) but may reflect coordinated activity among far-flung brain areas, through synchronization of spikes, for example. The fourth law, related to the third one, is that qualia are always linked with attention.

The first and third laws of qualia are crucial. To get a clearer understanding of the first law (i.e., the irrevocable nature of qualia), I will use a concrete example. If you shut one eye and aim your other eye's blind spot at a homogeneous yellow wall, you don't see a gap or dark region corresponding to the gap; it gets filled-in by the surrounding yellow. Indeed, you can even have a yellow doughnut that surrounds the blind spot (with its inner margin just overlapping the outer edge of the blind spot), and you will see a convincing homogeneous yellow disc rather than a ring. Furthermore, if this ring is surrounded by a field of identical rings, the filled-in inner ring "pops out" conspicuously from the background—without scrutiny. This observation calls into question some philosophers' claim that you simply ignore what's in your blind spot: How can something you ignore pop out at you? Thus, filling-in of the blind spot has a clear, irrevocable, "in your face" quality. The relevance of blind spot filling-in to understanding the idea of qualia becomes even clearer if it is compared with the failure to notice the huge gap in the visual field behind one's head. If you stand in a yellow room, you don't experience what you can't see behind you as a big, dark region or as a vacuum behind your head. Nor do you perceive a yellow wall behind you filling-in the missing part of the room. You simple assume, infer, or deduce that the walls behind you are also yellow. In some abstract sense, the deduction of yellow behind your head and the filling-in of yellow into the blind spot are similar, of course. Both are examples of *interpolation*, of the system guessing what is in the undersampled region based on what is in the surrounding region. Yet, phenomenologically, the two instances are utterly different. In the case of the blind spot, you literally see the yellow in the middle of the doughnut, whereas for the blind region behind your back, you infer or guess that it must be yellow without seeing any color localized there; it has no yellow qualia, you might say.

This distinction lies at the heart of the riddle of qualia. It takes us back to the question we started with: why do some neural events have sensory qualia associated with them, whereas others don't? In other words, what do qualia "buy" you in evolutionary terms? My hunch is that when sensory signals reach a certain preestablished criterion of certainty, the perceptual mechanism labels the event as being "beyond a reasonable doubt" in order to confer certainty and eliminate hesitation from subsequent decisions about processing. For example, when something is (say) 98% likely to be red, the brain pretends it is 100% certain that the thing is red and creates a corresponding sensory representation that allows you subsequent hesitation-free perceptual processing. The "pretend" representation also endures in short-term memory long enough to facilitate subsequent decisions and is resistant to tampering from top-down influences—that is, it is irrevocable. I suggest that in true instances of qualia-laden filling-in, the brain uses the surrounding information (or other relevant information) to say (in effect) "It is more than 98% likely that this line is actually passing through the blind spot (or that this yellow color extends right across the blind spot). Therefore, I will assume that the sensory support for it really exists in the outside world, and will activate the corresponding region in sensory cortical areas in a manner indistinguishable from genuine bottom-up sensory activation." Contrast this with the gap behind your head when the brain tentatively infers the presence of yellow or the tail of a cat sticking out from under the table, which causes you to infer the whole cat. In both instances, you use top-down influences to partially activate the sensory neurons corresponding to "yellow" or "cat," but you don't literally see the color or the animal (because the level of activation is still far less than what you could achieve with a real input). This is important because it allows you to say, in effect, "Maybe it's a cat but maybe it's a strange new species—so let me reserve judgment; indeed, I can just as readily imagine it to be a mutant pig with a cat's tail." This explains the biological function of genuine sensory filling-in in particular and of qualia in general. Their purpose is to highlight sensory activity as being certain in order to eliminate hesitation from subsequent decision making and confer stability on behavior (Ramachandran and Hirstein, 1997). When stimuli around the blind spot are yellow, it makes sense to experience yellow qualia in the region corresponding to the blind spot, because very likely the physical stimulus inside the blind spot is indeed yellow. For the region behind your head, you don't fill-in with qualia because there is a fair chance that you will be wrong (the wall behind you might be red) and the penalty will be too high (there might be a lion behind you). In short, for the region behind your head, you create tentative representations that you are allowed to change your mind about, but you are stuck with the qualia in your blind spot. Note that from an evolutionary perspective, it makes sense not to attach qualia to an interpolation process over areas so large that the outcome cannot be certain.

## The Human Rabbit

To sharpen the above argument further, let us perform a thought experiment. You have a blind spot in your eye and a big gap behind your head; you fill-in the blind spot but merely guess what is behind you. Now imagine that as the human species evolves, the two eyes migrate progressively backward so that your visual field starts expanding, and encroaches further and further upon the gap behind your head, as in a rabbit. Eventually the gap is almost closed, and what remains is a small blind spot of the same size as the original blind spot in front. Would there be a certain threshold size of the blind spot below which you would suddenly experience indubitable, irrevocable qualia in this new blind spot? My answer is that once a certain criterion level of certainty is reached (a gap smaller than perhaps 5–10 degrees?), evolution will insert a sensory representation that is identical to the one produced by a real sensory event, just as is the case for the natural blind spot. Such evolution would necessarily require new extensions of currently existing sensory maps and new back projections. The net result would be the creation of an irrevocable sensory representation that endures in short-term memory and allows the luxury of hesitation-free decisions about subsequent processing of the input (Ramachandran and Hirstein, 1997; Ramachandran and Blakeslee, 1998).

In sum, at a sufficiently abstract level of analysis, filling-in (e.g., across the blind spot) and finding out (e.g., what's behind your head) are indeed the same, but the neural representations differ to the extent that they fulfill different computational needs for subsequent processing. For further debate on these and other topics, I recommend an article by Pessoa et al. (1998), in which a consensus view emerges that Pat Churchland and I were essentially correct in suggesting that filling-in really does occur, in suggesting that it might be worthwhile to look for neural mechanisms underlying filling-in, and in suggesting that filling-in mechanisms are different from those involved in finding out.

In our view, Dennett's notion that you don't *need* to fill-in because there is no homunculus watching a screen is a red herring; the homunculus may correspond to higher-order decision-making mechanisms (which may need gap-free representations to function optimally). It is possible that this also applies to other, "higher" types of filling-in, such as in anosognosia, in which a patient is not only indifferent to his or her paralysis but actively inserts false beliefs (e.g., rationalizations) to explain away the paralysis. Such anosognosia occurs even in normal people to a limited extent; when we miss the flight to Paris, we use the "sour grapes" strategy when we say, "Oh, it's snowing there now. It's just as well that I missed the flight; it would have been unsafe landing there." There seems to be a need to fabricate false information in order to avoid the anxiety or anger that we would experience should we admit that our own bad decisions (e.g., leaving too late) were really the reason why we missed the plane. We have no inkling of what neural mechanisms might be involved in the confabulations (filling-in) seen in anosognosia, but meanwhile, at least the filling-in of blind spots and scotomas can be approached experimentally.

## Conclusions

The study of filling-in is instructive from (at least) four points of view. First, as noted above, it helps us sharpen our ideas about the philosophical question of qualia. Second—and more interesting to most scientists—it may provide key insights into the neural mechanisms underlying surface interpolation in normal vision. The relevance of filling-in for normal surface and object perception is one of the core themes in the first part of the book. Third, filling-in may be relevant to neuronal plasticity effects that follow peripheral damage, and to plasticity effects that contribute to certain types of perceptual and skill learning (see Ramachandran and Braddick, 1973; Ramachandran, 1976). And finally, there are strong hints that the dynamic receptive field changes that may underlie filling in may require the activity of anatomical back projections. The study of filling-in and related plasticity phenomena may entail a radical revision of our views of what receptive fields are and what they are really doing when we view natural visual scenes. The second and third parts of this book contain many speculations on these intriguing topics.

This book is testimony to the fact that the study of filling-in has reached a new level of maturity. Thanks largely to new psychophysical and physiological experiments that began a decade ago, the study of this fascinating phenomenon has moved from vague phenomenology and philosophical quibbles to detailed experimental research. This book represents a culmination of the substantial progress that has been made, and I am confident that it will provide impetus for new research. In an age of increasing specialization, the book is a breath of fresh air; it exemplifies precisely the convergence of ideas from many disciplines that the field of cognitive neuroscience badly needs.

## References

Brewster D (1832) *Letters in Natural Magic.* John Murray: London.
Churchland PS and Ramachandran VS (1993) Filling in: why Dennett is wrong. In: Dahlbom (ed), *Dennett and His Critics.* Oxford: Basil Blackwell, pp 28–52.

Crick F and Koch C (in press) In: Sejnowsky T (ed), *Twenty-three Unsolved Problems in Neuroscience*.

Dennett DC (1991) *Consciousness Explained*. Boston: Little, Brown and Co.

Dennett DC (1992) "Filling in" versus finding out: a ubiquitous confusion in cognitive science. In: Pick HL Jr, van den Broek P, and Knill DC (eds), *Cognition: Conceptual and Methodological Issues*. Washington, DC: American Psychological Association, pp 33–49.

Dennett DC and Kinsbourne M (1992) Time and the observer—the where and when of consciousness in the brain. *Behav Brain Sci* 15:183–201.

De Weerd P, Gattass R, Desimone R, and Ungerleider L (1995) Responses of cells in monkey visual cortex during perceptual filling-in of an artificial scotoma. *Nature* 377:731–734.

Durgin FH, Tripathy SP and Levi DM (1995). On the filling in of the visual blind spot: some rules of thumb. *Perception* 24:827–840.

Fiorani M, Rosa MGP, Gattass R, and Rocha-Miranda CE (1992) Dynamic surrounds of receptive fields in primate striate cortex: a physiological basis for perceptual completion. *Proc Natl Acad Sci USA* 89:8547–8551.

Gatass R, Fiorani M, Rosa MPG, Pinon MCF, Sousa APB, and Soares JGM (1992) Visual responses outside the classical receptive field, a possible correlate of perceptual completion. In: Lent R (ed): *The Visual System from Genesis to Maturity*. Boston: Birkhauser, pp 233–244.

Gilbert C and Wiesel T (1992) Receptive field dynamics in adult primary visual cortex. *Nature* 356:150–152.

Kanizsa G (1979) *Organization in Vision*. New York: Praeger.

Kapadia M, Gilbert C, and Westheimer G (1994) A quantitative measure of short term cortical plasticity in human vision *J Neurosci* 14(1):451–457.

Lettvin JY (1976) On seeing sidelong. *The Sciences* 16:10–20.

Paradiso MA and Nakayama K (1991) Brightness perception and filling-in. *Vis Res* 31:1221–1236.

Pessoa L, Thompson E and Noë A (1998) Finding out about filling-in: a guide to perceptual completion for visual science and the philosophy of perception. *Behav Brain Sci* 21:65–144.

Pettet MW and Gilbert CD (1992) Dynamic changes in receptive-field size in cat primary visual cortex. *Proc Natl Acad Sci USA* 89:8366–8370.

Ramachandran VS (1976) Learning-like phenomena in stereopsis. *Nature* 262:382–384.

Ramachandran VS (1992a) Blind spots. *Sci Am* 266:86–91.

Ramachandran VS (1992b) Filling in gaps in perception: part 1. *Curr Dir Psychol Sci* 1:199–205.

Ramachandran VS (1993) Filling in gaps in perception: part 2. *Curr Dir Psychol Sci* 2:56–65.

Ramachandran VS and Braddick OJ (1973) Orientation specific learning in stereopsis. *Perception* 2:371–376.

Ramachandran VS and Gregory R (1991) Perceptual filling in of artificially induced scotomas in human vision. *Nature* 350:699–702.

Ramachandran VS, Gregory R, and Aiken W (1993) Perceptual fading of visual texture borders. *Vis Res* 33:717–722.

Ramachandran VS and Hirstein W (1997) Three laws of qualia; what neurology tells us about the biological functions of consciousness. *J Consciousness Studies* 4:429–457.

Ramachandran VS and Blakeslee S (1998) *Phantoms in the Brain: Probing the Mysteries of the Human Mind.* New York: William Morrow.

Ramachandran VS and Hirstein W (1998). The perception of phantom limbs: the D. O. Hebb lecture. *Brain* 121:1603–1630.

Sergent J (1988) An investigation into perceptual completion in blind areas. *Brain* 111:347–373.

Weiskrantz L, Warrington EK, Sanders MD, and Marshall J (1974) Visual capacity in the hemianopic field following a restricted occipital ablation. *Brain* 97(4):709–728.

Yarbus AL (1967) *Eye Movements and Vision.* New York: Plenum Press.

# Contributors

YUZO M. CHINO, Ph.D.
College of Optometry
University of Houston
Houston, Texas

CHRISTINE E. COLLINS, Ph.D.
Department of Psychology
Vanderbilt University
Nashville, Tennessee

GREG DAVIS, Ph.D.
School of Psychology
Birkbeck College
London, UK

LETICIA DE OLIVEIRA, Ph.D.
Biophysics Institute Carlos Chagas Filho
Federal University of Rio de Janeiro
Rio de Janeiro, Brazil

PETER DE WEERD, Ph.D.
Department of Psychology
University of Arizona
Tucson, Arizona

JULIEN DOYON, Ph.D.
Department of Psychology
University of Montreal
Montreal, Canada

JON DRIVER, Ph.D.
Institute of Cognitive Neuroscience
University College London
London, UK

THOMAS ELBERT, Ph.D.
Department of Psychology
University of Konstanz
Konstanz, Germany

MARIO FIORANI, JR., M.D., Ph.D.
Biophysics Institute Carlos Chagas Filho
Federal University of Rio de Janeiro
Rio de Janeiro, Brazil

HOWARD S. FRIEDMAN, Ph.D.
Krieger Mind/Brain Institute
Johns Hopkins University
Baltimore, Maryland

RICARDO GATTASS, M.D.
Biophysics Institute Carlos Chagas Filho
Federal University of Rio de Janeiro
Rio de Janeiro, Brazil

STEPHEN GROSSBERG, Ph.D.
Department of Cognitive and Neural
    Systems Center for Adaptive Systems
Boston University
Boston, Massachusetts

JON H. KAAS, Ph.D.
Department of Psychology
Vanderbilt University
Nashville, Tennessee

VICTOR W. MARK, M.D.
Departments of Physical Medicine and Rehabilitation
Veterans Affairs Medical Center
Birmingham, Alabama

JASON B. MATTINGLEY, Ph.D.
Department of Psychology
School of Behavioral Science
University of Melbourne
Parkville, Australia

JANINE MENDOLA, Ph.D.
Center for Advanced Imaging
West Virginia University School of Medicine
Morgantown, West Virginia

HEIKO NEUMANN, Ph.D.
Faculty for Informatics
Ulm University
Ulm, Germany

CHRISTO PANTEV, Ph.D.
Rotman Research Institute for Neuroscience
University of Toronto
Toronto, Canada

MICHAEL A. PARADISO, Ph.D.
Department of Neuroscience
Brown University
Providence, Rhode Island

LUIZ PESSOA, Ph.D.
Laboratory of Brain and Cognition
National Institute of Mental Health
Bethesda, Maryland

RAPHAEL PINAUD, M.SC.
Department of Psychology
University of Arizona
Tucson, Arizona

V.S. RAMACHANDRAN, M.D., Ph.D.
Department of Psychology
University of California, San Diego
La Jolla, California

CARLOS EDUARDO ROCHA-MIRANDA, M.D.
Brazilian Academy of Sciences
Rio de Janeiro, Brazil

ANDREW F. ROSSI, Ph.D.
Laboratory of Brain and Cognition
National Institute of Mental Health
Bethesda, Maryland

MICHAEL SCHULTE, Ph.D.
Institute of Experimental Audiology
University of Münster
Münster, Germany

LOTHAR SPILLMANN, Ph.D.
Arbeitsgruppe Hirnforschung
Freiburg University
Freiburg, Germany

EDWARD TAUB, Ph.D.
Department of Psychology
University of Alabama at Birmingham Center
Birmingham, Alabama

LIISA A. TREMERE, Ph.D.
Department of Psychology
University of Arizona
Tucson, Arizona

LESLIE G. UNGERLEIDER, Ph.D.
Laboratory of Brain and Cognition
National Institute of Mental Health
Bethesda, Maryland

ELIANE VOLCHAN, M.D., Ph.D.
Biophysics Institute Carlos Chagas Filho
Federal University of Rio de Janeiro
Rio de Janeiro, Brazil

RÜDIGER VON DER HEYDT, Ph.D.
Krieger Mind/Brain Institute
Johns Hopkins University
Baltimore, Maryland

ROBIN WALKER, Ph.D.
Royal Holloway
University of London
Egham, Surrey, UK

NATHAN WEISZ, Ph.D.
Department of Psychology
University of Konstanz
Konstanz, Germany

HONG ZHOU, Ph.D.
Krieger Mind/Brain Institute
Johns Hopkins University
Baltimore, Maryland

# Filling-In

# 1

## Introduction:
### Filling-In: More Than Meets the Eye

PETER DE WEERD AND LUIZ PESSOA

Under particular conditions, the visual system perceptually fills-in restricted regions in space with surrounding information. This perceptual filling-in process, which we also refer to as *perceptual completion*, has become a topic of extensive research in the last several decades. Perhaps the best-known example of perceptual completion is the filling-in across the blind spot during the use of monocular vision (see Chapter 8). The blind spot corresponds to a small region in the eye devoid of photoreceptors, where the optic nerve leaves the eye. The blind spot is not perceived as a *void* or a dark region in space. Instead, it is perceived as having the same brightness, color, or texture as the surrounding background (hence the expression *filling in*).

In parallel with psychophysical research on filling-in and related perceptual phenomena, physiological evidence has accumulated showing that the activity of neurons in sensory cortex can be influenced by stimuli presented outside their classical receptive field (RF) in the RF surround (see Chapter 15). The term *receptive field* will be used exclusively to refer to the classical receptive field, as determined by an isolated bar stimulus. The term *surround* or *RF surround* will be used to refer to the region outside the classical RF where a bar stimulus presented alone does not activate the neuron, but where a stimulus can modulate the response to a second stimulus presented inside the classical RF. The existence of extra-RF (surround) influences has been associated with various types of contextual perception, including perceptual filling-in phenomena.

A separate tradition of physiological research has led to the insight that the representation of sensory space in sensory cortex can be modified by experience. These changes in sensory representations have been demonstrated following systematic changes in sensory input—for instance, due to injury or during the learning of a new skill. This book takes the view that influences from the RF surround, which form the basis of perceptual completion and other forms of contextual perception, under some circumstances can become the engine of a remapping of sensory space upon cortex (Chapter 15).

This book brings together evidence collected at a systems level from research traditions in visual, somatosensory, and auditory modalities. These sensory systems share a number of striking organizational features. One such feature is that sensory space is represented topographically in primary sensory cortex, as well as in lower-order cortex receiving input from the primary cortex. This topographic representation reflects an orderly anatomical projection in which sensory information impinging on neighboring points of a receptor sheet is transmitted to neighboring points of the primary sensory area through the thalamus. In addition to strong inputs arriving via primary (thalamic) afferents forming the basis for the classical RF, cortical sensory neurons also receive weaker inputs from other cortical neurons. These inputs arrive via feedback connections from higher-order cortical areas, or via lateral connections within areas, and they form the basis for the RF surround. Changes in cortico-cortical connections can lead to modifications of RF structure and surround, which we suggest can be the first sign of a remapping of sensory space onto cortex (see below).

In the visual system, there is an extensive body of knowledge on the contribution of extra-RF influences to contextual perception. In Part I of this book, we will highlight two types of visual contextual perception: the perception of illusory contours and the perceptual filling-in of surfaces. Both perceptual phenomena exemplify the *interpolation* of visual information across regions where that information is not present. Furthermore, visual scientists have gained important insights into the mechanisms of cortical reorganization induced by retinal or cortical damage. This topic will be explored in Part II and will lead to the idea that the modulation of surround influences, which normally are involved in contextual perception, can lead to a remapping of visual space onto retinotopically organized visual cortical areas. Remapping in sensory modalities other than vision is explored in Part III, and it will be shown that under some circumstances similar reorganizations can take place in motor cortex. Reorganization will be discussed not only in the context of peripheral injury (deafferentation), but also in the context of skill learning.

In the concluding chapter (Chapter 15), an integrative approach will be taken to various perceptual completion phenomena, taking place on a faster time scale and to cortical reorganization in sensory and motor cortex induced by peripheral damage or skill learning, taking place on a slower time scale. We propose that systematic changes in the interplay between inhibitory and excitatory inputs from the RF surround permit cortical neurons to become driven by new sources of input, which, in addition to the initial functional (perceptual) consequences, can lead to a long-term structural reorganization of cortex. Below, a more detailed overview of the different parts of the book is given.

## Part I: Perceptual Completion (Filling-In) in the Visual System

Chapter 1 presents a conceptual and computational motivation for the existence of filling-in mechanisms in vision. In natural visual scenes, one's view of an object is often occluded by other objects, which leads to an interrupted, incomplete projection of that object's contours and surfaces onto the retina. Because occlusion is the rule rather than the exception, the visual system has evolved mechanisms that interpolate contours and surfaces on the basis of incomplete local cues.

The idea that the perception of contours and surfaces relies on mechanisms that interpolate local information has been the source of several interesting and controversial questions: Are there explicit representations of completed contours in the visual cortex? Does the perception of a surface mean that there is neural activity somewhere in the brain *representing* the surface's feature (e.g., brightness, or color)? Where in the visual system might neural activity associated with filling-in be observed? To understand these questions, the associated controversy, and the neural mechanisms that might underlie interpolation, it is necessary to review some basic aspects of the organization of the visual system.

The visual system consists of several largely parallel anatomical pathways, which tend to process different aspects of the visual input (Desimone and Ungerleider, 1989; Distler et al., 1993). This specialization can in part be traced back to two main classes of retinal ganglion cells. Essentially, parvocellular cells (which have small RFs) are specialized in fine spatial analysis of object features, while magnocellular cells (which have larger RFs) are specialized in motion detection. Ultimately, these two different retinal signals form the basis for a subdivision into two cortical systems: a ventral one, extending into the temporal lobe and specialized in object processing, and a dorsal one, extending into the parietal lobe and specialized in the processing of motion and spatial relations between objects. Furthermore, anatomical and physiological evidence suggests that contours and surfaces may be analyzed by different processing streams within the occipitotemporal pathway (see Fig. 1-1 in Chapter 2).

Physiological and anatomical studies show evidence of a strong hierarchical component in the way visual information is processed within the different streams. In the primary visual cortex (V1), located posteriorly in the brain, neurons have small RFs and code simple features of the visual input, such as the orientation of edges. In addition, neighboring points in the retinal image are projected onto neighboring points of cortex. This type of topographic projection is referred to as *retinotopy*, which is analogous to somatotopy in the somatosensory system and tonotopy in the auditory system. In visual areas at increasingly higher levels of visual processing, and more anterior in the brain, increasingly complex features of stimuli are processed, RFs become larger, and retinotopy breaks down. This physiological evidence is complemented by data from anatomical tracer experiments that suggest serial, or feedforward, anatomical connections from more posterior visual areas (e.g., V1) to more anterior ones (e.g., V2) (Ungerleider and Desimone, 1989; Distler et al., 1993). A similar hierarchy of processing exists in other sensory systems.

The retinotopic projection of the visual field onto early visual areas such as V1 and V2 raises the possibility that an interpolation between local measurements will generate neural activity in retinotopically organized cortex that is *isomorphic* (Todorovic, 1987) with the perception of a completed contour or surface. In other words, there may be a one-to-one correspondence between the perceived spatial distribution of contours or surfaces and the neural activity in a given brain region, or bridge locus (Teller, 1994; see also Pessoa et al., 1998).

The paradigmatic example of contour interpolation is the perception of illusory contours. Illusory contours are contours that are perceived in the absence of any physical discontinuities. They are induced by an appropriate arrangement and alignment of local elements (inducers), suggesting one surface overlaying or occluding another (see Fig. 1-2 in Chapter 2). The perception of illusory contours was originally interpreted as the result of top-down cognitive operations providing the best interpretation for the arrangement of local elements in the stimulus (Gregory, 1965). This proposal was challenged by findings that neurons in V2, and possibly even in V1, are selective for the orientation of illusory contours (von der Heydt et al., 1984; Grosof et al., 1993). These neural responses were observed while the inducing elements were kept well outside the classical RF. Hence, the responses correlated with a perceived contour that was not physically present inside the RF. Such responses indicate that some visual neurons can interpolate a contour between local elements outside their RF, which, because of their alignment, suggests the likely presence of a contour. Thus, when local two-dimensional (2D) cues are likely to correspond to a contour that is occluded, the visual system is highly biased to *assume* the presence of contours (and surfaces) in regions of the image where the contour is not physically present. The presence of a topographically organized correlate of illusory contours in visual areas as early as V1 and V2 has cast serious doubt on the interpretation that those contours are the result of a *cognitive interpretation* of 2D displays. Rather, illusory contours in 2D displays are likely to be a consequence of contour interpolation mechanisms that are heavily biased to interpret 2D cues in a three-dimensional (3D) fashion.

Whether surfaces are represented in an isomorphic fashion in retinotopic areas, analogous to the isomorphic representation of contours, remains controversial. The large majority of neurons in early visual areas are most effectively stimulated by discontinuities and contours in the image, which raises the question of how homogeneous regions within surfaces are represented. Dennett (1991) suggested that surfaces might be symbolically filled-in by high-level operations in higher-order cortex. As an example, consider the blind spot again. According to Denett (1991), the filling-in of information across the blind spot would not be the result of an active low-level process, but rather could follow from symbolically *tagging* the associated region of space with *more of the same*. Several studies, however, have demonstrated physiological correlates of completion across the blind spot. These correlates were observed in visual areas as low in the visual hierarchy as V1 (see Chapter 9). Moreover, a number of psychophysical and neurophysiological findings support the general idea of topographic representations of filled-in surface properties within bounded regions in retinotopically organized cortex (Chapters 4 and 5; see also Chapters 2 and 8). On the other hand, neural activity in retinotopically organized visual areas during perceptual filling-in of color does not appear to be isomorphic with the percept (Chapter 6). Color perception may have evolved primarily to evaluate the desirability or quality of relevant items in the environment (e.g., food, mating partners, predators). Compared to brightness, for example, color may contribute significantly more to the processing of the *meaning* of objects and less to the processing of contours and surfaces. As a consequence, the processing of object color may depend to a large extent on high-level nonretinotopic brain regions that are involved in the recognition and evaluation of objects. Studies demonstrating that lesions in inferotemporal cortex significantly impair color perception support this notion (Heywood et al., 1995; Huxlin et al., 2000; Cowey et al., 2001). Thus, the question of whether the perceptual filling-in of surfaces is associated with isomorphic neural filling-in processes may be answered differently for different surface features.

Isomorphic neural correlates of perceptual completion phenomena are related to the neurophysiological finding that the responses to stimuli inside the classical RF of neurons in V1 and other areas can be modulated by stimuli presented in the RF surround, outside the classical RF. This property is commonly referred to as the *context sensitivity* of visual neurons, and among its purposes may be the completion of contours (figure–ground segregation) and the filling-in of the surfaces bounded by those contours. Chapters 2 to 8 explore the mechanisms of completion in the visual system, as well as cognitive factors, such as attention (Chapter 7), influencing them. Data collected with psychophysical (Chapters 4, 5, and 7), neurophysiological (Chapters 4, 5, and 6), neuroimaging (Chapter 3), and computational (Chapters 2 and 8) approaches will be discussed. An important idea that underlies all chapters in Part I is that interpolation depends on (a modulation of) surround influences, and that the existence of those mechanisms is essential for the *appropriate* perception of objects. Indeed, if an occluded object cannot be perceived as complete behind the occluder, it can never be a target for appropriate action. In Part I, the terms *completion* and *filling-in* are often used interchangeably (as in this Introduction), but some authors (Chapter 2) use the term *completion* to refer to contour interpolation based on contour segments and the term *filling-in* to refer to the spread of a given feature (e.g., color, brightness, or texture) within surfaces.

## Part II: Modulation of Extra-RF Effects and Cortical Reorganization in Visual Cortex

Modulations of extra-RF (surround) effects can lead to rapid changes in RF structure. Changes in RF structure and surround can be caused by peripheral injury to the receptor sheet or by cortical damage. RFs of neurons in deafferented cortical zones in V1 (e.g., due to retinal injury) expand within minutes of developing a retinal scotoma. Such RF expansions could form the basis of long-term changes in the mapping of the visual environment onto early cortical areas. This remapping may influence perceptual completion across a retinal scotoma (Chapter 5) such that the properties of completion at the beginning and at the end of reorganization may differ. In Part II, RF changes induced by retinal lesions are explored and long-term effects of retinal damage upon the mapping of visual space upon cortex are discussed (Chapter 10). Two special cases of completion are discussed as well: the perceptual completion of stimuli across the blind spot (Chapter 9), and the perceptual completion of stimuli across cortical lesions and into hemianopic hemifields (Chapter 11).

## Part III: Long-Term Cortical Remapping Induced by Peripheral Injury and Skill Learning

Long-term and persistent reorganization of sensory cortex in adult organisms as a result of altered sensory input has been documented most thoroughly in the somatosensory system. Many studies of somatotopic organization have reported that the amputation or anesthesia of a body part leads to an invasion of its cortical representation by representations of other body parts. As in the visual domain (Pettet and Gilbert, 1992), the initial effect of amputation or anesthesia is an expansion of the RFs of neurons in the deafferented cortical region, which start to respond to inputs from neighboring body parts to which they were not responsive originally (Merzenich et al., 1983; Rasmusson and Turnbull, 1983). In cases where the deafferentation was permanent, significant alterations in somatosensory representations have been reported. Perhaps the most massive rearrangement of somatotopic organization has been reported by Pons and colleagues (Pons et al., 1991). In normal primates, the regions of somatosensory cortex that are stimulated by the arm and hand, and by the face, lie next to each other. In several experimental monkeys, a dorsal rhizotomy was carried out, which severs the nerve fibers carrying sensory information from the arm and hand to the spinal cord. Eleven years later, Pons and colleagues studied the somatotopic organization of somatosensory cortex in their experimental monkeys, and found that neurons in the region of cortex that in normal animals receives information from arm and hand now could be stimulated by touching the face (Pons et al., 1991). This type of reorganization may be responsible for the *phantom limbs* reported in human patients after limb amputation (Ramachandran and Blakeslee, 1998). The experience of phantom limbs is an example of perceptual completion comparable to the completion through the blind spot or long-term retinal scotomas. Reorganization in the somatosensory cortex has been reported by a large number of investigators in a variety of species (e.g., Rasmusson, 1982; Merzenich et al., 1984; Borsook et al., 1988; Weiss et al., 1998). Further, in motor cortex it has been shown that motor representations are altered by peripheral nerve damage (Donoghue and Sanes, 1987; Sanes et al., 1988), and it has been shown that partial cochlear damage can modify tonotopic organization in primary auditory area A1 (Robertson and Irvine, 1989).

Significant alterations in cortical organization can be induced not only by deafferentation, but also by skill learning. In the somatosensory domain, a number of studies (Jenkins et al., 1990; Recanzone et al., 1992a–c) have demonstrated that the representations of digits involved in a tactile discrimination task expand as a consequence of carrying out that task. Some studies in the motor domain suggest relatively fast reorganization in the primary motor area, M1 (Classen et al., 1998), which can acquire a more permanent character after long-term training of the skill (Karni et al., 1995). Similar cortical reorganizations have been reported as a function of behavioral experience or training in auditory cortex (Recanzone et al., 1993; Sceich et al., 1993; Weinburger, 1993). Part III offers an in-depth discussion of the changes in cortical representations in several sensory modalities after peripheral injury (Chapter 14), during skill learning in normal subjects (Chapters 12 and 13), and during remedial training after injury (Chapter 14).

## Relationships Between Extra-RF Effects, Perceptual Filling-In, and Cortical Plasticity

This book presents a review of a wide array of interpolation effects taking place on widely varying time scales. All of these phenomena, however, imply a remapping of sensory (or motor) space onto cortex. Perceptual completion across the blind spot or across permanent scotomas, as well as the perception of illusory contours and surfaces, take place on a time scale of milliseconds. These phenomena represent the action of fast extra-RF mechanisms that have evolved to deal with likely aspects of sensory stimulation, possibly through experience-dependent mechanisms during early development. Initial RF effects following deafferentation take several minutes to develop, and the reorganization of the sensory or motor cortex due to injury or induced by skill learning typically takes place on a time scale of weeks or months. We consider these latter effects to be slow interpolation effects that lead to longer-lasting alterations in the mapping of sensory space or motor action onto cortex.

The principal hypothesis advanced in this volume is the idea that fast and slow interpolation effects represent successive stages in a chain of plastic events that can result in long-term changes in cortical organization, or remapping (Chapter 15). In the visual system, we propose that fast-acting disinhibition in the RF surround can lead not only to perceptual completion across the RF, through the action of ordinarily ineffective excitatory inputs from the RF surround, but also to a slow remapping of visual space onto cortex when the disinhibition is maintained. Thus, under particular conditions, fast disinhibition, and the associated neural interpolation and perceptual completion effects, may signify the beginning of long-term cortical remapping. Furthermore, we propose that the link between fast interpolation effects induced by disinhibition and long-term plasticity can be applied outside the domain of vision. We hypothesize that specific perceptual conditions (e.g., retinal stabilization), cortical deafferentation due to injury, and skill learning can each be a cause of disinhibition in a region of sensory and/or motor cortex, and that when these causes persist, weak excitatory inputs to neurons inside the disinhibited cortical region can become strengthened by Hebbian learning mechanisms. The resulting changes in neuronal connectivity are hypothesized to lead to long-term changes in RF structure and cortical representations.

The data reviewed in this volume indicate that interpolation mechanisms contributing to normal perception in adult sensory systems are subject to tremendous modifications when new perceptual and behavioral conditions emerge. These modifications reflect the enhanced or decreased importance of a subset of sensory inputs. In the motor system, modifications of neuronal connections within M1 and other motor regions will serve the purpose of linking movement components together (interpolation) into an effective motor action. These modifications reflect the enhanced or decreased importance of particular (subsets of) motor movement components. According to the idea that appropriate motor actions are often targeted to parts of stimuli that are perceptually completed (i.e., not directly present in the sensory input), the ultimate purpose of interpolation mechanisms and their plasticity in sensory systems may be to guarantee a continuous representation of objects under varying perceptual conditions, varying conditions of behavioral relevance, and even varying states of integrity of the sensory apparatus itself. By extending the concept of filling-in beyond the domain of visual perception, we hope to highlight its general role and purpose in sensory and motor systems. In this way, this volume aims to contribute to the discussion of the basic principles and cortical mechanisms that organize the brain in response to the world in which we live.

## References

Borsook D, Becerra L, Fishman S, Edwards A, Jennings CL, Stojanovic M, Papinicolas L, Ramachandran VS, Ganzales RG, and Breitner H (1988) Acute plasticity in the human somatosensory cortex following amputation. *Neuroreport* 9:1013–1017.

Classen J, Liepert, J, Wise SP, Hallett M, and Cohen LG (1998) Rapid plasticity of human cortical movement representation induced by practice. *J Neurophysiol* 79:1117–1123.

Cowey A, Heywood CA, and Irving-Bell L (2001) The regional cortical basis of achromatopsia: A study on macaque monkeys and an achromatopsic patient. *Eur J Neurosci* 14:1555–1566.

Denett D (1991) *Consciousness Explained*. Boston: Little, Brown and Company.

Desimone R and Ungerleider LG (1989) Neural mechanisms of visual processing in monkeys. In: Boller F and Grafman J (eds), *Handbook of Neuropsychology*, Vol 2. Amsterdam: Elsevier Science Publishers B.V. (Biomedical Division), pp 267–299.

Distler C, Boussaoud D, Desimone R, and Ungerleider LG (1993) Cortical connections of inferior temporal area TEO in macaque monkeys. *J Comp Neurol* 334:125–150.

Donoghue JP and Sanes JN (1987) Peripheral nerve injury in developing rats reorganizes representation pattern in motor cortex. *PNAS USA* 84:1123–1126.

Gregory RL (1965) Seeing in depth. *Nature* 207:16–19.

Grosof DH, Shapley, RM, and Hawken RM (1993) Macaque V1 neurons can signal "illusory" contours. *Nature* 365:550–552.

Grosof DH, Shapley RM, and Hawken MJ (1993) Macaque V1 neurons can signal "illusory" contours. *Nature* 365:550–552.

Heywood CA, Gaffa D, and Cowey A (1995) Cerebral achromatopsia in monkeys. *Eur J Neurosci* 7:1064–1073.

Huxlin KR, Saunders RC, Marchionini D, Pham HA, and Merigan WH (2000) Perceptual deficits after lesions of inferotemporal cortex in macaques. *Cereb Cortex* 10:671–683.

Jenkins WM, Merzenich MM, Ochs MT, Allard T, and Guic-Robles E (1990) Functional reorganization of primary somatosensory cortex in adult owl monkeys after behaviorally controlled tactile stimulation. *J Neurophysiol* 63:82–104.

Karni A, Meyer G, Jezzard P, Adams M, Turner R, and Ungerleider LG (1995) Functional MRI evidence for adult motor cortex plasticity during motor skill learning. *Nature* 377:155–158.

Merzenich MM, Kaas JH, Wall JT, Sur M, Nelson RJ, and Felleman DJ (1983) Progression of change following median nerve section in the cortical representation of the hand in areas 3b and 1 in adult owl and squirrel monkeys. *Neuroscience* 10:639–665.

Merzenich MM, Nelson RJ, Stryker MP, Cynader MS, Schoppmann A, and Zook JM (1984) Somatosensory cortical map changes following digit amputation in adult monkeys. *J Comp Neurol* 224:591–605.

Pessoa L, Thompson E, and Noë, A (1998) Finding out about filling-in: A guide to perceptual completion for visual science and the philosophy of perception. *Behav Brain Sci* 21:723–802.

Pettet MW and Gilber CD (1992) Dynamic changes in receptive-field size in cat primary visual cortex. *Proc Natl Acad Sci USA* 89:8366–8370.

Pons TP, Garraghty PE, Ommaya AK, Kaas JH, Taub E, and Mishkin M (1991) Massive cortical reorganization after sensory deafferentation in adult macaques. *Science* 252:1857–1860.

Ramachandran VS and Blakeslee S (1998) *Phantoms in the Brain*. New York: William Morrow and Company, Inc.

Rasmusson DD (1982) Reorganization of raccoon somatosensry cortex following removal of the fifth digit. *J Comp Neurol* 205:313–326.

Rasmusson DD and Turnbull BG (1983) Immediate effects of digit amputation on SI cortex in the raccoon: Unmasking of inhibitory fields. *Brain Res* 288:368–370.

Recanzone GH, Jenkins WM, Hradek GT, and Merzenich MM (1992a) Progressive improvement in discriminative abilities in adult owl monkeys performing a tactile frequency discrimination task. *J Neurophysiol* 67:1015–1030.

Recanzone GH, Merzenich MM, and Jenkins WM (1992b) Frequency discrimination training engaging a restricted skin surface results in an emergence of a cutaneous response zone in cortical area 3a. *J Neurophysiol* 67:1057–1070.

Recanzone GH, Merzenich MM, Jenkins WM, Grajski KA, and Dinse HR (1992c) Topographical reorganization of the hand representation in cortical area 3b of owl monkeys trained in a frequency discrimination task. *J Neurophysiol* 67:1031–1056.

Recanzone GH, Schreiner GE, and Merzenich MM (1993) Plasticity in the frequency representation of primary auditory cortex following discrimination training in adult owl monkeys. *J Neurosci* 13:87–103.

Robertson D and Irvine DRF (1989) Plasticity of frequency organization in auditory cortex of guinea pigs with partial unilateral deafness. *J Comp Neurol* 282:456–471.

Sanes JN, Suner S, Lando JF, and Donoghue JP (1988) Rapid reorganization of adult rat motor cortex somatic representation patterns after motor nerve injury. *PNAS USA* 85:2003–2007.

Scheich H, Simonis C, Ohl F, Tillein J, and Thomas H (1993) Functional organization and learning-related plasticity in auditory cortex of the Mongolian gerbil. *Prog Brain Res* 97:135–143.

Teller DY (1994) Linking propositions. *Vision Res* 24:1233–1246

Todorovic D (1987) The Craik-O'Brien-Cornsweet effect: New varieties and theoretical implications. *Percept Psychophys* 42:545–600.

von der Heydt R, Peterhans E, and Baumgartner G (1984) Illusory contours and cortical neuron responses. *Science* 224:1260–1262.

Weinberger NM (1993) Learning-induced changes of auditory receptive fields. *Curr Opin Neurobiol* 3:570–577.

Weiss T, Mitner WHR, Dillman J, Meissner W, Honker R, and Nowak H (1998) Reorganization of the somatosensory cortex after amputation of the index finger. *Neuroreport* 9:213–216.

# I

# FAST-ACTING FILLING-IN IN NORMAL VISION

# 2

## Filling-In the Forms:
## Surface and Boundary Interactions in Visual Cortex

### STEPHEN GROSSBERG

In order to discuss filling-in in the brain, it is helpful to caste this issue within a larger framework that clarifies more global properties of brain organization. This is useful because filling-in can be fully understood only within such a global perspective. In one traditional view, our brains are proposed to possess independent modules, as in a digital computer. In this view, we see by processing perceptual qualities such as visual form, color, and motion using different modules. This view's supporters sometimes turn to the fact that the brain is organized into parallel processing streams. Figure 2-1 schematizes how at least three such streams within the visual cortex are activated by light impinging on the retina. One stream goes from retina through the lateral geniculate nucleus (LGN) parvo stage (classified due to its *parvocellular* cell type) to the cortical processing stages V1 blob, V2 thin stripe, V4, and then inferotemporal cortex. Another stream goes from retina through LGN parvo, V1 interblob, V2 interstripe, V4, and again on to inferotemporal cortex. Still another stream goes from retina through LGN magno (classified due to its *magnocellular* cell type) to cortical processing layer 4B in area V1, V2 thick stripes, MT, and then parietal cortex. More will be said below about the role that these streams play in vision and, more specifically in filling-in.

The existence of such streams certainly supports the idea that brain processing is specialized, but it does not, in itself, imply that these streams are independent modules that are able to fully compute their particular processes on their own. In fact, much perceptual data argue against the existence of independent modules, because strong interactions are known to occur between perceptual qualities. For example, changes in the perceived form or color of an object can cause changes in its perceived motion, and vice versa, while changes in the perceived brightness of an object can cause changes in its perceived depth, and vice versa (Egusa, 1983; Kanizsa, 1974; Faubert and von Grunau, 1995; Smallman and McKee, 1995; Pessoa et al., 1996). The existence of such interactions suggests

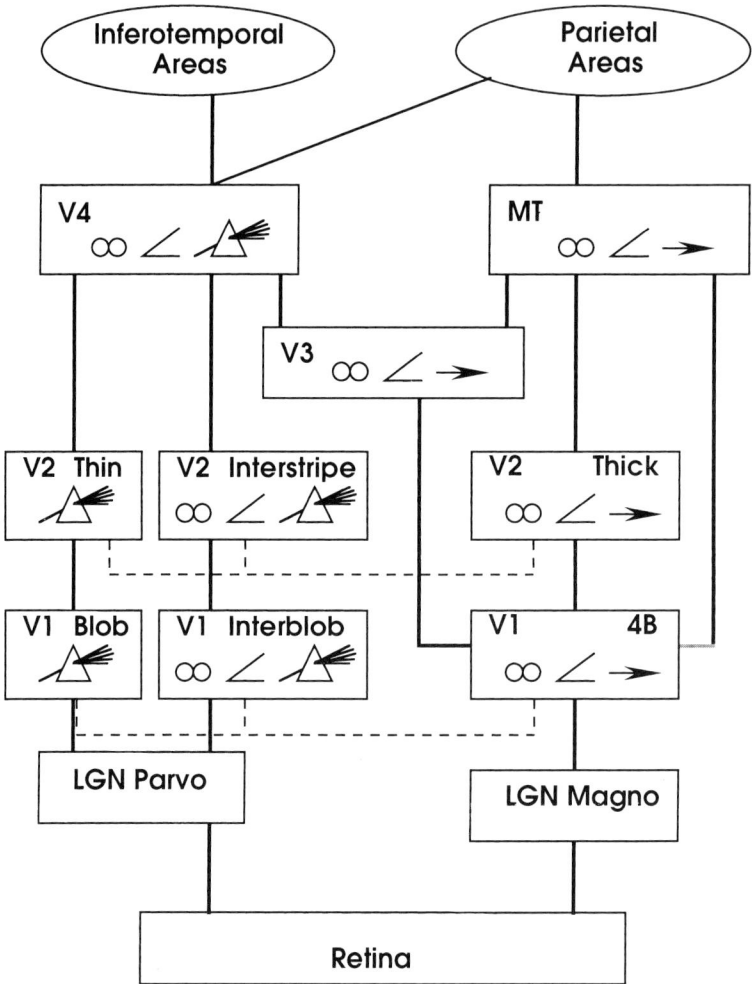

**Figure 2-1.** Schematic diagram of anatomical connections and neuronal selectivities of early visual areas in the macaque monkey brain. Icons indicate the response selectivities of cells at each processing stage: rainbow = wavelength selectivity, angle symbol = orientation selectivity, spectacles = binocular selectivity, and right-pointing arrow = selectivity to motion in a prescribed direction. LGN = lateral geniculate nucleus. (*Source:* Adapted with permission from EA DeYoe and DC van Essen. 1988. Concurrent processing streams in monkey visual cortex. *Trends Neurosci* 11:219–226)

that the mechanisms whereby we perceive the geometry of the world do not obey the classical geometrical axioms on which a lot of mathematics is based. How and why do these qualities interact? What is the geometry by which we really see the world? Answers to these questions are needed to determine the functional and computational units that govern behavior as we know it.

A great deal of theoretical and experimental evidence suggests that the brain's processing streams compute *complementary* properties. Each stream's properties are related to those of a complementary stream much as a lock fits its key or two pieces of a puzzle fit together. We are all familiar with complementarity principles in physics, such as the famous Heisenberg Uncertainty Principle of quantum mechanics, which notes that precise measurement of a particle's position forces uncertainty in measuring its momentum, and vice versa. As in physics, the mechanisms that enable each stream in the brain to compute one set of properties prevent it from computing a complementary set of properties. Due to the complementarity of the brain's processing streams, each stream exhibits complementary strengths and weaknesses. How, then, do these complementary properties get synthesized into a consistent behavioral experience? It is proposed that *interactions* between these processing streams overcome their complementary deficiencies and generate behavioral properties that realize the unity of conscious experiences. In this sense, *pairs* of complementary streams are the functional units of perception because only through their interactions can key behavioral properties be competently computed. Said in another way, one needs to study how pairs of complementary streams interact together in order to understand how the brain computes unambiguous information about various aspects of the world. These interactions may be used to explain many of the ways in which perceptual qualities are known to influence each other. Thus, although analogies like a key fitting its lock or puzzle pieces fitting together are suggestive, they do not fully capture the interactive dynamism of what complementarity means in the brain.

It is also well known that each stream can possess multiple processing stages. For example, in Figure 2-1, there are distinct processing stages in the LGN followed by the cortical areas V1, then V2, and then V4 on their way to the inferotemporal and parietal cortices. Why is this so? Accumulating evidence suggests that these stages realize a process of *hierarchical resolution of uncertainty. Uncertainty* here means that computing one set of properties at a given stage can suppress information about a different set of properties at that stage. In the brain, these uncertainties are proposed to be overcome by using more than one processing stage to form a stream. Overcoming informational uncertainty utilizes both hierarchical interactions within the stream and the parallel interactions between streams that overcome their complementary deficiencies. The computational unit is thus not a single processing stage; it is, rather, an ensemble of processing stages that interact within and between complementary processing streams.

According to this view, the organization of the brain obeys principles of uncertainty and complementarity, as does the physical world with which brains interact and of which they form a part. These principles reflect each brain's role as a self-organizing measuring device *in* the world and *of* the world, and may explain the brain's functional organization better than the simpler view of computationally independent modules. How filling-in is controlled in the brain provides an excellent example of such complementary computing. It is within this context that the capability of the visual system will be discussed to interpolate information across regions where that information is physically absent. This capability is a direct consequence of the architecture of the visual system.

## FACADE Theory: Boundary Grouping and Surface Filling-In

### All Boundaries Are Invisible

To begin, let us recall that visual processing provides excellent examples of parallel processing streams (Fig. 2-1). What evidence is there to suggest that these streams compute complementary properties, and how is this done? A neural theory, called *FACADE* (Form-And-Color-And-DEpth) theory (e.g., Grossberg, 1994, 1997), proposes that perceptual *boundaries* are formed in the LGN-interblob-interstripe-V4 stream, while perceptual surfaces are formed in the LGN-blob-thin stripe-V4 stream. Many experiments have supported this prediction (e.g., Elder and Zucker, 1998; Rogers-Ramachandran and Ramachandran, 1998; Lamme et al., 1999).

FACADE theory suggests how and why perceptual boundaries and perceptual surfaces compute complementary properties. Filling-in is proposed to occur within the surface processing stream. Due to the proposed complementarity of the boundary and surface streams, one needs to analyze both streams to understand fully the way in which either stream normally functions. One also needs to analyze how the streams interact to understand the properties of the filling-in process per se. Figures 2-2a and 2-2b illustrate three pairs of complementary properties using visual illusions that are induced by variants of a Kanizsa square. For example, in response to viewing Figure 2-2a, our brains construct a percept of a square even though the image contains only four black pacman, or pie-shaped, figures on a white background. As noted below, this percept is due to an interaction between the processing streams that form perceptual boundaries and surfaces.

You might immediately wonder why our brains construct a square where there is none in the image. There are several functional reasons why our brains have developed strategies to construct complete representations of boundaries and surfaces on the basis of incomplete information. One is that there is a *blind spot* in our retinas, namely, a region where no light-sensitive photoreceptors exist. This region is blind because of the way in which the pathways from retinal photoreceptors are collected together to form the optic nerve that carries them from the retina to the LGN in Figure 2-1. We are not usually aware of this blind spot because our brains complete boundary and surface information across it. The actively completed parts of these percepts are visual illusions, because they are not

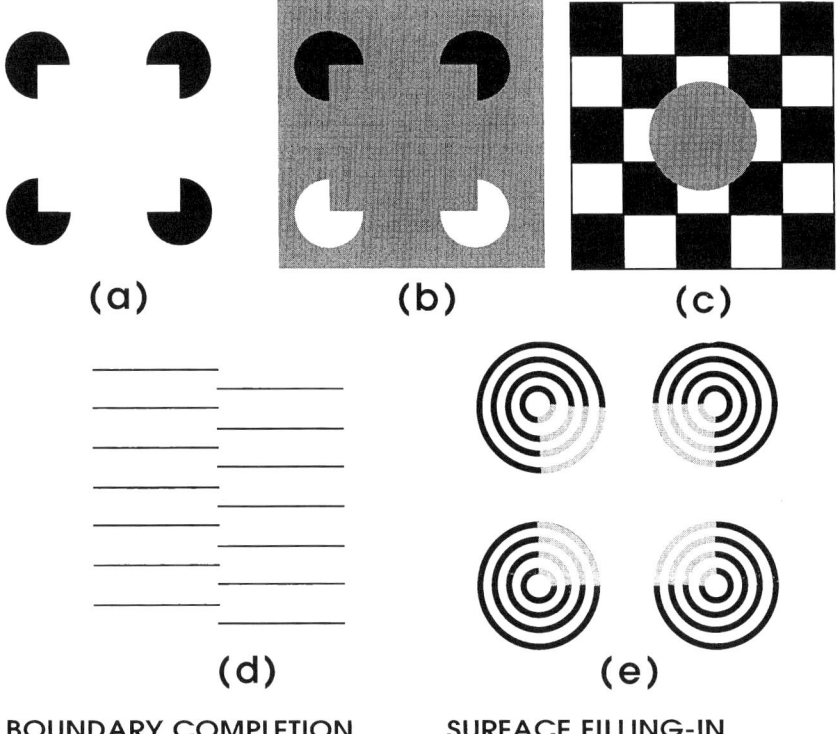

**BOUNDARY COMPLETION**

oriented
inward
insensitive to contrast polarity

**SURFACE FILLING-IN**

unoriented
outward
sensitive to contrast polarity

**Figure 2-2.** Visual boundary and surface interactions. (a) The emergent Kanizsa square can be seen and recognized because of the enhanced illusory brightness within the illusory square relative to the background brightness outside the square. (b) The reverse-contrast Kanizsa square can be recognized but not seen. We are aware of the square boundary even though the gray color inside and outside the square is approximately the same. (c) The boundary of the gray disk can form around its entire circumference, even though the relative contrast between the disk and the white and black background squares reverses periodically along the circumference. (d) The vertical illusory contour that forms at the ends of the horizontal lines can be consciously recognized even though it cannot be seen by virtue of any contrast difference between it and the background. (e) In this example of neon color spreading, the color in the gray contours spreads in all directions until it fills the square illusory contour. This percept illustrates the three complementary properties of boundary completion and surface filling-in that are summarized below the figure: The boundaries can form *inwardly* and in an *oriented* manner between pairs or greater numbers of image inducers. The output of this boundary system is also *insensitive* to contrast polarity because it pools signals from opposite contrasts at each position, as illustrated by Figures 2-2b and 2-2c. The gray surface color fills-in the square *outwardly* and in an *unoriented* fashion. It is *sensitive* to contrast polarity because it creates visible percepts of brightness and color. Boundaries are predicted to form within the interblob stream, whereas surfaces are predicted to form within the blob stream; see Figure 2-1.

derived directly from visual signals on our retinas. Thus many of the percepts that we believe to be "real" are visual illusions whose boundary and surface representations just happen to look real. What we call a visual illusion may thus be just an unfamiliar combination of boundary and surface information. This hypothesis is illustrated by the percepts generated in our brains from the images in Figure 2-2.

In response to the images in Figures 2-2a and 2-2b, illusory contours form *inwardly* between cooperating pairs of colinear edges of the four pacman, or pie-shaped inducers in the image. Four such contours form the boundary of the perceived Kanizsa square. (If boundaries formed outwardly from a single inducer, then any speck of dirt in an image could crowd all of our percepts with an outwardly growing web of boundaries.) This boundary completion process is *oriented* to form only between (almost) like-oriented and (almost) colinear inducers. Both of these properties are useful to complete edges in a scene that are not fully detected at the retina due to the blind spot, or due to other retinal imperfections such as retinal veins and scotomas. The square boundary in Figure 2-2a can be both seen and recognized because of the enhanced illusory brightness of the Kanizsa square relative to its background; see the explanation below. In contrast, the square boundary in Figure 2-2b can be recognized even though it is not visible; that is, there is no brightness or color difference on either side of the boundary. Figure 1-2b shows that *some* boundaries can be recognized even though they are perceptually unseen or invisible. Such percepts are sometimes said to be *amodal*. FACADE theory predicts that *all boundaries are invisible* within the boundary stream, which is proposed to be the interblob cortical processing stream (Fig. 2-1).

Why are all boundaries invisible within the boundary stream? The invisible boundary in Figure 2-2b can be traced to the fact that its vertical boundaries form between black and white inducers that possess opposite contrast polarity with respect to the gray background; that is, the black inducers have a black-to-gray, or dark-to-light, polarity with respect to the background, whereas the white inducers have a white-to-gray, or light-to-dark, polarity with respect to the background. The same is true of the boundary around the gray circular disk in Figure 2-2c. In this figure, the gray disk lies in front of a black and white textured background whose contrasts with respect to the disk reverse along its perimeter. In order to build a boundary around the entire disk, despite these contrast reversals, the boundary system pools, or adds, signals from pairs of *simple cells* that are sensitive to the same orientation and position but to opposite contrast polarities. This pooling process occurs in the V1 interblob stream at the *complex cells*. This is how the square boundary in response to Figure 2-2b, and the circular boundary in response to Figure 2-2c, start to form in our brains. This pooling process renders the boundary system output *insensitive* to contrast polarity. The boundary system hereby loses its ability to represent visible colors or brightnesses: Because it pools light/dark and dark/light contrasts at each position, its output cannot signal the difference between dark and light. It is in this sense that "all boundaries are invisible." The *inward* and *oriented* boundary completion process that forms the illusory square is activated by these pooled signals in the V2 interstripe area (Von der Heydt et al., 1984; Peterhans and Von der Heydt, 1989). These three properties of boundary completion (oriented, inward, insensitive to contrast polarity) are summarized at the bottom of Figure 2-2. Figure 2-2d illustrates another invisible boundary that can be consciously recognized.

Such a boundary formation process in the brain is a key mechanism whereby we perceive geometrical objects such as lines, curves, and textured objects. Rather than being defined in terms of such classical units as points and lines, these boundaries arise as a coherent pattern of excitatory and inhibitory signals across a feedback network that describes the cellular interactions from the retina through the LGN and the V1 interblob and V2 interstripe areas (Gove, et al., 1995; Grossberg, 1999b; Grossberg and Raizada, 2000; Grossberg and Williamson, 2001). In such a network, spatially long-range excitatory, or cooperative, interactions try to build the boundaries across space while interacting with shorter-range inhibitory, or competitive, interactions that suppress incorrect boundary groupings. These interactions select the best boundary grouping from among many possible interpretations of a scene. The winning grouping is represented either by an approach to equilibrium or by a synchronous oscillation of the system, until the grouping is reset to enable a subsequent grouping to form (Francis et al., 1994; Francis and Grossberg, 1996). The same system can approach either an equilibrium or an oscillation, depending upon how its parameters are chosen, notably the relative rate at which excitatory and inhibitory signals are processed. Classical geometry is hereby replaced by nonlinear neural networks that do a type of on-line statistical inference to select and complete the statistically most favored boundary groupings of a scene while suppressing noise and incorrect groupings. Our model for how such perceptual boundaries are formed has been called the *Boundary Contour System* (BCS). The word *boundary* was selected to acknowledge that groupings may form in response to edges, texture gradients, shading, stereo, and other scenic cues where "contours" occur.

## *Surfaces Are for Seeing*

If boundaries are invisible, then how do we see anything? FACADE theory predicts that visible properties of a scene are represented by a surface processing system, which is predicted to occur within the blob cortical stream (Fig. 2-1). A key step in representing a visible surface is the filling-in process. What is filling-in, and why and how does it occur? An early stage of surface processing compensates for variable illumination or *discounts the illuminant*. Otherwise, illuminant variations, which can change from moment to moment, could seriously distort all percepts. Discounting the illuminant attenuates color and brightness signals except near regions of sufficiently rapid surface change, such as edges or texture gradients, which are relatively uncontaminated by illuminant variations. The discounting process hereby selects *feature contours* at positions where luminance or color changes quickly. These feature contours are relatively uncontaminated by illumination gradients.

Neural models have proposed how later stages of surface formation fill in the attenuated regions with these relatively uncontaminated color and brightness signals (Cohen and Grossberg, 1984; Grossberg and Todorovic, 1988; Gove et al., 1995; Pessoa et al., 1995; Grossberg and Kelly, 1999). Remarkably, the filling-in process can also allocate brightness and color signals to their perceived depths on a three-dimensional (3D) surface through a process called *surface capture*, whereby the boundaries formed within the V2 interstripes interact with the V2 thin stripes and area V4 (see Fig. 2-1) to trigger depth-selective filling-in processes there (Grossberg, 1994, 1997; Grossberg and McLoughlin, 1997; Grossberg and Pessoa, 1998; Kelly and Grossberg, 2000). This multistage filling-in process is an example of hierarchical resolution of uncertainty, because the later filling-in stage overcomes uncertainties about brightness and color that were caused by discounting the illuminant at an earlier processing stage. How surface capture may occur in the brain is summarized below.

Before discussing depthful surface capture, we need to understand a more basic property: How do the illuminant-discounted signals fill-in an entire region? Filling-in behaves like a diffusion of brightness across space. For example, consider the percept of *neon color spreading* that is elicited by Figure 2-2e (Redies and Spillmann, 1981). This figure consists of circular annuli, part of which are black and part gray. In response to this figure, we can see an illusory square filled with a gray color. FACADE theory suggests that this percept is due to an interaction between the boundary and surface systems. In particular, the black boundaries cause small breaks, called *end gaps*, in the gray boundaries where they join; see Grossberg and Mingolla (1985) and Grossberg (1994, 1999a) for further discussion of how this happens. The gray color can hereby spread through these breaks from the annuli into the illusory square. In this percept, filling-in spreads *outward* from the individual gray inducers in all directions. Its spread is thus *unoriented*. How is this spread of activation contained? FACADE theory predicts that signals from the boundary stream to the surface stream define the regions within which filling-in is restricted within the surface stream. These boundaries surround the annuli (except for their small breaks) and also form the square illusory contour. Thus, filling-in is a form of anisotropic diffusion in which boundary signals nonlinearly gate, or inhibit, the diffusive flow of signal. Without these boundary signals, filling-in would dissipate across space, and no surface percept could form. Invisible boundaries hereby indirectly ensure their own visibility through their interactions with the surface stream, within which all visible percepts are predicted to form.

With these ideas in mind, we can better understand finer aspects of the other percepts that form in response to the images in Figure 2-2. In Figure 2-2a, the square boundary is induced by four black pacmen that are all less luminant than the white background. In the surface stream, discounting the illuminant causes these pacmen to induce local brightness enhancements adjacent to the pacmen and just within the boundary of the square. At a subsequent processing stage, these enhanced brightness signals spread within the square boundary, thereby causing the entire interior of the square to look brighter. The square is visible because the filled-in activity level within the square is higher than the filled-in activity level of the surrounding region. Filling-in can hereby lead to visible percepts because it is *sensitive* to contrast polarity. These three properties of surface filling-in (unoriented, outward, sensitive to contrast polarity) are summarized at the bottom of Figure 2-2. They are complementary to the corresponding properties of boundary completion.

In Figure 2-2b, the opposite polarities of the two pairs of pacmen with respect to the gray background lead to approximately equal filled-in activities inside and outside the square, since the black pacmen cause enhanced brightness signals but the white pacmen cause enhanced darkness signals. As a result, the effects of these opposite inductions can approximately cancel out after filling-in if the relative contrasts, and sizes of the pacmen and the square, are chosen correctly. When this happens, the boundary can be recognized but not seen. In Figure 2-2d, the white background can fill-in uniformly on both sides of the vertical boundary, by filling-in around the horizontal black lines, so no visible contrast difference is seen on the two sides of the vertical boundary.

In addition to explaining percepts such as those arising from Figure 2-2, filling-in clarifies how our brains can see brightnesses and colors within the boundaries that span retinal imperfections like the blind spot. Thus the same mechanisms can complete surface representations across spatial gaps like the blind spot, as well as across spatial gaps caused by discounting the illuminant. Similar considerations help to explain how we see continuous blue surfaces (Grossberg, 1987a, Section 31) despite the fact that the spatial distribution of blue cones on the retina is very sparse (Tansley and Boynton, 1976, 1978; Boynton et al., 1985).

These remarks just begin to illustrate the importance of filling-in and how it seems to be organized in the brain. Even in the seemingly simple case of the Kanizsa square, one often perceives a square hovering in front of four partially occluded circular disks, which seem to be completed behind the square, even though they are invisible there. FACADE theory predicts how surface filling-in helps such figure–ground percepts to occur in response to both two-dimensional (2D) pictures and 3D scenes; see below for an introductory discussion, and Grossberg (1994, 1997), Grossberg and McLoughlin (1997), and Kelly and Grossberg (2000) for more detailed examples and explanations.

In summary, boundary completion and surface filling-in illustrate two key principles of brain organization: hierarchical resolution of uncertainty and complementary interstream interactions. Figure 2-2 summarizes three pairs of complementary properties of the boundary and surface streams. Hierarchical resolution of uncertainty is illustrated by surface filling-in: Discounting the illuminant creates uncertainty by suppressing surface color and brightness signals except near surface discontinuities. Higher stages of filling-in complete the surface representation using properties that are complementary to those whereby boundaries are formed, guided by signals from these boundaries. This reduces the uncertainty that was originally created by discounting the illuminant. Our model for how surfaces are formed is called the *Feature Contour System* (FCS) because it clarifies how the *features* that we consciously see are processed into visible 3D surface percepts. This happens through filling-in operations that are activated by the *feature contours* that are extracted when the illuminant is being discounted. FACADE theory attempts to characterize how the BCS and FCS are internally organized and how they interact to overcome their complementary deficiencies.

Boundary-gated filling-in is a type of anisotropic diffusion that differs strongly from the classical view of how a surface is formed, that has often been adopted in computer vision, in terms of surface normals or differential forms. The mathematical analysis of surface filling-in has hardly begun, even though its remarkable properties have already been successfully used in processing complex imagery in technology (e.g., Waxman et al., 1995). Another important problem on which a great deal of work remains to be done concerns the origin of the complementarity of boundaries and surfaces. One prediction is that this property arises through a process of symmetry-breaking as the embryonic brain bifurcates into its parallel cortical processing streams.

## Brightness Constancy, Contrast, and Assimilation

Controversy persists about whether or not a physical filling-in interaction exists; for example, see Dennett (1991) and Pessoa et al. (1998). This question can be answered only by direct experimental testing and by showing how neural models that include filling-in can explain many data that cannot be explained by models that omit it. In the Dennett (1991) critique of the physical existence of filling-in as a process in the brain, no explanations of the parametric properties of the percepts that have been used to support the filling-in concept were attempted, despite the fact that modeling articles had already explained and simulated key perceptual data by using a neural filling-in process; for example, see Cohen and Grossberg (1984), Grossberg and Mingolla (1985), Grossberg (1987a, 1987b), and Grossberg and Todorovic (1988). Psychophysical data that directly support a filling-in process by studying its temporal dynamics have also been reported (Paradiso and Nakayama, 1991) and have been quantitatively simulated by Arrington (1994) using the brightness perception model of Grossberg and Todorovic (1988).

Since that time, many other data have been explained and simulated by FACADE theory with the help of filling-in. These include data about 3D figure–ground perception (Grossberg, 1994, 1997; Grossberg and McLoughlin, 1997; Kelly and Grossberg, 2000), texture perception (Grossberg and Pessoa, 1998), brightness perception (Gove et al., 1995; Grossberg and Kelly, 1999), negative aftereffects (Francis and Grossberg, 1996), and long-term aftereffects like the McCollough effect (McCollough, 1965; Grossberg et al., 2001). Most of these data have no other mechanistic explanation at this time. Any vision theory that purports to do without filling-in now needs to explain these data in order to be competitive. In particular, any such theory needs to provide principled explanations of how basic phenomena like discounting the illuminant and filling-in across the blind spot can occur.

One of the lessons from these modeling studies is that filling-in cannot be studied adequately outside the context of a more comprehensive vision model, if only because of the complementarity of boundary and surface computations. Another lesson is that different combinations of mechanisms may be rate-limiting in giving rise to the different percepts that depend in part on filling-in. For example, Grossberg and Todorovic (1988) showed that the following simple mechanisms are sufficient to explain many, but not all, data properties of brightness perception. A few of these data properties are illustrated in Figure 2-3. They can be explained by interactions of (1) an on-center/off-surround network of cells that obey shunting, or membrane, equations, (2) a boundary formation network, and (3) a surface filling-in network. The cells of the shunting on-center/off-

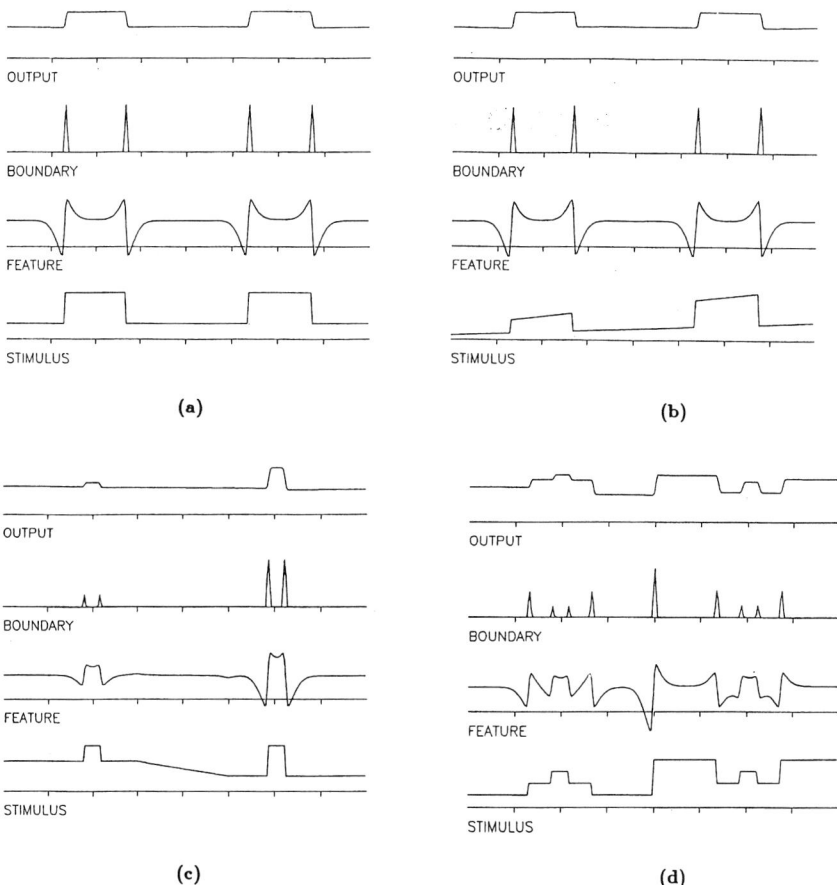

**Figure 2-3.** How filling-in can explain examples of brightness constancy (a and b), brightness contrast (c), and brightness assimilation (d) using mechanisms that discount the illuminant (FEATURE) from a pattern of image luminances (STIMULUS) and use the discounted activity pattern to compute a BOUNDARY representation within which the FEATURE pattern fills-in to generate an OUTPUT brightness pattern. See text for details. (*Source:* Adapted with permission from Grossberg and Todorovic, 1988)

surround network preprocess visual inputs by discounting the illuminant and computing Weber law–modulated estimates of image reflectances that are sensitive to the local context of luminance signals, thereby contrast-normalizing input intensities. These contrast-normalized cell activities then input to the boundary formation and surface filling-in networks.

Figure 2-3 gives four examples of how the simplest filling-in network works. The lowest row of each panel in the figure shows a one-dimensional (1D) cross section of image luminance. The next-lowest row shows how a shunting on-center/off-surround network of cells can transform these image intensities. A comparison of (a) and (b) shows that such a network can compensate for a gradient of illumination; see the patterns labeled FEATURE in the figure. In so doing, the network can also distort the true pattern of image reflectances by generating cusps and dips in the profile of cell activities across space. One of these distortions is the attenuation of image reflectances away from object edges or other rapidly changing luminance gradients across space. This is the key mechanism whereby the illuminant is discounted. Boundary and surface interactions help to compensate for these distortions by exploiting the information that survives the discounting process. The boundaries create a frame within which the illuminant-discounted signals can fill-in within the surface processing stream; see the patterns labeled BOUNDARY in the figure. Thus, in Figures 2-3a and 2-3b, boundaries form at the luminance discontinuities of the image because the boundary system is sensitive to discontinuities in the activity profile of discounted signals. The pattern of these discounted signals is topographically mapped into filling-in domains (FIDOs) within the surface stream, or FCS. Here the discounted signals can begin to spread across space. This spreading process has many of the properties of diffusion. The signal spread is contained within boundary signals that are topographically mapped from the BCS into the FIDOs. The result is given in the top row of each panel, namely, the patterns labeled OUTPUT.

Figures 2-3a and 2-3b show how these simple mechanisms can discount the illuminant and recover the original pattern of image reflectances under some circumstances. This is an example of *brightness constancy*. However, due to the discounting process, image reflectances are not always veridically recovered. For example, the STIMULUS in Figure 2-3c contains two steps of equal luminance on a background that varies so gradually between them that no boundary is detected. In the OUTPUT profile, *brightness contrast* obtains; that is, the right step is more active than the left step in the OUTPUT activity profile. This is due to the sensitivity of the on-center/off-surround network to image contrasts; see the FEATURE pattern. Remarkably, however, the luminance gradient that caused the brightness contrast is not visible in the final percept. The background has uniform brightness in the OUTPUT because there is no boundary to restrict the filling-in process between the two luminance steps, as also occurs in vivo under such conditions. In addition to showing how brightness contrast can occur due to the discounting process, this is a philosophically interesting example because it demonstrates a *visible effect of an invisible cause*.

Figure 2-3d shows that the same mechanisms can also cause the opposite of brightness contrast, namely, *brightness assimilation* (Helson, 1963). This figure simulates an effect that was reported by Shapley and Reid (1986). The luminance profile here is derived from a standard brightness contrast profile by the introduction of two additional test regions. These test luminance steps are the same and are placed on equally but less luminant backgrounds. A simple brightness contrast explanation would suggest that the two steps should have the same brightness. However, humans report that the left step looks brighter than the right one, as also occurs in the OUTPUT activity profile of the model. The perceived brightness of the background has been assimilated into the brightness of the steps. How this happens in the model can be inferred from Figure 2-3d, which shows that a spatial pattern of activity cusps and dips is caused by the discounting process. These cusps and dips are broader than the boundaries that they induce. When this FEATURE profile fills-in within its narrower boundaries, assimilation obtains in the OUTPUT as an emergent property of network interactions.

The same model can explain many other brightness data in a unified way, including variants of the Craik-O'Brien-Cornsweet effect, the Koffka-Benussi ring, Kanizsa-Minguzzi anomalous brightness differentiation, the Hermann grid, a Land Modrian viewed under constant and gradient illumination that cannot be explained by Retinex theory, impossible staircases, bull's-eyes, and various nested combinations of luminance profiles. That such a simple combination of discounting-and-normalizing, boundary, and surface interactions can explain such a large body of brightness data, with a fixed set of parameters, is a challenge to other models of filling-in and brightness perception. Properties like lightness scission and anchoring require further structure to be understood. See Grossberg (1999a) for an example of scission during neon color spreading, and see Grossberg et al. (1995) for examples of how contrast and luminance channels, working together, may contribute to anchoring.

## *Three-Dimensional Vision and Figure–Ground Separation*

Although the mechanisms illustrated in Figure 2-3 may be necessary for explaining how filling-in works within the brain, they are certainly not sufficient. In particular, the mechanisms in Figure 2-3 are not sufficient to explain how two eyes work together to generate 3D percepts of surfaces in depth, notably how percepts of occluding and occluded objects are generated in depth. The struggle to understand such 3D vision and figure–ground perception has been a key motivation for the further development of FACADE theory; see, for example, Grossberg (1994, 1997). Multiple problems need to be solved in order to understand 3D vision and figure–ground perception.

*Three-Dimensional Surface Capture and Filling-In*
How are the luminance and color signals received by the two eyes transformed into 3D surface percepts? FACADE theory posits that multiple depth-selective boundary representations exist and interact with multiple depth-selective surface filling-in domains to determine which surfaces in depth can be seen. The same

filling-in processes that enable us to see perceptual qualities like brightness and color are predicted to also determine the relative depth of these surfaces. In particular, depth-selective boundaries selectively *capture* brightness and color signals at their own FIDOs to support depthful visual percepts. FACADE theory predicts how perceived depth and brightness can interact. In fact, brighter surfaces can look closer (Egusa, 1983).

*Binocular Fusion, Grouping, and da Vinci Stereopsis*
Granted that surface capture can achieve depth-selective filling-in, how are the depth-selective boundaries formed that control surface capture? Our two eyes view the world from slightly different perspectives. Their different views lead to relative displacements, or disparities, on the two retinas of the images that they register. These disparate retinal images are binocularly matched at disparity-sensitive cells. The disparity-sensitive cells are used to form depth-selective boundaries, which capture surface filling-in signals at the corresponding depth-selective FIDOs.

When two eyes view the world, part of a scene may be seen by only one eye. No disparity signals are available at these locations by which to determine the depth of the monocularly viewed features, yet they are seen at the correct depth (Nakayama and Shimojo, 1990). FACADE theory proposes how depth-selective filling-in of a nearby binocularly viewed region propagates into the monocularly viewed region to impart the correct depth. This proposal also explains related phenomena like the *equidistance tendency*, whereby a monocularly viewed object in a binocular scene seems to lie at the same depth as the retinally most contiguous binocularly viewed object (Gogel, 1965). This work leads to a number of new hypotheses, including how horizontal and monocularly viewed boundaries are added to all boundary representations, and how an *asymmetry between near and far* distributes boundaries from nearer to farther surface representations. Without these mechanisms, all occluding objects would look transparent.

*Multiple Scales into Multiple Boundary Depths*
When a single eye views the image of an object in depth, the same size of the retinal image may be due to either a large object far away or a small object nearby. How is this ambiguity overcome to activate the correct disparity-sensitive cells? The brain uses multiple receptive field sizes, or scales, that achieve a *size–disparity correlation* between retinal size and binocular disparity. It has often been thought that larger scales code nearer objects and smaller scales more distant objects. For example, a nearer object can lead to a larger disparity that can be binocularly fused by a larger scale. In fact, each scale can fuse multiple disparities, although larger scales can fuse a wider range of disparities (Julesz and Schumer, 1981). This ambiguity helps to explain how higher spatial frequencies in an image can sometimes look closer, rather than more distant, than lower spatial frequencies in an image, and how this percept can reverse during prolonged viewing (Brown and Weisstein, 1988). FACADE theory explains these reversals by analyzing how multiple spatial scales interact to form depth-selective boundary groupings (Grossberg, 1994).

Multiple spatial scales also help to explain how shaded surfaces are seen. In fact, if boundaries were sensitive only to the bounding edge of a shaded surface, then shaded surfaces could look uniformly bright and flat after filling-in occurs. Recall that boundaries respond to shading gradients as well as to edges. Different scales react differently to different regions of the shading gradients, leading to a multiple-depth *boundary web* of small boundary compartments. Such a boundary web traps contrasts locally and leads to a shaded surface percept.

*Recognizing Objects versus Seeing Their Unoccluded Parts*
In many scenes, some objects lie partially in front of other objects and thereby occlude them. How do we know which features belong to the different objects in both 3D scenes and 2D pictures? If we could not make this distinction, then object recognition would be severely impaired. FACADE theory predicts how the mechanisms that solve this problem when we view 3D scenes also solve the problem when we view 2D pictures.

Figure 2-4 clarifies some of the issues that need to be understood. In the Bregman-Kanizsa image of Figure 2-4a, the gray B shapes can be readily recognized even though they are partially occluded by the black snakelike occluder. In Figure 2-4b, the black occluder is replaced by white. Although the same amount of gray is shown in both images, the B shapes are much harder to recognize in Figure 2-4b. This difference is attributed to the fact that the boundaries shared by the black occluder and the gray B shapes in Figure 2-4a are assigned by the brain to the black occluder. These boundaries are formed at a boundary representation that is perceived to be closer to the viewer than the boundary representation of the gray shapes. With the shared boundaries removed from the gray B shapes, the B boundaries can be completed at a farther boundary representation, behind the position of the black occluder, in much the same way that the Kanizsa square

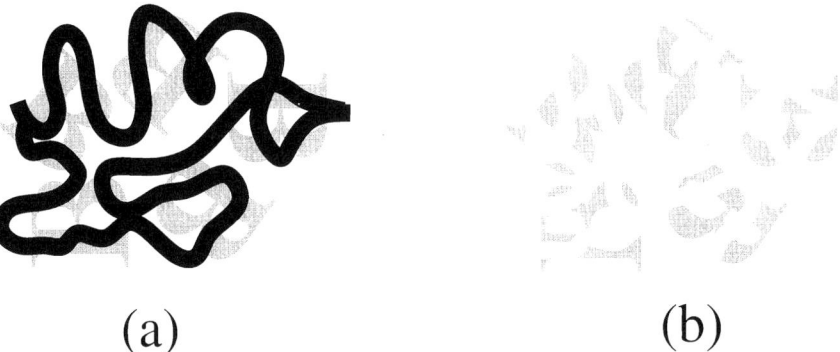

**Figure 2-4.** (a) Uppercase gray B letters are partially occluded by a black snakelike occluder. (b) Same B shapes as in (a), except that the occluder is white and therefore merges with the remainder of the white background. (*Source:* Adapted with permission from Nakayama et al., 1989)

boundary is completed in Figure 2-2a. These completed boundaries help us to recognize the B's at the farther depth. In Figure 2-4b, the shared boundaries are not removed from the gray shapes, and they prevent the completion of the gray boundaries.

To actually do this, the brain needs to solve several problems. First, it needs to figure out how geometrical and contrast factors work together. In Figure 2-4a, for example, the T-junctions where the gray shapes intersect the black occluders seem to be a cue for signaling that the black occluder looks closer than the gray shapes. However, if you imagine the black occluder gradually getting lighter until it matches the white background in Figure 2-4b, it is clear that when the occluder is light enough, the gray shapes will no longer appear behind the occluder. Thus, geometrical factors like T-junctions are not sufficient to cause figure–ground separation. They interact with contrast relationships within the scene too.

The brain also needs to figure out how to complete the B boundaries "behind" the occluder in response to a 2D picture. In particular, how are different spatial scales differentially activated by a 2D picture as well as by a 3D scene so that the occluding and occluded objects can be seen in depth? Moreover, if the B boundaries can be completed and thereby recognized, then why do we not *see* completely filled-in B shapes too, including in the regions behind the black occluder? This situation demonstrates that there is a design tension between the properties needed to recognize opaque objects, including where they are occluded, and our ability to see only their unoccluded surfaces. Here again, *the asymmetry between near and far* plays a key role, as noted below.

*From Boundary–Surface Complementarity to Consistency*
The very existence of such subtle data might fill one with wonder about how the brain evolved to behave in this way. FACADE theory predicts how a small number of simple mechanisms that realize a few new perceptual principles can, when they interact together, explain figure–ground data. The need for one of these principles can be seen in Figure 2-2, which illustrates that boundary and surface computations are complementary. How, then, do we see a single percept wherein boundaries and surfaces are consistently joined? How does *complementarity* become *consistency*? FACADE theory proposes how consistency is achieved by a simple kind of feedback that occurs between the boundary and surface streams. Remarkably, this feedback can also explain many facts about figure–ground perception. The remainder of the chapter sketches some of these principles and mechanisms.

## FACADE Principles and Mechanisms

Figure 2-5 is a macrocircuit of FACADE theory in its present form. Monocular processing of left-eye and right-eye inputs by the retina and the LGN discounts the illuminant and generates parallel signals to the BCS and FCS. These signals

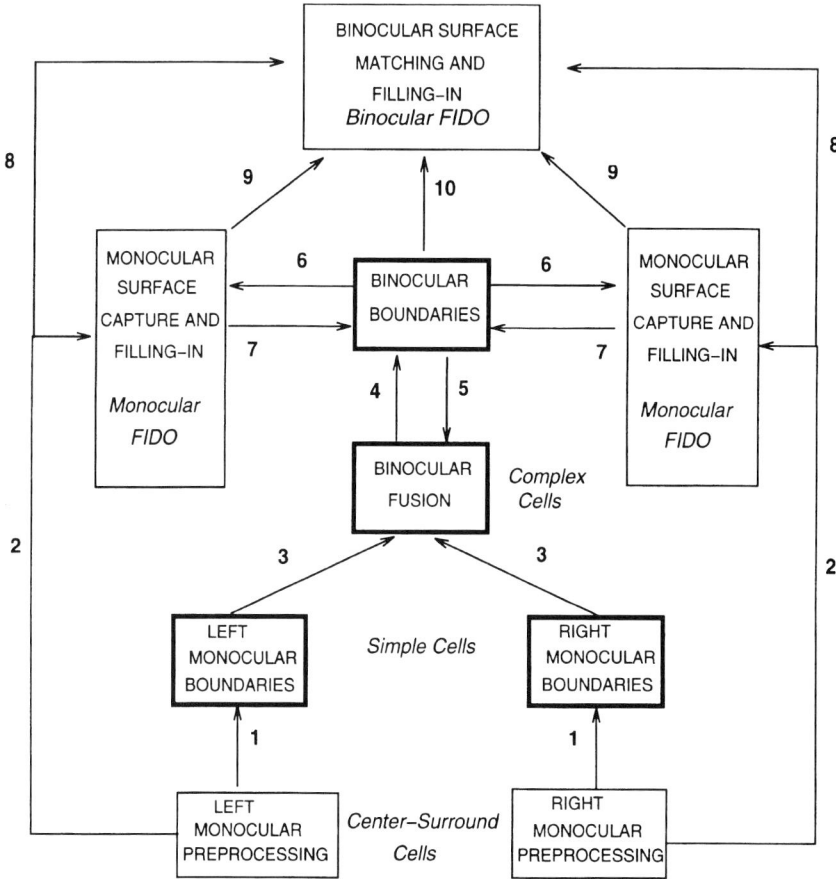

**Figure 2-5.** FACADE macrocircuit showing interactions of the Boundary Contour System (BCS) and Feature Contour System (FCS). FIDO = filling-in domain. See text for details. (*Source:* Reprinted with permission from Kelly and Grossberg, 2000)

go to model cortical simple cells via pathways 1 in Figure 2-5, and to monocular FIDOs via pathways 2. Model simple cells have oriented receptive fields and come in multiple sizes. Simple cell outputs are binocularly combined at disparity-sensitive complex and complex end-stopped (or hypercomplex) cells via pathways 3. Complex cells with larger receptive fields can binocularly fuse a broader range of disparities than can cells with smaller receptive fields, thereby realizing a *size-disparity correlation* (Smallman and MacLeod, 1994). Competition across disparity at each position and among cells of a given size scale sharpens complex cell disparity tuning (Fahle and Westheimer, 1995). Spatial competition (end-stopping) and orientational competition convert complex cell responses into spatially and orientationally sharper responses at hypercomplex cells.

How are responses from multiple receptive field *sizes* combined to generate boundary representations of relative *depths* from the observer? FACADE theory proposes that hypercomplex cells activate bipole cells via pathway 4. These bipole cells carry out long-range grouping and boundary completion via horizontal connections that occur in layer 2/3 of area V2 interstripes. Bipole grouping collects together outputs from hypercomplex cells of all sizes that are sensitive to a given depth range. The bipole cells then send excitatory feedback signals via pathways 5 back to all hypercomplex cells that represent the same position and orientation, and send inhibitory feedback signals to hypercomplex cells at nearby positions and orientations. The feedback binds together, or groups, cells of multiple *sizes* into a BCS representation, or copy, that is sensitive to a prescribed range of *depths*. Multiple BCS copies are formed, each corresponding to different (but possibly overlapping) depth ranges.

This grouping process also play a a key role in figure–ground separation. Each bipole cell has an oriented receptive field with two branches (Fig. 2-6). Each branch receives inputs from a range of almost colinear orientations and positions. When the bipole cell does not receive direct bottom-up activation of its cell body, it can fire only if both receptive field branches are simultaneously active. This ensures that the cells do not complete boundaries beyond a line end unless there is another line end that provides evidence for such a linkage. The bipole cell thus behaves like a statistical AND gate. Such cells were first used by Cohen and Grossberg (1984) and Grossberg and Mingolla (1985) to model data about perceptual grouping and filling-in. Cells with similar properties in cortical area V2 were first reported by von der Heydt et al. (1984). Bipole cell properties are also consistent with many subsequent psychophysical data; for example, see Field et al. (1993) and Shipley and Kellman (1992). Grossberg and Raizada (2000) and Grossberg and Williamson (2001) have simulated how bipole properties may develop and are anatomically realized in layer 2/3 of cortical areas V1 and V2.

How does the bipole grouping process contribute to figure–ground separation? Long-range excitatory bipole signals combine with shorter-range inhibitory signals to make the system sensitive to T-junctions (Fig. 2-6), without the use of explicit T-junction operators. In particular, horizontally oriented bipole cells that are located where the top of the T joins its stem receive excitatory inputs to both of their receptive field branches. Vertically oriented bipole cells that process the stem of the T where it joins the top receive excitatory support only in the one branch that is activated by the stem. Because of this excitatory imbalance, inhibition of the stem by the top can cause a gap in the stem boundary (Fig. 2-6), termed an *end-gap*. During filling-in, boundaries contain the filling-in process. Where end-gaps occur, brightness or color can flow out of a figural region. FACADE theory predicts that this escape of color or brightness via filling-in is a key step that initiates figure–ground separation; see Grossberg (1994, 1997), Grossberg and McLoughlin (1997), and Kelly and Grossberg (2000) for examples.

How do multiple depth-selective BCS copies capture brightness and color signals within depth-selective FCS surface representations? This happens in at

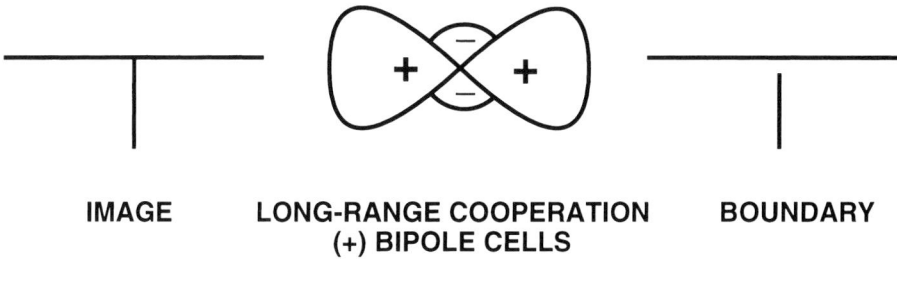

**Figure 2-6.** T-junction sensitivity in the Boundary Contour System (BCS). (a) T-junction in an image. (b) Bipole cells provide long-range cooperation (+), whereas hypercomplex cells provide short-ranger competition (−). (c) An end-gap in the vertical boundary arises due to this combination of cooperation and competition. (*Source:* Reprinted with permission from Grossberg, 1997)

least two stages. The first stage of *monocular FIDOs* may exist in V2 thin stripes. Each monocular FIDO is broken into three pairs of opponent FIDOs (black/white, red/green, and blue/yellow) that receive achromatic and chromatic signals from a single eye. A pair of monocular FIDOs, one for each eye, corresponds to each depth-selective BCS copy and receives its strongest boundary-gating signals from this BCS copy. Each monocular FIDO may also receive weaker boundary signals from BCS copies that represent depths close to that of its primary BCS copy. In this way, a finite set of FIDOs can represent a continuous change in perceived depth.

*Surface capture* is triggered when BCS boundary-gating signals interact with illuminant-discounted FCS signals. Pathways 2 in Figure 2-5 input discounted monocular FCS signals to *all* monocular FIDOs. Only some FIDOs will selectively fill-in these signals, and thereby lift monocular FIDO signals into depth-selective surface representations for filling-in. The boundary signals along pathways 6 in Figure 2-5 determine which FIDOs will fill-in. These boundary signals selectively capture FCS inputs that are spatially coincident and orientationally aligned with them. Other FCS inputs are suppressed. These properties follow when double-opponent, boundary-gating, and filling-in processes interact. How this happens, and how it can explain data about binocular fusion and rivalry, among other percepts, are discussed in Grossberg (1987b).

Because these filled-in surfaces are activated by depth-selective BCS boundaries, they inherit the depths of their boundaries. Three-dimensional surfaces may hereby represent depth as well as brightness and color. This link between depth, brightness, and color helps to explain *proximity–luminance covariation*, or why brighter surfaces tend to look closer; see, for example, Egusa (1983).

Not every filling-in event generates a visible surface. Because activity spreads until it hits a boundary, only surfaces that are surrounded by a *connected* BCS boundary are effectively filled-in. Otherwise, the spreading activity can dissipate across the FIDO. This property helps to explain data ranging from neon color spreading to how T-junctions influence 3D figure–ground perception (Grossberg,1994).

An analysis of how the BCS and FCS react to 3D images shows that too many boundary and surface fragments are formed as a result of the size-disparity correlation (Richards and Kaye, 1974; Tyler, 1975; Kulikowski, 1978; Julesz and Schumer, 1981; Schor et al., 1984). As noted above, larger scales can fuse a larger range of disparities than can smaller scales. How are the surface depths that we perceive selected from this range of possibilities across all scales? FACADE's proposed answer to this question follows from its answer to the more fundamental question: How is perceptual *consistency* derived from boundary–surface *complementarity*? FACADE predicts how this may be achieved by feedback between the boundary and surface streams, which is predicted to occur no later than V2. This mutual feedback also helps to explain why blob and interblob cells share so many receptive field properties even though they carry out such different tasks. In particular, boundary cells, which summate inputs from both contrast polarities, can also be modulated by surface cells, which are sensitive to just one contrast polarity.

Boundary–surface consistency derives from a contrast-sensitive process that detects the contours of successfully filled-in regions within the monocular FIDOs. Only successfully filled-in regions *can* activate such a contour-sensitive process; other regions either do not fill-in at all or their filling-in dissipates across space. These filled-in contours activate FCS-to-BCS feedback signals (pathways 7 in Fig. 2-5) that strengthen boundaries at their own positions and depths while inhibiting redundant boundaries at farther depths. This inhibition from near-to-far is called *boundary pruning*. It illustrates a perceptual principle called the *asymmetry between near and far*. The operation of this principle is reflected in many data, including 3D neon color spreading (Nakayama et al., 1990). Grossberg (1994, 1999a) discusses how to explain such data.

How does boundary pruning influence figure–ground separation? Boundary pruning spares the closest surface representation that successfully fills-in a region, and inhibits redundant copies of occluding object boundaries that would otherwise form at farther depths. When these redundant occluding boundaries are removed, the boundaries of partially occluded objects can be completed behind them within BCS copies that represent farther depths, as in response to Figure 2-4a but not Figure 2-4b. Moreover, when the redundant occluding boundaries collapse, the redundant surfaces that they momentarily supported at the monocular FIDOs also collapse. Occluding surfaces hereby form in front of occluded surfaces. Boundary pruning also helps to explain data properties about depth/brightness interactions such as: Why do brighter Kanizsa squares look closer (Kanizsa, 1955, 1974; Bradley and Dumais, 1984; Purghé and Coren, 1992)? Why is boundary pruning relevant here? A Kanizsa square's brightness is an emergent property that is determined after *all* brightness and darkness inducers fill-in within the square. This emergent brightness within the FIDOs then influences the square's perceived depth. Within FACADE, this means that the FIDO's brightness influences the BCS copies that control relative depth. This occurs via the FCS-to-BCS feedback signals, including pruning, that ensure boundary–surface consistency (Grossberg, 1997, Section 22).

Visible brightness percepts are not represented within the monocular FIDOs. Model V2 representations of binocular boundaries and monocular filled-in surfaces are predicted to be *amodal*, or perceptually invisible. These representations are predicted to directly activate object recognition mechanisms in inferotemporal cortex and beyond, since they accurately represent occluding and occluded objects. In particular, boundary pruning enables boundaries of occluded objects to be completed within the BCS, which makes them easier to recognize, as in the Bregman-Kanizsa display of Figure 2-4. The monocular FIDO surface representations fill-in an occluded object within these completed object boundaries, even behind an opaque occluding object. We can hereby *know* the color of occluded regions without *seeing* them. How do we *see* opaque occluding surfaces? How does the visual cortex generate representations of occluding and occluded objects that can be easily recognized, yet also allow us to consciously see, and reach for, only the unoccluded parts of objects?

FACADE theory proposes that the latter goal is achieved at the binocular FIDOs using a different combination of boundary and surface representations than is found at the monocular FIDOs. The surface representations at the monocular FIDOs are depth-selective, but they do not combine brightness and color signals from both eyes. Binocular combination of brightness and color signals takes place at the binocular FIDOs, which are predicted to exist in cortical area V4. It is here that *modal*, or visible, surface representations occur, and we see only unoccluded parts of occluded objects, except when transparent percepts are generated by special circumstances.

For this to happen, monocular FCS signals from both eyes (pathways 8 in Fig. 2-5) are binocularly matched at the binocular FIDOs. These matched signals are redundantly represented on multiple FIDOs. The redundant binocular signals are pruned by inhibitory contrast-sensitive signals from the monocular FIDOs (pathways 9 in Fig. 2-5). As in the case of boundary pruning, these *surface pruning* signals arise from surface regions that successfully fill-in within the monocular FIDOs. These signals inhibit the FCS signals at their own positions and farther depths. As a result, occluding objects cannot redundantly fill-in surface representations at multiple depths. Surface pruning is another example of the *asymmetry between near and far*.

As in the monocular FIDOs, FCS signals to the binocular FIDOs can initiate filling-in only where they are spatially coincident and orientationally aligned with BCS boundaries. BCS-to-FCS pathways 10 in Figure 2-5 carry out depth-selective surface capture of the binocularly matched FCS signals that survive surface pruning. In all, binocular FIDOs fill in FCS signals that (1) survive within-depth binocular FCS matching and across-depth FCS inhibition; (2) are spatially coincident and orientationally aligned with BCS boundaries; and (3) are surrounded by a connected boundary (web).

One further property completes this summary: At the binocular FIDOs, nearer boundaries are added to FIDOs that represent their own and farther depths. This asymmetry between near and far is called *boundary enrichment*. Enriched boundaries prevent occluding objects from looking transparent by blocking filling-in of occluded objects behind them. The total filled-in surface representation across all binocular FIDOs represents the visible percept. It is called a FACADE representation because it multiplexes the properties of Form-And-Color-And-DEpth that give FACADE theory its name.

## Conclusion

This chapter outlines how filling-in may play a key role in surface perception, ranging from lower-level uses, such as recovering surface brightness and color after discounting the illuminant and filling-in the blind spot, to higher-level uses, such as completing depthful modal and amodal surface representations during 3D vision and figure–ground separation. Surface filling-in plays a central role in visual percepts because boundary and surface computations are complementary. Boundaries and surfaces need to interact reciprocally to merge these complementary properties into a consistent visual percept. Boundaries help to trigger depth-selective surface filling-in, and successfully filled-in surfaces reorganize the global patterning of boundary and surface signals via feedforward and feedback signals. Within FACADE theory, a small number of perceptual principles and mechanisms achieve such interactions and help to explain and predict a large body of perceptual and neural data, including the Weisstein effect; 3D neon color spreading; 3D Kanizsa-Varin percepts; Bregman-Kanizsa figure–ground separation; Kanizsa stratification; various lightness percepts, including the Munker-White, Benary cross, and checkerboard percepts (Grossberg, 1994, 1997; Kelly and Grossberg, 2000); and da Vinci stereopsis (Grossberg, 1994; Grossberg and Howe, 2002; Grossberg and McLoughlin, 1997). Without a filling-in process, many of these explanations would not have been possible. This fact represents a challenge to all perceptual models that omit filling-in from their explanatory toolbox.

*Acknowledgments*

Supported in part by the Air Force Office of Scientific Research (AFOSR F49620-01-1-0397), the Defense Advanced Research Projects Agency and the Office of Naval Research (ONR N00014-95-1-0409), and the Office of Naval Research (ONR N00014-95-1-0657 and ONR N00014-01-1-0624). The author wishes to thank Robin Amos for his valuable assistance in the preparation of the manuscript.

## References

Arrington KF (1994) The temporal dynamics of brightness filling-in. *Vision Res* 34:3371–3387.
Boynton RM, Eskew RT Jr, and Olson CX (1985) Research note: Blue cones contribute to border distinctness. *Vision Res* 25:1349–1352.

Bradley DR and Dumais ST (1984) The effects of illumination level and retinal size on the depth stratification of subjective contour figures. *Perception* 13:155–164.

Brown JM and Weisstein N (1988) A spatial frequency effect on perceived depth. *Percept Psychophys* 43:53–56.

Cohen MA and Grossberg S (1984) Neural dynamics of brightness perception: Features, boundaries, diffusion, and resonance. *Percept Psychophys* 36:428–456.

Dennett D (1991) *Consciousness Explained.* Boston: Little, Brown and Company.

Egusa H (1983) Effects of brightness, hue, and saturation on perceived depth between adjacent regions in the visual fields. *Perception* 12:167–175.

Elder JH and Zucker SW (1998) Evidence for boundary-specific grouping. *Vision Res* 38:143–152.

Fahle M and Westheimer G (1995) On the time-course of inhibition in the stereoscopic perception of rows of dots. *Vision Res* 35:1393–1399.

Faubert J and von Grünau M (1995) The influence of two spatially distinct primers and attribute priming on motion induction. *Vision Res* 36:149–173.

Field DJ, Hayes A, and Hess RF (1993) Contour integration by the human visual system: Evidence for a local "association field." *Vision Res* 33:173–193.

Francis G and Grossberg S (1996) Cortical dynamics of boundary segmentation and reset: Persistence, afterimages, and residual traces. *Perception* 25:543–567.

Francis G, Grossberg S, and Mingolla E (1994) Cortical dynamics of feature binding and reset: Control of visual persistence. *Vision Res* 34:1089–1104.

Gogel WC (1965) Equidistance tendency and its consequences. *Psychol Bull* 64:153–163.

Gove A, Grossberg S, and Mingolla E (1995) Brightness perception, illusory contours, and cortiogeniculate feedback. *Vis Neurosci* 12:1027–1052.

Grossberg S (1987a) Cortical dynamics of three-dimensional form, color, and brightness perception: I. Monocular theory. *Percept Psychophys* 41:87–116.

Grossberg S (1987b) Cortical dynamics of three-dimensional form, color, and brightness perception: II. Binocular theory. *Percept Psychophys* 41:117–141.

Grossberg S (1994) 3–D vision and figure–ground separation by visual cortex. *Percept Psychophys* 55:48–120.

Grossberg S (1997) Cortical dynamics of 3-D Figure-ground perception of 2-D pictures. *Psychol Rev* 104:618–658.

Grossberg S (1999a) A comment on "Assimilation of achromatic color cannot explain the brightness effects of the achromatic neon effect" by Marc K Albert. *Perception* 28:1291–1302.

Grossberg S (1999b) How does the cerebral cortex work? Learning, attention, and grouping by the laminar circuits of visual cortex. *Spatial Vision* 12:163–186.

Grossberg S and Howe PDL (2002) A laminar cortical model of stereopsis and 3-D surface perception. Tech Rept CAS/CNS-2002–002. Submitted.

Grossberg S, Hwang S, and Mingolla E (2001) Thalamocortical dynamics of the McCollough effect: Boundary-surface alignment through perceptual learning. *Vision Res* 42:1259–1286.

Grossberg S and Kelly F (1999) Neural dynamics of binocular brightness perception. *Vision Res* 39:3796–3816.

Grossberg S and McLoughlin N (1997) Cortical dynamics of 3–D surface perception: Binocular and half-occluded scenic images. *Neural Networks* 10:1583–1605.

Grossberg S and Mingolla E (1985) Neural dynamics of form perception: Boundary completion, illusory figures, and neon color spreading. *Psychol Rev* 92:173–211.

Grossberg S, Mingolla E, and Williamson JR (1995) Synthetic aperture radar processing by a multiple scale neural system for boundary and surface representation. *Neural Networks* 8:1005–1028.

Grossberg S and Pessoa L (1998) Texture segregation, surface representation, and figure–ground separation. *Vision Res* 38:2657–2684.

Grossberg S and Raizada RDS (2000) Contrast-sensitive perceptual grouping and object-based attention in the laminar circuits of primary visual cortex. *Vision Res* 40:1413–1432.

Grossberg S and Todorovic D (1988) Neural dynamics of 1–D and 2–D brightness perception: A unified model of classical and recent phenomena. *Percept Psychophys* 43:241–277.

Grossberg S and Williamson JR (2001) A neural model of how horizontal and interlaminar connections of visual cortex develop into adult circuits that carry out perceptual grouping and learning. *Cereb Cortex* 11:37–58.

Helson H (1963) Studies of anomalous contrast and assimilation. *J Opt Soc Am* 53:179–184.

Julesz B and Schumer RA (1981) Early visual perception. *Annu Rev Psychol* 32:572–627.

Kanizsa G (1955) Margini quasi-percettivi in campi con stimolazione omogenea. *Rev Psicologia* 49:7–30.

Kanizsa G (1974) Contours without gradients or cognitive contours. *Ital J Psychol* 1:93–113.

Kelly F and Grossberg S (2000) Neural dynamics of 3–D surface perception: Figure-ground separation and lightness perception. *Percept Psychophys* 62:1596–1618.

Kulikowski JJ (1978) Limit of single vision in stereopsis depends on contour sharpness. *Nature* 275:126–127.

Lamme VAF, Rodriguez-Rodriguez V, and Spekreijse H (1999) Separate processing dynamics for texture elements, boundaries, and surfaces in primary visual cortex of the macaque monkey. *Cereb Cortex* 9:406–413.

McCollough C (1965) Color adaptation of edge-detectors in the human visual system. *Science* 149:1115–1116.

Nakayama K and Shimojo S (1990) Da Vinci stereopsis: Depth and subjective occluding contours from unpaired image piont. *Vision Res* 30:1811–1825.

Nakayama K, Shimojo S, and Ramachandran VS (1989) Stereoscopic depth: Its relation to image segmentation, grouping, and the recognition of occluded objects. *Perception* 18:55–68.

Nakayama K, Shimojo S, and Ramachandran VS (1990) Transparency: Relation to depth, subjective contours, luminance, and neon color spreading. *Perception* 19:497–513.

Paradiso MA and Nakayama K (1991) Brightness perception and filling-in. *Vision Res* 31:1221–1236.

Pessoa L, Beck J, and Mingolla E (1996) Perceived texture segregation in chromatic element-arrangement patterns: High luminance interference. *Vision Res* 36:1745–1761.

Pessoa L, Mingolla E, and Neumann H (1995) A contrast- and luminance-driven multiscale network model of brightness perception. *Vision Res* 35:2201–2223.

Pessoa L, Thompson E, and Noë A (1998) Finding out about filling in: A guide to perceptual completion for visual science and the philosophy of perception. *Behav Brain Sci* 21:723–802.

Peterhans E and von der Heydt R (1989) Mechanisms of contour perception in monkey visual cortex, II: Contours bridging gaps. *J Neurosci* 9:1749–1763.

Purghé F and Coren S (1992) Amodal completion, depth stratification, and illusory figures: A test of Kanizsa's explanation. *Perception* 21:325–335.

Redies C and Spillmann L (1981) The neon color effect in the Ehrenstein illusion. *Perception* 10:667–681.

Richards WA and Kaye MG (1974) Local versus global stereopsis: Two mechanisms. *Vision Res* 14:1345–1347.

Rogers-Ramachandran DC and Ramachandran VS (1998) Psychophysical evidence for boundary and surface systems in human vision. *Vision Res* 38:71–77.

Schor CM, Wood I, and Ogawa J (1984) Binocular sensory fusion is limited by spatial resolution. *Vision Res* 24:661–665.

Shapley R and Reid RC (1986) Contrast and assimilation in the perception of brightness. *Proc Natl Acad Sci USA* 82:5983–5986.

Shipley TF and Kellman PJ (1992) Perception of partly occluded objects and illusory figures: Evidence for an identify hypothesis. *J Exp Psychol Hum Percept Perform* 18:106–120.

Smallman HS and MacLeod DIA (1994) Size–disparity correlation in stereopsis at contrast threshold. *J Opt Soc Am A* 11:2169–2183.

Smallman HS and McKee SP (1995) A contrast ratio constraint on stereo matching. *Proc R Soc Lond B* 260:265–271.

Tansley BW and Boynton RN (1976) A line, not a space, represents visual distinctness of borders formed by different colors. *Science* 191:954–957.

Tansley BW and Boynton RN (1978) Chromatic border perception: The role of the red- and green-sensitivity cones. *Vision Res* 18:683–697.

Tyler CS (1975) Spatial organization of binocular disparity sensitivity. *Vision Res* 15:583–590.

Von der Heydt R, Peterhans E, and Baumgartner G (1984) Illusory contours and cortical neuron responses. *Science* 224:1260–1262.

Von Tschermak-Seysenegg A (1952) *Introduction to Physiological Optics* (P. Boeder, trans.). Springfield, IL: Charles C Thomas.

Waxman AM, Seibert MC, Gove A, Fay DA, Bernardon AM, Lazott C, Steele WR, and Cunningham RK (1995) Neural processing of targets in visible, multispectral IR and SAR imagery. *Neural Networks* 8:1029–1051.

# 3

## Contextual Shape Processing in Human Visual Cortex:
### Beginning to Fill-In the Blanks

JANINE MENDOLA

A fundamental task of our visual system is to extract the contours and surfaces in an image, and to determine which contours represent the edge of object surfaces. As a rule, the retinal image of contours and surfaces is obstructed, due to imperfections and gaps in the receptor array, and due to objects occluding one another. The visual system, however, possesses the ability to appreciate the physical presence of contours and surfaces of which parts are not visible, which is referred to as *perceptual completion* or *filling-in*. In this chapter, evidence will be reviewed indicating that the human visual system creates a neural signal for many such completed contours and surfaces.

A classic example of the visual system's capacity to ignore obstructions or gaps in the receptor array is its ability to ignore the natural blind spot (corresponding to the optic disc). Subjects will fill-in the blind area with a copy of the nearest input that is available, around the edges of the blind spot (e.g., Ramachandran, 1992). This phenomenon is a specific example of interpolation of information across regions of visual space where that information is not physically present, which is the general definition of the filling-in (completion) process studied in this chapter. There is considerable evidence to suggest that a similar process contributes to the perception of contours and surfaces. Contour completion is evident in the Kanisza square figure (Figure 3-1A), in which the alignment of edges in the pacman inducing elements contributes to the illusion of a contour spanning the gaps between the inducers (e.g., Petry and Meyer, 1987). A process of surface completion is suggested by the brightness filling-in of the interior of the square induced by the pacman elements, which makes the square look brighter than the background (e.g., Halpern and Salzman, 1983; Dresp et al., 1990). This type of filling-in is referred to as *modal completion*, and it may play a role in the normal perception of surfaces and contours (Paradiso and Nakayama, 1991; Grossberg, 1994; Lesher, 1995; Nakayama et al., 1995). The

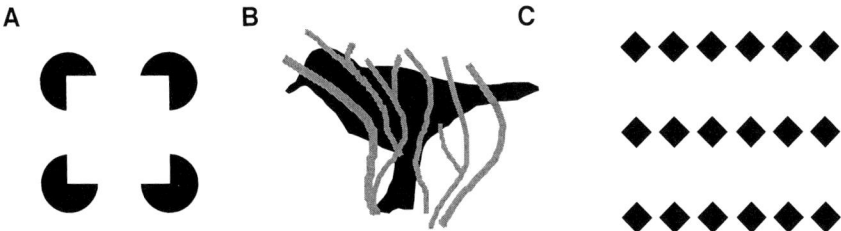

**Figure 3-1.** Examples of object occlusion and Gestalt grouping. (A) Illusory shapes illustrate contour interpolation (between the pacman edges) and surface interpolation (the interior of the perceived square) (B) The recognition process needs to fill-in the missing parts of an occluded object and connect the visible segments to indicate a bird behind the grasslike occluders. (C) The proximity relations between the elements makes grouping of the elements horizontally more likely, for example, favoring an interpretation of horizontal rather than vertical branches of a tree.

filling-in of contours and surfaces that are occluded by other objects is referred to as *amodal completion*. Despite superficial resemblances, the modal and amodal completion of surfaces and their contours probably relies on a number of different neural mechanisms (see Chapters 2 and 7). In general, however, the rules that govern perceptual completion are thought to reveal spatial context-dependent mechanisms contributing to normal visual perception. Examples of perceptual context dependency other than perceptual completion include the perception of Gestalt groupings, luminance contrast, color constancy, depth planes, coherent motion, and texture contrast (Spillmann and Werner, 1996).

Perceptual completion is beneficial because it usually results in accurate scene interpretation. In natural images, line ends, corners, and collinear line segments in the retinal input are two-dimensional (2D) cues that are often related to occlusion of one object by another. As a result, the visual system has a strong bias to interpret these 2D cues in a three-dimensional (3D) manner, which in 2D images can lead to illusory perceptions of complete contours and surfaces ordered in depth. This bias towards 3D interpretations reveals mechanisms that estimate the presence of complete contours and surfaces on the basis of incomplete information during daily perception (Fig. 3-1B) and that may reflect a cumulative record (memory) of the most likely stimuli given particular types of retinal input (Mumford, 1994).

The process of finding the "real" contours and surfaces in an image is critically intertwined with object recognition. Many computational models of object recognition have found it necessary to incorporate filling-in processes to find contours, and to estimate the depth ordering and occlusion of surfaces (e.g., Sadja and Finkel, 1995). Even in unusually sparse images without object occlusions, there are contextual effects acting across long distances in visual space that help to govern contour extraction and grouping of object constituents into perceptual wholes (Fig. 3-1C). There may be a close relationship between these so-called Gestalt principles and filling-in processes. Ultimately, the presence of mechanisms that calculate estimates of surfaces and contours that go beyond spatially local and temporally brief sensory measurements may reflect the fact that the physical laws of cause and effect that define our world act over space and time. Any brain that does not accommodate that fact would be at a hopeless disadvantage compared to one that does.

## Literature Review

This review will start with a brief discussion of contextual effects in the physiological responses of single neurons in cats and primates. The following section will review the physiological investigations of contextual visual phenomena in human visual cortex made possible by noninvasive functional neuroimaging techniques. The review is organized to address two important topics concerning filling-in and related contextual effects. First, what are the contributions of feedforward, feedback, and lateral anatomical connections? Second, how large is the neural network that contributes to particular classes of contextual effects? Given the excellent temporal and spatial resolution of single unit recordings, this technique is best suited to answer the first question. The large field of view in functional magnetic resonance imaging makes that methodology better suited to answer the second question. Of course, physiological approaches are increasing their field of view by doing ensemble recordings, and fMRI approaches are now rapidly increasing their temporal and spatial resolution. However, considering these complementary techniques together is currently the best strategy. The final section will discuss how single-neuron properties can be related to population indices and how the organization of the primate visual system may impact our thoughts about filling-in.

### Single-Neuron Properties in Macaque Cortex

Since the first single-cell recordings in visual cortex in the 1960s, visual neurobiologists have conceptualized neurons primarily as local filters that break down visual scenes by extracting particular features from small regions of space (Hubel and Wiesel, 1968). Hubel and Wiesel proposed that filters with increasingly complex properties are built through convergent input from filters with more elementary properties. This has led to a hierarchical view of the visual system, which is supported by the abundance of feedforward connections between visual areas, as well as by decreases in retinotopy, increases in receptive field (RF) size, and increases in response latency as one ascends the hierarchy of cortical areas (Ungerleider and Desimone, 1986; Maunsell and Newsome, 1987; Felleman and Van Essen, 1991).

The presence of horizontal and feedback connections, however, is not well accounted for by classical feedforward models (Gilbert, 1992), nor do these models agree with evidence from physiological studies starting in the 1970s. Those studies demonstrated that the response to a stimulus placed inside the classical

RF of a neuron could be modulated by a surrounding stimulus placed far outside the RF, although no response was obtained to the surrounding stimulus presented alone. This finding was first reported in primary visual cortex (V1), but it is now known that this property exists in all retinotopically organized cortex (e.g., Maffei and Fiorentini, 1976; Nelson and Frost 1978; Allman et al., 1985). These contextual effects could reflect lateral connectivity between neurons within areas or feedback connections from higher-tier areas. Lateral mechanisms in early visual areas such as V1 have been proposed to contribute to contextual effects, including the grouping of collinear line segments, and the segregation of such groups from a random background (Kapadia et al., 1995). Feedback effects on contextual mechanisms have been demonstrated directly by reversible deactivation of area MT in the monkey. Hupe et al. (1998) found that feedback connections from MT enhance the sensitivity of center-surround mechanisms in V1, V2, and V3 contributing to figure–ground segregation. Related findings have been reported in the cat (Rivadulla and Sur, 2000). In the following paragraphs, contextual mechanisms contributing to contour and surface completion will be discussed.

Fiorani et al. (1992) reported a contextual property in V1 related to *contour interpolation*. When a line was moved behind an occluder, neurons whose RFs overlapped with the occluder were sensitive to the coherently moving line ends even though they remained outside the RF. The same property was shown for neurons with RFs (determined through the ipsilateral eye) within the blind spot of the contralateral eye. When the ipsilateral eye was closed, these neurons responded to coherent stimulation of parts of the contralateral retina around the blind spot (see Chapter 9).

A remarkable physiological finding indicating contextual completion of contours was reported by von der Heydt and colleagues (1984). In that study, an illusory bar induced by aligned corners placed outside the classical RF of V2 neurons yielded significant responses, just as if a real bar had been presented inside the RF. Subsequent experiments in cats and monkeys showed that neurons in V1 and V2 carry signals related to illusory contours, and that the signals in V2 are more robust than those in V1 (Redies et al., 1986; von der Heydt et al., 1989; Grosof et al., 1993; Sheth et al., 1996; see also Ramsden et al., 1999). Recent results indicate that responses to illusory contours occur earlier in V2 (70–95 ms) than in V1 (100–200 ms) (Lee and Nguyen, 2001). In addition, some neurons in V2, V3, and V4 (rarely, in V1) signal border ownership (Baumann et al., 1997; Zhou et al., 2000). When the edge of a shape was presented in the RF of such neurons, their activity depended on whether the shape was presented to the left or right of the length axis of the RF rather than on the contrast polarity at the edge.

Other studies have shown that neurons signal the presence of contours occluded in depth (amodal completion) in V2 (Bakin et al., 2000) and perhaps on a limited scale in V1 (Sugita, 1999). Neurons responded to these locally invisible or ambiguous borders almost as rapidly as to physical contours (20–30 ms after stimulus onset). Such rapid responses favor models based on local connections as opposed to distant feedback connections, and put constraints on the overall length and synaptic complexity of the underlying neural connections. These data thus suggest a contribution of early visual areas to contour integration (e.g., Hess and Field, 1999).

While most neurophysiological studies have focused on the completion of boundaries, some recent studies have tackled the issue of *surface completion* (Chapters 2, 4–8). Komatsu et al. (2000) examined the responses of V1 neurons with RFs in the blind spot, in an awake monkey, using homogeneous patches or *surface* stimuli. Neurons that responded to monocular contralateral patch stimuli generally had unusually large RFs (~8 degrees) exceeding the size of the blind spot. Interestingly, these neurons showed longer response latencies for monocular contralateral (blind spot) stimulation than for ipsilateral stimulation, consistent with additional contributions from feedback or lateral connections in the former case. In 1996, Rossi et al. reported that V1 neurons were modulated in a way that correlated with illusory brightness changes in a homogeneous patch that covered the classical RF. This dynamic illusion was created by modulating the luminance surrounding the patch, quite distant from the classical RF, indicating a contribution from feedback or lateral connections (Chapter 4).

Lamme and colleagues (1998b) have reported enhanced responses in V1 neurons when the classical RF was covered by textured figures of various sizes but not homogeneous backgrounds (Zipser et al., 1996, but see Rossi et al., 2001). In 1999, Lamme et al. investigated whether this enhancement was related to a filling-in process. They recorded from neurons when classical RFs were centered on the interior of figures, the figure–ground border, or the background and found distinct population responses in each condition. Interestingly, the response enhancement triggered by the figure's interior was delayed by about 80 ms compared to the response to the border, suggesting that border detection enabled a filling-in process that propagated from the edge to the figure's center. The delayed enhancement of responses inside the figure may reflect a slow speed in texture propagation, or it may be due in part to a slow process of figure–ground assignment following a more rapid detection of boundaries (see Chapters 2, 5 and 8). Figure–ground assignment may require an iterative process involving multiple areas, and surface filling-in may have to await the completion of that process. This idea is supported by findings that the delayed (~80 ms) enhancement of V1 responses inside the figure, but not the fast boundary signals, is disrupted after extrastriate lesions, as well as by anesthesia (Lamme et al., 1998a, 1998b).

The surface filling-in that occurs during normal, free-viewing, surface perception, and that could have some correlates in neural activity in V1, occurs faster than the filling-in process that has been observed behaviorally for stabilized images. When images are stabilized on the retina by prolonged fixation, the background invades and fills in the figure after about 5–15 seconds (De Weerd et al., 1998). This delay suggests that filling-in must await the completion of a separate process associated with adaptation to the stabilized figure–ground border. De Weerd et al. (1995) have observed a potential physiological substrate for this delayed filing-in percept in the responses of single neurons (whose activity increased during filling-in) in areas V2 and V3 but not V1. The possibility that this type of filling-in might contribute to the perception of real surfaces is discussed in Chapter 5. Another mechanism that could contribute to the neural coding of surfaces is neural synchronization. In fact, synchrony has been offered as a candidate for the coding of surface segmentation (Sadja and Finkel 1995; Usher and Donnelly, 1998; Tallon-Baudry and Bertrand, 1999; Castelo-Branco et al., 2000) and, therefore, a role for temporal mechanisms in filling-in is plausible. However, this temporal mechanism may not operate universally, as the delayed figure–ground signals in V1 for texture patterns do not seem to involve synchronous firing (Lamme and Spekreijse, 1998).

The reviewed studies suggest that lateral and feedback connections can both contribute to the completion of contours and surfaces. In the following section, data from imaging studies will be discussed relevant to the second topic addressed in this chapter: How large is the network contributing to contextual perception in general and to the completion of contours and surfaces in particular?

## Functional Neuroimaging of Human Visual Cortex

Functional magnetic resonance imaging (fMRI) has emerged as the dominant technique for human brain imaging. In this technique, endogenous, activity-dependent changes in local oxygenation and/or blood flow are measured while subjects perform experimental tasks (Bandettini et al., 1992; Kwong et al., 1992; Ogawa et al., 1992). Although the source of the fMRI signal is hemodynamic rather than neural, activity maps can be obtained with spatial resolution of at least 1 mm. The hemodynamic response to discrete inputs is delayed (~4 seconds) and protracted in time (~18 seconds) Early fMRI studies were limited by this slow hemodynamic response and made comparisons of "blocked" events that changed kind only every 12–30 seconds. Newer event-related designs, which exploit the essentially linear properties of the fMRI response (Buckner, 1998), permit an effective temporal resolution of at least 1–2 seconds.

Compared to the single-cell electrophysiological methods that have dominated visual neuroscience for decades, the neural field of view in fMRI is large, whereas the temporal and spatial resolution is poor. The large field of view is a great advantage for functional brain imaging, when contrasted with extracellular electrophysiological methods, because RF properties indicate only a subset of the interactions between neurons within and across areas. On the other hand, the poor temporal resolution of fMRI, even in event-related designs, is a disadvantage; it rarely permits the measurement of temporal dynamics. Future breakthroughs in human brain imaging are likely to be catalyzed by the combination of fMRI with electrophysiological techniques that supply the missing temporal information (e.g., Martinez et al., 1999). In addition, spatial resolution in fMRI, although excellent compared to that of positron emission tomography (PET), is limited compared to the spatial resolution of single-cell neurophysiology. Because averaging activity that maps across subjects reduces resolution, the best way to take full advantage of the spatial resolution of fMRI is to analyze individual subjects, preferably with visualization aids such as cortical flattening (Fig. 3-2).

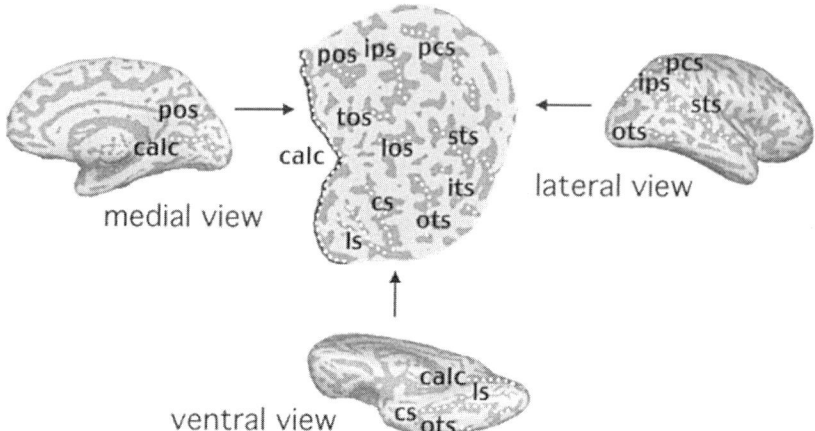

**Figure 3-2.** Location of cortical sulci on a flat map (subject JM). For the right hemisphere, the normally folded cortical surface has been inflated so that sulci and gyri are equally visible and are shown in the medial, ventral, and lateral views. Cortical gyri and sulci are uniformly light and dark gray, respectively. The central image shows the posterior third of the cortex in a flattened format. The inflated posterior pole, which is approximately cone-shaped in its normal folded state, has been opened along the calcarine sulcus and unfolded. The relationship between the various inflated views and the flattened patch can be appreciated. Some of the notable sulci are labeled with abbreviations on the flattened patch: pos = parieto-occipital sulcus; ips = intraparietal sulcus; pcs = postcentral sulcus; tos = transverse occipital sulcus; los = lateral occipital sulcus; sts = superior temporal sulcus; its = inferior temporal sulcus; ots = occipitotemporal sulcus; cs = collateral sulcus; ls = lingual sulcus.

The following overview of neuroimaging studies of contextual mechanisms is focused on Gestalt grouping and symmetry, and on (illusory) contour and shape perception. Different properties of interpolation mechanisms involved in these various perceptual phenomena will be discussed. Higher-order factors that influence contextual processes, such as attention and learning, will be discussed as well.

Different contextual phenomena recruit visual areas at different levels of the hierarchy of the human visual system, which is partly reviewed here. Visual areas in the human occipital lobe include V1, V2, up to area V8/TEO, in approximate hierarchical order. Anterior to these visual areas in the occipital lobe is the lateral occipital complex (LOC), described first in a pioneering study by Malach et al. (1995). The LOC is a fairly large cortical region anterior to retinotopic areas V7 and V8/TEO, and posterior to MT on the lateral aspect of the occipital lobe (the superior-inferior extent of this area is not well specified) (Fig. 3-3). Because of its response to structured images, a working definition and a diagnostic test for the LOC has been its greater response to globally structured (natural) images versus globally unstructured images (textures or scrambled versions of the

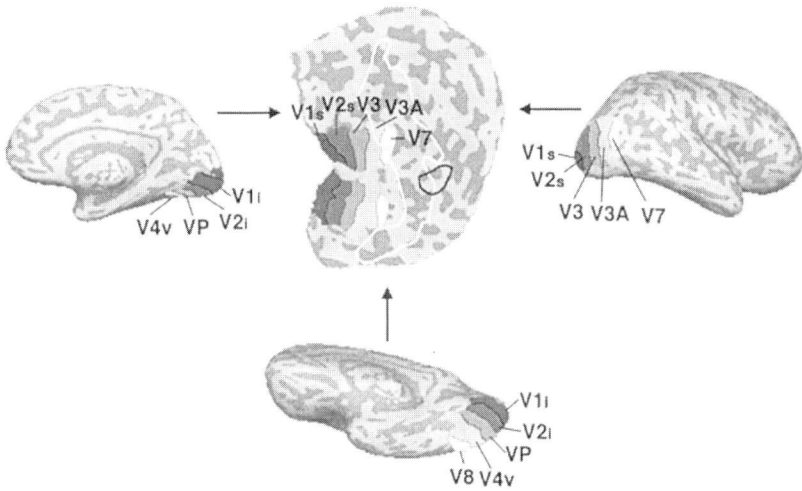

**Figure 3-3.** Location of retinotopic areas on a flat map (subject JM). Conventions are as described for Figure 2-1. The location of eight retinotopic areas—V1 (superior and inferior), V2 (superior and inferior), VP, V3, V4v, V3A, V8/TEO, and V7—are indicated. Also shown with a white outline is the location of the lateral occipital complex (LOC), estimated in this case by a separate experiment in which natural colored scenes were compared with scrambled versions of the same scenes. The black outline indicates the location of MT+ as indexed by a scan comparing low-contrast, moving rings with stationary rings.

original images). Although some crude retinotopy may be present, there is evidence that RFs are large and bilateral (Tootell et al., 1998). Further, the LOC almost certainly contains multiple visual areas (Vanduffel et al., 1997), and more work is required to divide it into functional subdivisions.

*Elemental Gestalt Grouping and Symmetry*
Few neuroimaging studies have looked specifically at perceptual grouping phenomena. Marois et al. (n.d., unpublished manuscript) have studied dot arrays that were aligned based on the principles of collinearity or proximity. They found more activity in V1 for stimulus arrays that could be perceptually grouped (experimental stimulus) compared to similar arrays that did not group (control). In these types of studies, however, there are unavoidable (retinotopic) differences between experimental and control stimuli, which makes the interpretation of the results difficult. Some studies have attempted to avoid this difficulty by using the same stimulus in experimental and control conditions and by directing attention to global (grouping) versus local aspects of hierarchical Navon figures (e.g., a PET study by Fink et al., 1996). In such figures, small letters are arranged into larger global patterns that correspond to either the same letter or a different letter. Selective attention to local or global levels appeared to activate distinct occipitotemporal regions, including what is probably area V4v, in both attention

conditions. Strong claims about the lateralization of activation were made, linking the left and right hemispheres to local and global processing, respectively, but these results seem to depend on the use of letters (shapes tend to reverse the lateralization) and have not been universally replicated (Heinze et al., 1998; Sasaki et al., 2001; Mangun et al., 2000). Nevertheless, the data taken together are suggestive of a role of lower-level, retinotopically organized cortex in grouping operations.

Studies of texture segregation may also reveal a contribution of grouping mechanisms. Kastner et al. (2000) recently reported an experiment that compared the visual areas activated by the presence versus absence of boundaries in oriented line-segment textures (checkerboard alternation of a 90 degree orientation difference). The results showed a gradient of increasing activation from lower-tier to higher-tier areas, with a significant signal in V4, V8/TEO, and V3A but not V1 or V2 (see Fig. 3-3). The absence of signal in V1 and V2 may reflect limited signal-to-noise ratio of the fMRI signal or specific aspects of the stimulus. Related results have been reported by Braddick et al. (2000). The data in these studies confirm that relatively simple grouping and segregation processes can recruit several retinotopically organized visual areas.

An important form of elemental grouping is the perception of symmetrical relations between object components or image features. The perception of symmetry may be a particularly important task due to the striking prevalence and significance of these patterns in biology (Tyler, 1995). Furthermore, many simple stimuli that are used to study grouping phenomena (e.g., Kanizsa squares) contain bilateral symmetry, so it is crucial to distinguish grouping relations from symmetry per se.

Tyler and colleagues used fMRI to study the visual cortical response to static random-dot patterns with one vertical axis, one horizontal axis, and two or four axes of symmetry (compared to similar patterns with no symmetry (Tyler and Baseler, 1998). They found activation in the LOC, especially the dorsal portion (middle occipital gyrus). This pattern of activation was very similar to the pattern reported for the comparison of illusory Kanizsa squares versus control images with rotated inducers (Mendola et al., 1999) (e.g., Fig. 3-5C), using flattened-cortex visualization (Figs. 3-2 and 3-3). Furthermore, this pattern was different from the one produced by equivalent luminance-defined shapes, which showed greater signals in lower-tier retinotopic areas. The similarity between the symmetry and illusory shape results raised the possibility that symmetry was in fact the defining characteristic of the Kanizsa stimuli. However, making the Kanizsa-type shape asymmetrical did not significantly alter the results (Fig. 3-4A). A comparison within the same subject confirmed a striking overlap of activity patterns in visual cortical regions during presentation of illusory shapes and symmetrical dot patterns (Fig. 3-4B). Thus, symmetry may be a sufficient but not a necessary condition for robust activation of the LOC. In sum, the data suggest that the LOC is recruited during the perception of illusory shapes and symmetry but not during more elemental Gestalt grouping. It is possible that the per-

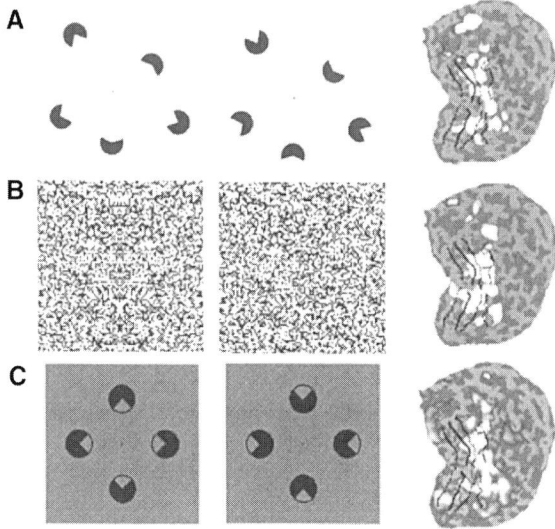

**Figure 3-4.** Stimulus comparisons and single-subject flat map results for three experiments. Panels A–C show data from the right hemisphere of subject JM. (A) The representation of an asymmetrical illusory shape was probed with a comparison between aligned and rotated inducer versions of a Kanizsa-type stimulus. Regions of cortex that respond more to the the aligned than to the rotated inducers are shown with a scale ranging from $p \leq 10^{-2}$ to $p \leq 10^{-6}$ in the right hemisphere. Visual area borders from the same subject have been overlaid. Horizontal meridian representations are drawn with solid lines; vertical meridians are shown by dotted lines. This pattern is quite similar to that obtained for a standard, symmetrical illusory square shown in Figure 2-5C in that both cases activated V3A, and the lateral occipital region anterior to it (i.e., to the right in this figure), to a greater degree than the lower-tier retinotopic areas. (B) The stimulus comparison was between a vertically symmetrical dot pattern and a random dot pattern. The resulting pattern of activation is very similar to that shown in (A). (C) The representation of amodal completion was explored with a stimulus comparison that suggested object occlusion versus one that did not. The experimental condition was seen as a gray diamond shape viewed through four circular apertures, that is, the gray diamond was amodally completed. The control condition was seen as four separate shapes in the same depth plane. The extent of overlapping regions of activation with (A) and (B) is impressive, with the lateral occipital region a dominant focus. This stimulus amodal comparison did yield more activation in the ventral occipotemporal region, which has been linked with recognition of faces and other objects. Other conventions are as described in previous figure legends.

ception of illusory shapes and symmetry requires integration over particularly long ranges, and that this recruits the LOC.

*Surface and Shape*
Even the relatively simple illusory shape stimuli used to study the LOC (Hirsch et al., 1995; Ffytche and Zek; 1996; Mendola et al., 1999) can contain multiple

cues, and their contribution to LOC activity and their mutual interactions remain poorly understood. Cues to depth, which are present in many of these stimuli, have been reported to influence the perception of (illusory) surfaces and shapes. Below, the relationship between fMRI activity related to illusory shapes and several cues to depth (including stereopsis and interposition) is discussed.

Mendola et al. (1999) compared illusory contour-defined shapes with stereo-defined shapes on the premise that implied depth was a critical feature of the illusory shape. They showed large overlap in the regions activated by illusory and stereo-defined shapes. Furthermore, Moore and Engel (2001) have provided a convincing demonstration that the activity in LOC is modulated by perceived 3D structure. Modulation was found with both image-based and top-down variables that changed 3D percepts. We may conclude, as in the case of symmetry, that perceived depth may be sufficient but not necessary for LOC activation. Clarification of the anatomical relationship between the precise regions in the LOC modulated by 3D structure and those sensitive to symmetry is needed. Finally, it may be significant that symmetry itself can be a cue to depth relations (Kontsevich, 1996).

Another sensation that often co-occurs with perceived depth is amodal completion, which refers to the sense that occluded objects are filled-in behind their occluders, so that the visible pieces are connected. There have been suggestions that modal (in front) completion might be processed differently than amodal (behind) completion (Davis and Driver, 1997; Corballis et al., 1999; but see Kellman et al., 1998). Preliminary fMRI data are presented in a single subject in order to compare the cases of modal versus amodal completion. The results show an impressive degree of overlap in the brain regions activated by the two cases, but the overlap is not perfect (Fig. 3-4C). More work on this topic is necessary.

The evidence, taken together, suggests that a common feature of all stimuli that recruit the LOC is the requirement to group or structure local information into a global perception. One specific function of the LOC might be to contribute to interpolation processes relevant for the perception of contours and surfaces. Similar to symmetry perception, the perception of contours and surfaces may require long-range interpolation mechanisms, which may be an important general function of the LOC. Some evidence from Mendola et al. (1999) explicitly supports the role of LOC in long-range interpolation. They reported that activation strength in the LOC increased when the distance between inducing lines was *increased* in shifted-grating illusory shapes. Similarly, for Kanizsa-type shapes, activation increased with the number of inducing elements until a closed shape was evident (Fig. 3-5A–C). Hence, even though the presence of closure is formally an all-or-none property of shapes, the integration of increasingly long and curved contours from multiple elements may serve as an increasingly good trigger for LOC neurons sensitive to closure (Sadja and Finkel, 1995).

Despite its potentially general role in a variety of long-range interpolation processes, it remains important to tease apart the signal in LOC related to different global cues (stereo, symmetry, global motion cues, etc.) and to determine whether any of these cues is processed preferentially in subregions of the LOC (e.g., Van Oostende et al., 1997; Tyler & Baseler, 2000). This approach can fur-

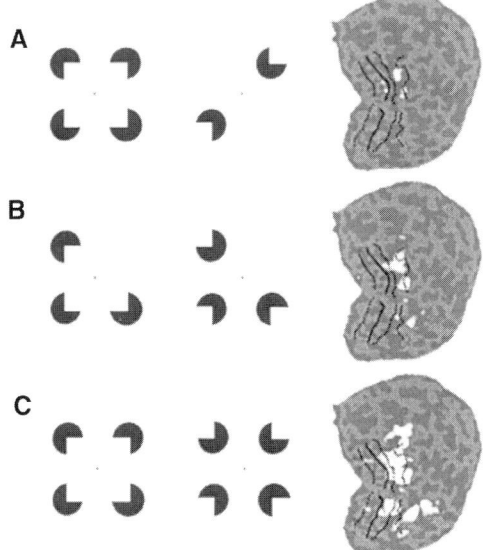

**Figure 3-5.** Functional magnetic resonance imaging (fMRI) response to increasingly complete illusory shapes. Panels A–C show data from the right hemisphere of subject JM. All stimulus comparisons are between aligned and rotated (Kanizsa) inducers. The activation maps are shown for three increasingly complete illusory shapes. Visual area borders are transposed from the field sign map in the same subject. Signal strength increases with increasing completeness in the lateral occipital region. Panel C shows the classical Kanizsa-type illusory square and a control image in which inducers have been rotated to destroy the illusory shape. The complete illusory square subtended 7.5 degrees. Other conventions are as described in previous figure legends.

ther our understanding of how different cues relevant to contour, surface, and object perception interact.

It is apparent from the above discussions that elemental grouping and global shape processing preferentially engage retinotopic and nonretinotopic areas, respectively. The distinction between retinotopic and nonretinotopic areas (a gradual distinction in practice) is relevant to debates about whether filling-in is primarily an *isomorphic* or a *symbolic* process (see the following Discussion). To date, no fMRI studies have reported a direct measurement of filling-in per se, but in the case of illusory Kanizsa shapes (Mendola et al., 1999), both contour completion and surface filling-in were probably critical processing steps. Retinotopically specific signals were detected in areas such as V1 and V2, and they could reflect an isomorphic (contour) filling-in process in those areas. At the same time, the results suggest that neural correlates of filling-in become much stronger in less retinotopically organized areas. It can be assumed that within these areas with large RFs, local neural interactions that do not maintain isomorphism with the retinal input can readily take place. Perhaps *symbolic* interpolations along nonspatial dimensions occur in such areas. The most important question, however, is how isomorphic and symbolic processes work together in the large, heavily interconnected cortical network that is typically activated during the processing of illusory contours and surfaces.

Part of the answer to that question may come from some intriguing data in the temporal domain from Halgren et al. (2002). In a magnetoencephalographic (MEG) study of illusory contour perception they found weak, early activity (110 ms) in V1 followed by major activation in the LOC (155 ms). Modulation then spreads back from this location toward the occipital pole, as well as ventrally to involve ventral occipital and temporal cortices for the next 180 ms. The late ventral temporal response (235 ms) is centered in the lingual and fusiform areas implicated in object identification. The V1/V2 modulation at this time likely reflects top-down modulation by lateral occipitotemporal and ventral temporal areas. These results clearly suggest the presence of a feedback effect in early retinotopic areas, and also suggest that isomorphic activity related to interpolation of contours and surfaces in those areas might be guided by the outcome of more symbolic processes in the LOC. As discussed, one of those symbolic processes might consist of the higher-order interpolation processes (*long-range* in a spatial sense) that extract the complex global structure of visual information. In addition, the explicit recognition of that structure as an object might interact with isomorphic processes in retinotopic cortex.

*Recognition*
It is difficult to study boundary extraction and figure–ground identification without acknowledging that *object recognition* is the ultimate goal. Although many aspects of surface perception indicate that it is not dependent on cognitive/semantic inferences and usually precedes object recognition per se (Nakayama et al., 1995), some scientists have proposed rather direct, bidirectional links between object recognition and boundary/surface mechanisms (e.g., Moore and Cavanagh, 1998). In agreement with that idea, there is growing evidence that activity in parts of the LOC is directly correlated with recognition performance (Grill-Spector et al., 2000). Furthermore, parts of the LOC (especially the ventral portion) seem to have a role in object identification that transcends the particular cues with which the object is defined (e.g., gray-scale luminance, outline, motion, texture) (Grill-Spector et al., 1998; Kourtzi et al., 2000). Thus, it is possible that symbolic operations in the LOC related to object recognition influence and guide spatial interpolation operations in retinotopic cortex.

*The Role of Attention*
An unresolved issue in the study of filling-in and related interpolation phenomena is the role of voluntary attention. Some grouping and filling-in mechanisms can occur without explicit awareness, as has been observed after certain cortical lesions (Mattingley et al., 1997; Vuilleumier and Landis, 1998). Likewise, when normal subjects are presented with stimuli that are completely unexpected, they may be aware of remarkably little global structure (Mack et al., 1992), yet still

show implicit evidence of processing (Moore and Egeth, 1997). On the other hand, because object recognition often requires attention, one might expect that processes that lead to object perception can be modulated by attention as well. This idea is supported by the finding that fundamental image properties like border ownership can be affected by explicit task instructions (e.g., Subirana-Vilanova and Richards, 1991) and by the finding that directed attention modulates the filling-in of *artificial scotomas* (see Chapter 11). A striking example of interactions between contour completion and attention was discovered by Roelfsema et al. (1998). They showed that responses of (monkey) V1 neurons to the various localized line segments of a target curve were simultaneously enhanced relative to responses evoked by a distractor curve, even if the two curves crossed each other. Future models will probably assign at least some role for attention in grouping and segmentation and, by extension, for some types of filling-in (see Grossberg, 2001; Chapters 2 and 8).

For attention and object recognition to influence more elementary sensory processes, one or more iterations of a number of feedback loops may be necessary (see Chapters 2 and 8). One recent imaging study has explicitly considered the role of attentional feedback connections by integrating electroencephalographic (EEG) and fMRI measures (Martinez, et al., 1999). These authors demonstrated elegantly that V1 activation during a visual attention paradigm is likely to be caused by *temporally* late EEG feedback signals from *hierarchically* higher brain regions. Note that it is important to make a distinction between the latency of response(s) in a particular area and that area's hierarchical position in a wiring scheme (Young and Scannell, 2000). This is related to the existence of multiple feedback loops with different time courses, which can interact dynamically (Lamme and Roelfsema, 2000; Hupe et al., 2001).

## Discussion

The visual system is organized as a set of sensory maps in which retinotopy decreases at increasingly higher levels of hierarchy. Neurons in any of these maps receive inputs via a mixture of feedforward, feedback, and lateral connections. This type of organization may provide the structural basis for neural activity that underlies various types of contextual perception, including filling-in. Because we have argued that some of the questions relevant to perceptual completion are best answered by comparing single-unit physiology in monkeys with neuroimaging data from humans, we will begin the discussion with an assessment of the extent to which both types of data can be directly compared.

### *How Relatable Are Single-Neuron Physiology and Whole Brain Neuroimaging?*

Rees et al. (2000) recently utilized the abundant data on single-neuron responses to global coherent motion in macaque area MT to directly interpret a linear increase in the fMRI signal to increased motion coherence in human cortex. By relating the previously documented linear rise in MT neuronal firing to the fMRI response, they calculated that a 1% signal change in human cortex was equivalent to an increase of nine spikes per second per neuron in monkey MT. Subsequently, another study reported a similar analysis with different stimuli for V1, and found a similar proportional relationship between BOLD and spikes (Heeger et al., 2000). This type of estimation is a first step toward a better interpretation of future imaging studies of completion phenomena and other sensory and cognitive functions. Other combinations of techniques will help connect fMRI results and neuronal properties. Promising strategies include combined optical imaging and single-unit electrophysiology in primates (e.g., Das and Gilbert, 1995; Ramsden et al., 1999), as well as combined fMRI and single-unit electrophysiology in primates (e.g., Logothetis et al., 1999).

## Contribution of Feedforward, Feedback, and Lateral Connectivity to Contextual Interpolation

Neurophysiological data seem to support a temporal distinction between contour and surface interpolation. Most of the contour integration data from areas V1 and V2 report responses with relatively short latency. Moreover, the horizontal connectivity in V1 provides a ready substrate for sensitivity to local contrasts in several domains (Knierim and van Essen, 1992; Zipser et al., 1996), which can contribute to contour perception. There may be a qualitative difference between V1 and V2, however, with the latter area capable of interpolation in more domains.

On the other hand, the context sensitivity related to surface completion displayed by neurons in V1, V2, and V3 has shown a tendency toward delayed neural response latencies. The MEG study of Halgren et al. (2002) explicitly demonstrated that for illusory shape perception, activity spreads from higher-tier areas with large RFs to lower-tier areas starting about 150 ms after stimulus onset. Perhaps surface filling-in results from a reentry of input from higher-tier areas with large RFs. A delayed reentry in areas like V1 could explain the temporal separation between neural activity related to local contrast and global surface integration (Zipser et al., 1996) and could provide a method of neuronal multiplexing. Thus, although interpolation may depend in part on lateral connectivity within retinotopically organized areas, feedback or reentry may play a role in enabling the interpolation. The large cortical network activated during perceptual completion, revealed by fMRI, is compatible with the idea that multiple interactions between a number of areas contribute to interpolation mechanisms.

Finally, neural synchrony remains a candidate mechanism for filling-in as opposed to the previously discussed rate mechanisms. An interesting question is to what extent synchrony (related to interpolation mechanisms and perceptual completion) in early visual areas is orchestrated by feedback. Direct electrophysiological measures of human visual cortex and ensemble recordings in animals might answer these questions in the future.

## Can Areas That Represent Surfaces Be Retinotopic?

The debate over isomorphic versus symbolic mechanisms of filling-in is interesting, not only from a philosohical point of view, but also because it focuses attention on the possible neural substrates of contour and surface filling-in (Pessoa et al., 1998). Only retinotopic areas seem likely to maintain isomorphism between the stimulus and the neural representation (see Chapters 2, 4–6, and 8). On the other hand, there is some evidence suggesting that illusory shapes may be processed by mechanisms that are largely scale invariant (Ringach and Shapley, 1996; Mendola et al., 1999). Possibly, long-range interactions contributing to filling-in might occur within different coordinate systems and over different spatial scales, depending on stimulus features (Gattass et al., 1999). This view keeps open the possibility that both retinotopic and less retinotopic areas can (possibly in concert) contribute to filling-in.

While isomorphism of activity in retinotopic areas with surface perception is an interesting idea, it oversimplifies the debate on mechanisms of surface perception. An accurate representation of surfaces (and contours) must take into account depth relations between surfaces, and any cortical representation that is purely isomorphic with physical or retinal input will therefore be insufficient. How can retinotopically organized areas represent occlusion, which entails the representation of two different entities at the same retinal location? This issue is related to the question of amodal completion, which might depend upon different mechanisms than modal completion (Chapter 7). Some formal models of brain function have proposed that surface relations in depth can be coded explicitly in retinotopic areas by using the temporal dimension (Sadja and Finkel, 1995).

Considered broadly, *filling-in* and *completion* serve as umbrella terms that bind several key threads in current visual neuroscience. The threads include contextual interactions that act over space, the role of feedback effects, the challenge of adding the third dimension back into 2D retinal input, the implications of retinotopic and nonretinotopic representations, and the potential contribution of mechanisms of attentional control and object recognition to filling-in. A better understanding of the interpolation processes that underlie filling-in should advance our concepts about many of these topics.

## References

Allman J, Miezin F, and McGuinness E (1985) Stimulus specific responses from beyond the classical receptive field. *Annu Rev Neurosci* 8:407–430.

Bakin JS, Nakayama K, and Gilbert CD (2000) Visual responses in monkey areas V1 and V2 to three-dimensional surface configurations. *J Neurosci* 20(21):8188–8198.

Bandettini PA, Wong EC, Hinks RS, Tikofsky RS, and Hyde JS (1992) Time course EPI of human brain function during task activation. *Magn Reson Med* 25:390–397.

Baumann R, van der Zwan R, and Peterhans E (1997) Figure–ground segregation at contours: A neural mechanism in the visual cortex of the alert monkey. *Eur J Neurosci* 9:1290–1303.

Braddick OJ, O'Brien JM, Wattam-Bell J, Atkinson J, and Turner R (2000) Form and motion coherence activate independent, but not dorsal/ventral segregated, networks in the human brain. *Curr Biol* 10:731–734.

Buckner RL (1998) Event-related fMRI and the hemodynamic response. *Hum Brain Mapp* 6:373–377.

Castelo-Branco M, Goebel R, Neuenschwander S, and Singer W (2000) Neural synchrony correlates with surface segregation rules. *Nature* 405:685–689.

Corballis PM, Fendrich R, Shapley RM, and Gazzaniga MS (1999) Illusory contour perception and amodal boundary completion: Evidence of a dissociation following callosotomy. *J Cogn Neurosci* 11:459–466.

Das A and Gilbert CD (1995) Long-range horizontal connections and their role in cortical reorganization revealed by optical recording of cat primary visual cortex. *Nature* 375:780–784.

Davis G and Driver J (1997) Spreading of visual attention to modally versus amodally completed regions. *Psychol Sci* 8:275–281.

De Weerd P, Desimone R, and Ungerleider LG (1998) Perceptual filling-in: A parametric study. *Vision Res* 38:2721–2734.

De Weerd P, Gattass R, Desimone R, and Ungerleider LG (1995) Responses of cells in monkey visual cortex during perceptual filling-in of an artificial scotoma. *Nature* 377:731–734.

Dresp B, Lorenceau J, and Bonnet C (1990) Apparent brightness enhancement in the Kanizsa square with and without illusory contour formation. *Perception* 19:483–489.

Felleman DJ and Van Essen DC (1991) Distributed hierarchical processing in the primate cerebral cortex. *Cereb Cortex* 1:1–47.

Ffytche DH and Zeki S (1996) Brain activity related to the perception of illusory contours. *Neuroimage* 3:104–108.

Fink GR, Halligan PW, Marshall JC, Frith CD, Frackowiak RS, and Dolan RJ (1996) Where in the brain does visual attention select the forest and the trees? *Nature* 382:626–388.

Fiorani Jr. M, Rosa MG, Gattass R, Rocha-Miranda CE. Dynamic surrounds of receptive fields in primate striate cortex: a physiological basis for perceptual completion? *Proc Natl Acad Sci USA* 1992;89:8547–8551.

Gattass R, Pessoa L, De Weerd P, and Fiorani M (1999) Filling-in in topographically organized distributed networks. *An Acad Bras Cienc* 71:997–1015.

Gilbert CD (1992) Horizontal integration and cortical dynamics. *Neuron* 9:1–13.

Grill-Spector K, Kushnir T, Edelman S, Itzcak Y, and Malach R (1998) Cue-invariant activation in object-related areas of the human occipital lobe. *Neuron* 21:191–202.

Grill-Spector K, Kushnir T, Hendler T, and Malach R (2000) The dynamics of object-selective activation correlate with recognition performance in humans. *Nat Neurosci* 3:837–843.

Grosof DH, Shapley RM, and Hawken MJ (1993) Macaque V1 neurons can signal "illusory" contours. *Nature* 365:550–552.

Grossberg S (1994) 3-D vision and figure–ground separation by visual cortex. *Percept Psychophys* 55:48–121.

Grossberg S (2001) Linking the laminar circuits of visual cortex to visual perception: Development, grouping, and attention. *Neurosci Biobehav* 25:513–526.

Grossberg S, Mingolla E, and Ross WD (1997) Visual brain and visual perception: How does the cortex do perceptual grouping? *Trends Neurosci* 20:106–111.

Halgren E, Mendola, JD, Chong CDR, Dale AM (2002) Cortical activation to illusory contours as measured with MEG. *Neuroimage* (in press).

Halpern DF and Salzman B (1983) The multiple determination of illusory contours: 1. A review. *Perception* 12:281–291.

Heeger DJ, Huk AC, Geisler WS, and Albrecht DG (2000) Spikes versus BOLD: What does neuroimaging tell us about neuronal activity? *Nat Neurosci* 3:631–633.

Heinze HJ, Hinrichs H, Scholz M, Burchert W, and Mangun GR (1998) Neural mechanisms of global and local processing. A combined PET and ERP study. *J Cogn Neurosci* 10:485–498.

Hess R and Field D (1999) Integration of contours: New insights. *Trends Cogn Sci* 3:480–486.

Hirsch J, DeLaPaz RL, Relkin NR, Victor J, Kim K, Li T, Borden P, Rubin N, and Shapley R (1995) Illusory contours activate specific regions in human visual cortex: Evidence from functional magnetic resonance imaging. *Proc Natl Acad Sci USA* 92:6469–6473.

Hubel DH and Wiesel TN (1968) Receptive fields and functional architecture of monkey striate cortex. *J Physiol* 195:215–243.

Hupe JM, James AC, Girard P, Lomber SG, Payne BR, and Bullier J (2001) Feedback connections act on the early part of the responses in monkey visual cortex. *J Neurophysiol* 85:134–145.

Hupe JM, James AC, Payne BR, Lomber SG, Girard P, and Bullier J (1998) Cortical feedback improves discrimination between figure and background by V1, V2 and V3 neurons. *Nature* 394:784–787.

Kapadia MK, Ito M, Gilbert CD, and Westheimer, G (1995) Improvement in visual sensitivity by changes in local context: Parallel studies in human observers and in V1 of alert monkeys. *Neuron* 15:843–856.

Kastner S, De Weerd P, and Ungerleider L (2000) Texture segregation in the human visual cortex: A functional MRI study. *J Neurophysiol* 83:2453–2457.

Kellman PJ, Yin C, and Shipley TF (1998) A common mechanism for illusory and occluded object completion. *J Exp Psychol Hum Percept Perform* 24:859–869.

Knierim JJ and van Essen DC (1992) Neuronal responses to static texture patterns in area V1 of the alert macaque monkey. *J Neurophysiol* 67:961–980.

Komatsu H, Kinoshita A, and Murakami I (2000) Neural responses in the retinotopic representation of the blind spot in the macaque V1 to stimuli for perceptual filling-in. *J Neurosci* 20:9310–9319.

Kontsevich LL (1996) Symmetry as a depth cue. In: Tyler CW (ed), *Human Symmetry Perception and Its Computational Analysis.* Utrecht: VSP, pp 331–359.

Kourtzi Z and Kanwisher N (2000) Cortical regions involved in perceiving object shape. *J Neurosci* 20:3310–3318.

Kwong KK, Belliveau JW, Chesler DA, Goldberg IE, Weisskoff RM, Poncelet BP, Kennedy DN, Hoppel BE, Cohen MS, Turner R et al. (1992) Dynamic magnetic resonance imaging of human brain activity during primary sensory stimulation *Proc Natl Acad Sci USA* 89:5675–5679.

Lamme VA and Roelfsema PR (2000) The distinct modes of vision offered by feedforward and recurrent processing. *Trends Neurosci* 23:571–579.

Lamme VA, Rodriguez-Rodriguez V, and Spekreijse H (1999) Separate processing dynamics for texture elements, boundaries and surfaces in primary visual cortex of the macaque monkey. *Cereb Cortex* 9:406–413.

Lamme VA and Spekreijse H (1998) Neuronal synchrony does not represent texture segregation. *Nature* 396:362–366.

Lamme VA, Super H, and Spekreijse H (1998a) Feedforward, horizontal, and feedback processing in the visual cortex. *Curr Opin Neurobiol* 8:529–555.

Lamme VA, Zipser K, and Spekreijse H (1998b) Figure–ground activity in primary visual cortex is suppressed by anesthesia. *Proc Natl Acad Sci USA* 95:3263–3268.

Lee TS and Nguyen M (2001) Dynamics of subjective contour formation in the early visual cortex. *Proc Natl Acad Sci USA* 98:1907–1911.

Lesher GW (1995) Illusory contours: Toward a neurally based peceptual theory. *Psychonom Bull Rev* 2:279–321.

Logothetis NK, Guggenberger H, Peled S, and Pauls J (1999) Functional imaging of the monkey brain. *Nat Neurosci* 2:555–562.

Mack A, Tang B, Tuma R, Kahn S, and Rock I (1992) Perceptual organization and attention. *Cogn Psychol* 24:475–501.

Maffei L and Fiorentini A (1976) The unresponsive regions of visual cortical receptive fields. *Vis Res* 16:1131–1139.

Malach R, Reppas JB, Benson RR, Kwong KK, Jiang H, Kennedy WA, Ledden PJ, Brady TJ, Rosen BR, and Tootell RB (1995) Object-related activity revealed by functional magnetic resonance imaging in human occipital cortex. *Proc Natl Acad Sci USA* 92:8135–8139.

Mangun GR, Heinze HJ, Scholz M, and Hinrichs H (2000) Neural activity in early visual areas during global and local processing: A reply to Fink, Marshall, Halligan and Dolan RJ. *J Cogn Neurosci* 12:357–359.

Marois R, Feineigle PA, and Gore JC (n.d., unpublished manuscript) An fMRI study of elementary perceptual grouping.

Martinez A, Anllo-Vento L, Sereno MI, Frank LR, Buxton RB, Dubowitz DJ, Wong EC, Hinrichs H, Heinze HJ, and Hillyard SA (1999) Involvement of striate and extrastriate visual cortical areas in spatial attention. *Nat Neurosci* 2:364–369.

Mattingley JB, Davis G, and Driver J (1997) Preattentive filling-in of visual surfaces in parietal extinction. *Science* 275:671–674.

Maunsell JHR and Newsome WT (1987) Visual processing in monkey extrastriate cortex. *Annu Rev Neurosci* 10:363–401.

Mendola JD, Dale AM, Fischl B, Liu AK, and Tootell RB (1999) The representation of illusory and real contours in human cortical visual areas revealed by functional magnetic resonance imaging. *J Neurosci* 19:8560–8572.

Moore C and Cavanagh P (1998) Recovery of 3D volume from 2–tone images of novel objects. *Cognition* 67:45–71.

Moore CM and Egeth H (1997) Perception without attention: Evidence of grouping under conditions of inattention. *J Exp Psychol Hum Percept Perform* 23:339–352.

Moore C and Engel SA (2001) Neural response to perception of volume in the lateral occipital complex. *Neuron* 1:277–286.

Mumford D (1994) Neuronal architectures for pattern-theoretic problems. In: Koch C and Davis JL (eds), *Large-Scale Neuronal Theories of the Brain*. Cambridge, MA: MIT Press, pp 125–152.

Nakayama K, He ZJ, and Shimojo S (1995) Visual surface representations: A critical link between lower level and higher level vision. In: Kosslyn SM and Osherson DM (eds), *Visual Cognition and Action*. Cambridge, MA: MIT Press, pp 1–70.

Nelson JI and Frost BJ (1978) Orientation-selective inhibition from beyond the classic visual receptive field. *Brain Res* 139:359–365.

Ogawa S. Tank DW, Menon R, Ellermann JM, Kim SG, Merkle H, and Ugurbil K. (1992) Intrinsic signal changes accompanying sensory stimulation: Functional brain mapping with magnetic resonance imaging. *Proc Natl Acad Sci USA* 89:5951–5955.

Paradiso MA and Nakayama K (1991) Brightness perception and filling-in. *Vision Res* 31:1221–1236.

Pessoa L, Thompson E, and Noe A (1998) Finding out about filling-in: A guide to perceptual completion for visual science and the philosophy of perception. *Behav Brain Sci* 21:723–802.

Petry S and Meyer E (1987) *The Perception of Illusory Contours.* New York: Springer.

Rabbel CD, Dale AM, Mendola J, and Halgren E (2000) Timing and localization of cortical activation to illusory contours with anatomically constrained MEG. *Neuroimage* 11:713.

Ramachandran VS (1992) Blind spots. *Sci Am* 266:8–91.

Ramsden BM, Hung CP, and Roe AW (1999) Activation of illusory contour domains in macaque area V2 is accompanied by relative suppression of real contour domains in area V1. *Soc Neurosci Abstr* 25:2060.

Redies C, Crook JM, and Creutzfelt OD (1986) Neural response to borders with and without luminance gradients in cat visual cortex and dorsal lateral geniculate nucleus. *Exp Brain Res* 61:49–81.

Rees G, Friston K, and Koch C (2000) A direct quantitative relationship between the functional properties of human and macaque V5. *Nat Neurosci* 3:716–723.

Ringach DL and Shapley R (1996) Spatial and temporal properties of illusory contours and amodal boundary completion. *Vision Res* 36:3337–3350.

Rivadulla C and Sur M (2000) Contribution of corticocortical connections to the generation of orientation maps in V1. *Soc Neurosci Abstr* 26:140.

Roelfsema PR, Lamme VA, and Spekreijse H (1998) Object-based attention in the primary visual cortex of the macaque monkey. *Nature* 395:376–381.

Rossi AF, Desimone R, and Ungerleider LG (2001) Contextual modulation in primary visual cortex of macaques. *J Neurosci* 21:1698–1709.

Rossi AF, Rittenhouse CD, and Paradiso MA (1996) The representation of brightness in primary visual cortex. *Science* 273:1104–1107.

Sadja P and Finkel FH (1995) Intermediate-level visual representation and the construction of surface perception. *J Cogn Neurosci* 7:267–291.

Sasaki Y, Hadjikhani N, Fischl B, Liu AK, Marret S, Dale AM, and Tootell RB (2001) Local and global attention are mapped retinotopically in human occipital cortex. *Proc Natl Acad Sci USA* 98:2077–2082.

Sheth BR, Sharma J, Rao SC, and Sur M (1996) Orientation maps of subjective contours in visual cortex. *Science* 274:2110–2115.

Spillmann L and Werner JS (1996) Long-range interactions in visual perception. *Trends Neurosci* 19:428–434.

Subirana-Vilanova JB and Richards W (1991) A.I. Memo No. 1218. Massachusetts Institute of Technology Artificial Intelligence Laboratory. Cambridge, MA.

Sugita Y (1999) Grouping of image fragments in primary visual cortex. *Nature* 401:269–272.

Tallon-Baudry C and Bertrand O (1999) Oscillatory gamma activity in humans and its role in object representation. *Trends Cogn Sci* 3:151–161.

Tootell RBH, Mendola JD, Hadjikhani NK, Liu AK, and Dale AM (1998) The representation of the ipsilateral visual field in human cerebral cortex. *Proc Natl Acad Sci USA* 95:818–824.

Tyler CW (1995) Empirical aspects of symmetry perception. *Spat Vis* 9:1–11.

Tyler CW and Baseler H (1998) FMRI signal from a cortical region specific for multiple pattern symmetries. *Invest Ophthamol Vis Sc* 39:S169.

Tyler CW and Baseler HA (2000) In search of the depth map. *Functional Brain Imaging in Vision*, 4th annual Vision Research Conference, Abstract Book, PS4-1. Oxford, UK: Elsevier Science.

Ungerleider LG and Desimone R (1986) Cortical connections of visual area MT in the macaque. *J Comp Neurol* 248:190–222.

Usher M and Donnelly N (1998) Visual synchrony affects binding and segmentation in perception. *Nature* 394:179–182.

Vanduffel W, Vogles R, Tootell RBH, and Orban GA (1997) Scrambling images of natural objects: II. A double-label deoxyglucose study. *Invest Ophthalmol Vis Sci* 38:S10001.

Van Oostende S, Sunaert S, Van Hecke P, Marchal G, and Orban G (1997) The kinetic occipital (KO) region in man: An fMRI study. *Cereb Cortex* 7:690–701.

von der Heydt R and Peterhans E (1989) Mechanisms of contour perception in monkey visual cortex. I. Lines of pattern discontinuity. *J Neurosci* 9:1731–1748.

von der Heydt R, Peterhans E, and Baumgartner G (1984) Illusory contours and cortical neuron responses. *Science* 224:1260–1262.

Vuilleumier P and Landis T (1998) Illusory contours and spatial neglect. *Neuroreport* 9:2481–2484.

Young MP and Scannell JW (2000) Brain structure–function relationships: Advances from neuroinformatics. *Philos Trans R Soc Lond B Biol Sci* 355:3–6.

Zhou H, Friedman HS, and von der Heydt R (2000) Coding of border ownership in monkey visual cortex. *J Neurosci* 20:6594–6611.

Zipser K, Lamme VA, and Schiller PH (1996) Contextual modulation in primary visual cortex. *J Neurosci* 16:7376–7389.

# 4

## Surface Completion:
## Psychophysical and Neurophysiological Studies of Brightness

### ANDREW F. ROSSI AND MICHAEL A. PARADISO

Aside from filling-in of the blind spot, the classic demonstrations of perceptual filling-in involved images stabilized on the retina by means of either special contact lenses or optical means. If a stimulus is entirely stabilized, its color and lightness fade until it is no longer seen (Riggs et al., 1953). For example, an artificial scotoma can be created in a normal observer by stabilizing a small opaque spot. The perceptual consequence of the stabilization is that the scotoma perceptually fades and the area fills-in with the color and lightness of the surrounding area (Gerrits et al., 1966; Yarbus, 1967). Similarly, if a disk of one color is surrounded by an annulus of a different color and the border between the two areas is stabilized on the retina, the color in the surrounding annulus *spills into* the central disk and the stimulus uniformly appears to have the lightness and color of the annulus (Krauskopf, 1963; Yarbus, 1967; Larimer and Piantanida, 1988). These observations with stabilized images demonstrate that perceptual filling-in can occur even in normal observers.

But what is *filling-in*? We take the term to mean a temporally progressive process by which a surface representation is constructed. The most straightforward implementation of filling-in would be a *flow* of activity from a surface's borders to its interior. There is considerable evidence that luminance and chromatic contrast strongly affect the responses of visual neurons. For this reason the representation of a surface, in terms of neural activity, appears to be biased toward borders. To date, there is no physiological evidence to support the idea that a surface of uniform lightness and color has an isomorphic representation in the brain that fills-in over time. This argues against the simplest isomorphic version of filling-in. However, other implementations that involve temporally changing activity, without an isomorphism, are still possible.

In the following discussion, we present data from psychophysical and physiological experiments that explored brightness perception and the possible involvement of filling-in. To frame the discussion, we pose four questions: (1) Is filling-in a part of normal (nonstabilized) visual perception? (2) Under what conditions is there a perceptual spread of lightness and color? (3) Is there an explicit neural representation of surface attributes such as lightness and color? (4) Is spreading activity observed in visual cortex, and does it correlate with filling-in?

We will first discuss psychophysical experiments that imply that there is a scale-dependent filling-in process always at work in the perception of lightness. This process is remarkably slow compared to feature detection, and it appears to be initiated near luminance-contrast boundaries. We will then move to a discussion of physiological data that suggest that there is an explicit representation of lightness, not in the retina, but in visual cortex. Lightness-correlated activity in striate cortex appears to result from extensive inhibitory and facilitatory interactions from outside the small classical receptive fields. In experiments with Mondrian stimuli, interactions between different spatial locations give rise to lightness-constant responses in striate cortex. Thus, there appears to be considerable consistency between lightness perception and V1 activity. Moreover, the temporal properties of the cortical lightness representation are consistent with the temporal aspects of lightness perception in the psychophysical experiments. This is not a direct demonstration of filling-in, but the similar temporal properties suggest a common cortical mechanism.

## Psychophysical Investigations of Brightness and Filling-In

### Backward Masking Appears to Disrupt Surface Completion

Let us suppose that brightness is perceived via a filling-in process initiated by luminance-contrast boundaries. In some way, a response initially biased toward the boundaries fills-in to represent the interiors of uniform surfaces. If this working hypothesis is correct, there should be a measurable time in which the surface representation is incomplete. Is it possible to interfere with the filling-in process, leaving the percept in the incomplete stage? This was the approximate logic behind a brightness masking experiment we conducted (Paradiso and Nakayama, 1991). The first stimulus presented was a large disk of uniform brightness on a black background. According to the working hypothesis, brightness would fill-in from the disk's border to its interior. The disk was briefly flashed and, after a variable stimulus offset asynchrony (SOA), a masking stimulus was presented. The mask consisted of a bright line or circle on a black background with the masking contours positioned within the boundaries of the large, uniform disk. The critical additional assumption was that the contours in the mask would interfere with the brightness filling-in of the uniform disk if the mask was presented at a time when the disk's filling-in was incomplete. In other words, luminance-contrast borders serve to start and stop filling-in, as suggested by some models of brightness perception (Walls, 1954; Gerrits and Vendrik, 1970; Cohen and Grossberg, 1985).

Subjects viewed multiple cycles of the disk followed by the mask at various SOAs. Their task was to indicate which element of a palette of gray tones was most simiiar to the brightness perceived at the center of the disk. As we expected, with a long SOA, the disk was perceived as filled-in before the mask was presented. However, as the SOA was decreased, the brightness of the disk was affected. It is informative to contrast the effect of a mask consisting of a single line with that of a circular mask. When the mask was a short, bright line (smaller than the diameter of the disk), with SOAs of 50–100 ms small areas to the sides of the line appeared darkened (Fig. 4-1A). Otherwise, the disk appeared filled-in. If the same line was bent to form a circle, the effect was quite different. Outside the masking circle, the disk appeared normal except for a small area of darkening just next to the outside of the circle. This appeared similar to masking next to a straight line. However, inside the circular mask, there was a much more dramatic effect: At SOAs between 50 and 100 ms, the entire area of the disk inside the circular mask was significantly darker or black (Fig. 4-1B). Under optimal conditions, the brightness matches made in the center of the disk were reduced as much as 2 log units relative to the condition in which no masking was observed (i.e., at long target/mask intervals). Evidently, the circular shape of the mask was responsible for the large asymmetry in the masking strength inside and outside the circle. The normal appearance of the disk outside the area of the circular mask was consistent with the hypothesis that the outside edge of the disk played a role in determining its interior brightness and that the masking circle could interfere with this process only inside its radius.

The brightness masking effect was even stronger with dichoptic than monoptic presentation (square symbols in Fig. 4-1B). When the target and mask were presented to different eyes, the interior of the target disk was absolutely black. The fact that the masking was effective dichoptically suggests that the stimuli interact in visual cortex where there are binocular neurons.

In terms of the filling-in hypothesis, the results might be explained as follows. The presentation of the target disk initiates a propagation of brightness away from the border. This process can be interrupted as long as the masking contour is presented before the propagation of brightness has proceeded past it. For this reason, the masking circle can be effective if it is presented after the target.

If there is in fact propagation of a signal related to surface brightness, one should be able to see masking at a later time if the masking contour is farther from the edge of the target disk. To test this prediction, targets with radii ranging from 1.2 to 3.4 degrees were used with a 2.0 degree radius masking ring. Consistent with the prediction, the suppressive effect of the masks was greater as the target disk increased in size (Fig. 4-1C). Also, masking remained effective at longer SOAs as the distance between the edges of the two stimuli increased. Based on the latest times at which masking was effective with different distances between the outer edge of the disk and the circular mask, a velocity for brightness propagation was calculated. The estimated velocity was 110–150 deg/sec. Using estimates of the human cortical magnification factor for primary visual cortex, this comes out to a roughly constant speed of 0.15–0.4 m/sec for the propagation (if it occurred in V1).

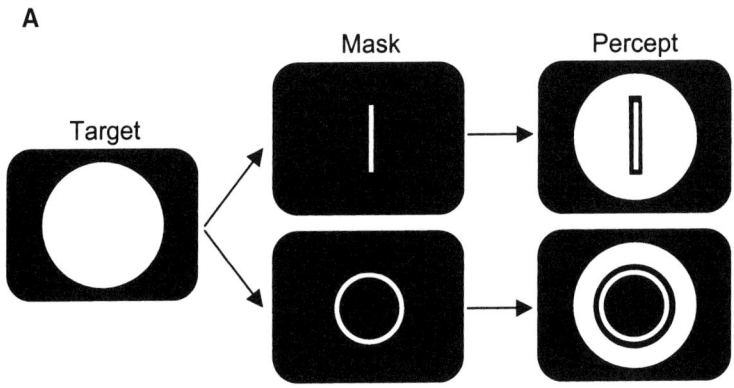
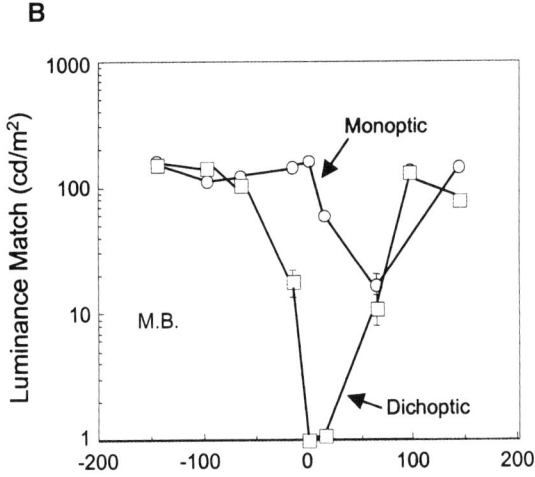
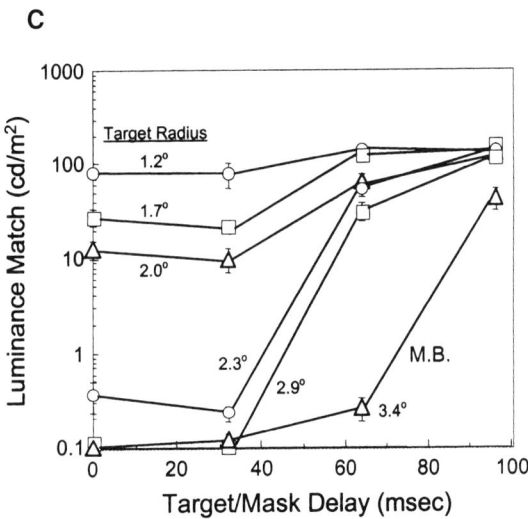

## Filling-In Percepts from Luminance Sweeps

If filling-in is a part of normal vision, we presumably don't notice it because the process is completed quickly. But perhaps it is possible to protract the duration of filling-in to make it visible. We conducted a number of experiments to explore this possibility by temporally modulating the luminance of a stimulus. Consider the following Gedanken experiment: On a dark computer screen, the luminance of a disk is gradually increased from dark to bright. Does the brightness increase simultaneously and equivalently everywhere throughout the disk? The answer is that under most conditions the brightness does appear to change uniformly. However, in some situations the disk's brightness is noticeably inhomogeneous as the luminance changes. Most commonly, it appears that brightness changes near the center of the uniform disk lag behind changes at the disk's edge. In other words, the center is a bit darker, and it looks as if brightness is moving inward from the edge of the disk. The central lag in brightness is even more pronounced when the entire computer screen is bright and a disk's luminance begins bright and gradually decreases (Fig. 4-2A). There is a striking percept that the center of the disk is brighter than the edge and that darkness sweeps into the center.

A critical determinant of these filling-in percepts is the rate at which the luminance is changed: The disk appears uniform if the luminance is changed rapidly or slowly but nonuniform if it is changed at intermediate rates. In exploring the phenomenon qualitatively, we tried a variety of stimulus configurations (squares, disks, etc.), stimulus sizes (0.5–10 degrees), and luminance modulation paradigms (linear, exponential, etc.). Generally speaking, the qualitative results did not depend critically on these parameters. For example, if the stimulus consisted of several simultaneously presented uniform patches, each patch would appear to fill-in independently from its own borders.

In quantitative experiments, the visual stimulus was a disk of uniform luminance and the luminance was temporally modulated in equally detectable steps (rather than equal steps in luminance). Controlled variables were the speed of the upward or downward luminance sweep and the dwell time spent at each luminance step. The parameter ranges that elicited the perception of brightness or darkness filling-in were comparable across observers. However, the appearance of the brightness spreading did not seem identical for all observers or on every

---

**Figure 4-1.** Suppression of brightness by backward masking. (A) Brief presentation of a disk-shaped target followed by a mask consisting of a thin line has little effect on the perception of the disk. If the mask is a white ring, the interior of the disk is darkened significantly. (B) If the disk and ring are shown to the same eye (monoptic), maximal brightness suppression occurs with a stimulus offset asynchrony (SOA) of 50–100 ms. With dichoptic masking, suppression is maximal at an SOA of zero. (C) With a fixed-size mask, brightness suppression increases as the target increases in size (and the distance between the edges of the target and the mask increases). Also, masking is obtained at longer delays as the target increases in size.

**A**

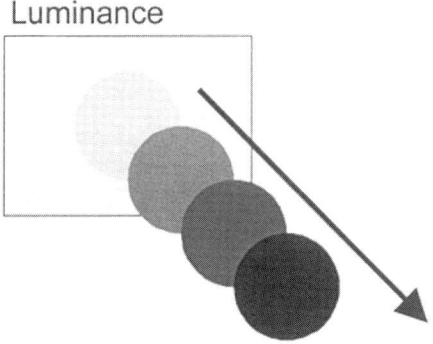

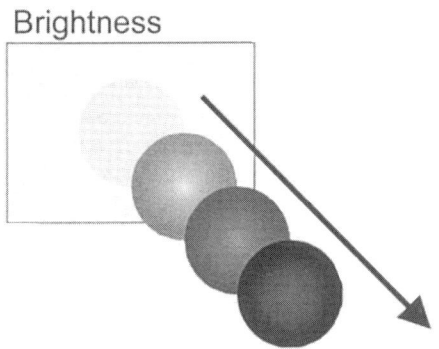

**B**

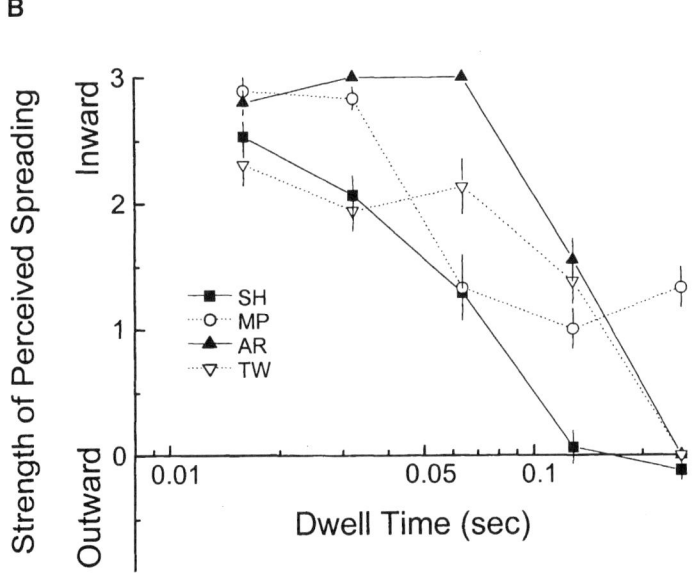

trial for the same observer. Sometimes the effect was a symmetrical inward spread of brightness or darkness, but in other cases there appeared to be a somewhat asymmetrical *winking* of brightness. Another interesting qualitative observation is that the sensation of darkness spreading obtained with downward luminance sweeps was almost always stronger than the sensation of brightness spreading in the upward sweeps.

The most important variable for the perception of brightness filling-in was the dwell time. Spreading brightness was seen with short dwell times, but as the dwell time increased above 50 ms, the darkness spreading effect decreased significantly (Fig. 4-2B). In other words, the perception of the modulated disk was nonuniform, and filling-in was lost if the luminance was held longer than 50–100 ms at each luminance step.

To determine whether the filling-in percepts might be based on mechanisms within the retina, we presented the luminance-modulated disk so that it surrounded the blind spot at the optic disk. In preliminary experiments, we were surprised to find that the perception of brightness or darkness filling-in was unaffected. For instance, in downward ramps, darkness appeared to sweep from the edge to the center of the modulated disk even though most of the disk's interior was imaged on a portion of the retina devoid of photoreceptors. The quantitative experiments confirmed this observation, showing that the luminance sweep speeds and dwell times that gave the strongest filling-in percepts were the same in the normal and blind spot versions of the experiment.

One interpretation of the results is that the edge and center of the stimuli have different brightness when the luminance is swept up or down because the sweep speed exceeds the rate of an underlying brightness process. It is known that the brightness of an area is strongly dependent on the luminance contrast at the area's border (Hess and Pretori, 1894; Heinemann, 1972). Perhaps there is a spread of activity in visual cortex underlying the perceptual filling-in. In order to account for the fact that inhomogeneities are not seen at fast luminance ramp speeds, one must postulate that the inhomogeneity exists for a period of time too short to be perceived. This would explain why we are not aware of any brightness nonuniformities in normal visual situations as we move our eyes about. Presumably, by stretching out the luminance ramp in time, an inhomogeneity can be maintained for a longer duration, making it perceptible. When the luminance ramp is very slow, each time the luminance is incremented, the filling-in process is completed before the next increment and the inhomogeneity is preserved for too short a time to be perceived.

**Figure 4-2.** Gradual luminance sweeps elicit filling-in percepts. (A) When the luminance of a uniform disk is progressively decreased, brightness changes toward the center appear to lag behind changes at the border. (B) The strength of the filling-in percept depends strongly on the dwell time spent at each luminance step. At short dwell times there are compelling filling-in percepts, but these are lost as the dwell time increases above about 50 msec. Data from four observers are shown.

## *Unique Spatiotemporal Dynamics of Lightness Revealed by Dynamic Induction*

In 1986, De Valois et al. published a surprising observation about the temporal characteristics of brightness induction that provides another piece of evidence suggesting that brightness processes are slow. The authors used a stimulus in which a static gray patch was surrounded by a larger area in which the luminance was modulated sinusoidally in time. The luminance modulation of the surround produced powerful brightness induction in the gray patch, roughly in antiphase to the surround modulation. Surprisingly, brightness modulation was induced in the gray patch only when the surround was modulated at quite low temporal frequencies (i.e., below about 2.5 Hz). When the surround was modulated at higher rates, the central patch appeared to be a static gray. This low cutoff for induced brightness modulation stands in stark contrast to the critical flicker fusion rate, which is an order of magnitude faster.

We extended the experiments of De Valois et al. to determine whether the properties of this dynamic form of brightness induction are consistent with the implications of the masking and luminance sweep experiments. The stimulus we used was a temporally modulated squarewave grating (Fig. 4-3A). The grating was modulated in a manner such that the luminance of every other stripe varied sinusoidally in time and the intervening stripes had constant luminance. Perceptually, the modulation produced brightness induction in the constant stripes, roughly in antiphase to the brightness of the luminance-modulated stripes. In light of the masking and luminance-sweep results, we were particularly interested in any dependence the temporal properties of brightness induction might have on spatial scale. Using the method of adjustment, we had observers find the highest temporal modulation rate at which induction was perceived at different spatial frequencies. We found that the lower the spatial frequency (i.e., the larger the areas of uniform brightness), the lower the cutoff temporal modulation rate (Fig. 4-3B). We also quantified the amplitude of the perceived brightness modulation that was induced. This showed that the amplitude of the brightness induction was greatest at low temporal modulation rates (Fig. 4-3C). The luminance matches to the peak and trough of the brightness modulation approach each other as the temporal frequency is increased, eventually becoming equal when there is no perceived brightness modulation. These results make it clear that below the cutoff modulation rate, the amplitude of brightness induction is graded relative to temporal frequency, and induction is not simply "off" and "on" above and below the cutoff rate, respectively.

The results of the dynamic induction experiments make two important points about the mechanisms involved in brightness perception. First, the process responsible for brightness changes due to induction is considerably slower than the process responsible for brightness changes from direct luminance modulation. Second, the time course of induction is scale-dependent. The low cutoff frequency for induction and the effect of modulation rate on the amplitude of induction suggest that induction is a slow process that simply cannot "keep up" with fast mod-

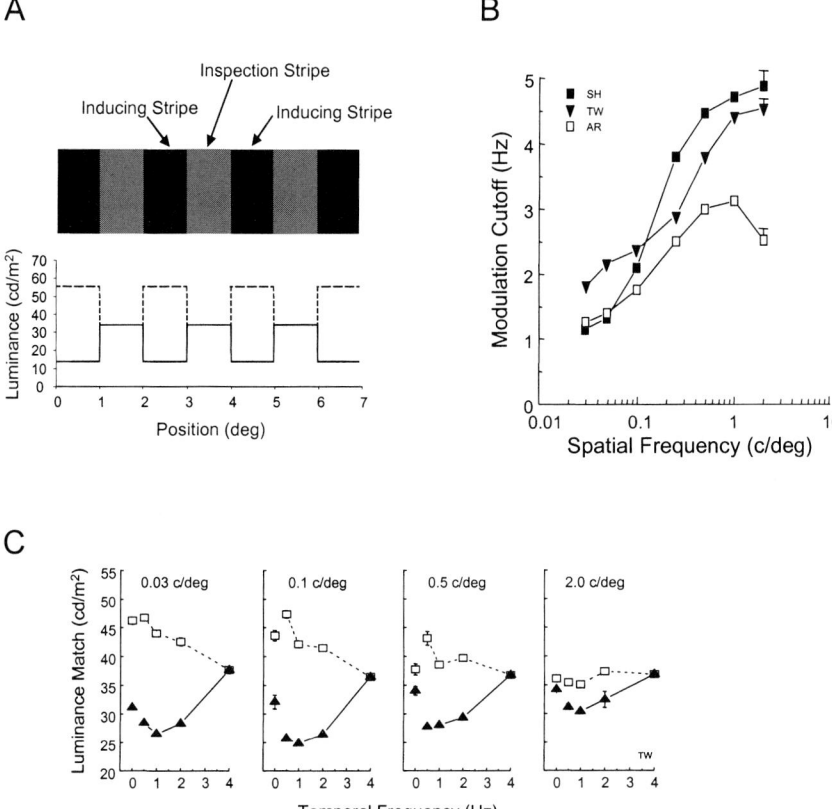

**Figure 4-3.** Temporal dynamics of brightness induction. (A) Upper: schematic view of the squarewave stimulus as it appeared to the observers. The luminance of the inducing stripes was modulated sinusoidally in time to induce brightness modulation in the static intervening stripes. Observers made judgments based on the appearance of the inspection stripe in the center of the grating. Lower: luminance profile of the squarewave grating. The solid and dashed lines represent the extreme luminance values of the inducing stripes. The static stripes had a luminance equal to the time-average luminance of the modulated stripes. (B) Temporal frequency cutoff for induced brightness modulation as a function of the spatial frequency of the squarewave grating. Data from three observers are shown. Error bars on the highest spatial frequency data points represent the average standard error of the mean (SEM), across frequency, for each observer. (C) Luminance matches to the maximum (open symbols) and minimum (solid symbols) of the induced brightness changes for one observer. Each graph shows the matches plotted as a function of the temporal frequency of the luminance modulation for a given spatial frequency of the squarewave grating. Data points at zero temporal frequency represent matches made when the inducing stripes were static (maximum or minimum luminance). Error bars represent ± SEM.

ulation rates. Said another way, it appears that larger spatial areas take more time to induce. Besides the fact that the cutoff rates for "real" and induced brightness changes differ by more than a factor of 10, they depend on spatial scale in opposite ways. While the critical flicker fusion rate increases with stimulus size, the cutoff frequency in our induction experiments decreases with size. The results indicate that there is a major difference between the mechanisms limiting perception of modulation with real and induced brightness.

Filling-in provides a possible account of the temporal properties of dynamic induction. Many studies have shown that brightness induction is largely based on the contrast at the edges of a uniform region rather than on the total amount of light in neighboring areas (e.g., Wallach, 1948; Heinemann, 1955). For instance, while the brightness of a gray patch depends on the luminance of a neighboring area, the induction effect quickly saturates as the neighboring area is stretched from a thin band to a wide band (Diamond 1955). If induction were initiated at edges and propagated inward, this would explain why it takes longer to induce a larger area and why the cutoff frequency decreases with increasing size. We measured the spatial phase of induced brightness across spatial scale, and this led to an estimate of 140–180 deg/sec for the induction process. This estimate is in rough agreement with the filling-in velocities estimated in the brightness masking and luminance sweep experiments.

To reconcile filling-in with the high cutoff frequency, we have proposed that brightness involves two mechanisms—a fast process that is relatively unaffected by the size of a uniformly luminous area and a slow filling-in process with a duration that increases with the size of a uniformly luminous area. A fast process largely based on luminance appears to be necessary to explain the high cutoff frequency for luminance modulation and the fact that this frequency does not decrease with the size of the modulated area. A slow process driven mainly by contrast appears to be required to account for the induction results, as well as results in the masking and luminance-sweep experiments. We hypothesize that when the luminance of an area is modulated, both the fast and slow processes are involved in determining the final brightness percept of that area. Previous experiments suggest that slow filling-in occurs with luminance modulation (Paradiso and Nakayama, 1991; Paradiso and Hahn, 1996), but the fast process presumably determines the cutoff frequency. The situation is different when brightness modulation occurs solely because of induction. In this case, we suggest that only the slow filling-in process is responsible for the perceived brightness modulation of the induced area. Thus, the velocity of the filling-in process would determine the cutoff frequency for induced modulation.

## Summary and Conclusions

A filling-in model of normal brightness perception can explain the psychophysical experiments described above. Most importantly, filling-in provides a possible account of the unusual spatiotemporal dynamics of brightness. Brightness mechanisms are slow and scale-dependent. While there are limits to the precision of the estimates, each of the three types of experiments discussed above suggests that brightness fills-in with a speed of approximately 150 deg/sec. We now proceed to a consideration of the physiological mechanisms underlying perceived brightness. Indeed, a critical question is whether there exists an explicit representation of brightness rather than an inference of brightness derived from edge responses.

## The Representation of Brightness in Primary Visual Cortex

Early studies of primary visual cortex emphasized the important role that luminance contrast plays in exciting neurons. Without a doubt, contrast is required to produce a significant response in many cells. Perhaps this means that there is not an explicit representation of brightness (or of surfaces in general) because an area of uniform brightness has no contrast. We will show below that this inference is incorrect, as many cells do respond to surfaces in the absence of contrast. Moreover, in some situations, many cortical neurons fire in a manner better correlated with brightness than with luminance or luminance contrast. The basis for these brightness-correlated responses appears to be extensive lateral interactions either within striate cortex or between cortical areas. It has not been established whether there is a neural correlate of the perceptual filling-in described above. However, spreading activity has been observed in primary visual cortex.

### Neural Responses Correlated with Perceived Brightness in an Induction Paradigm

For there to be a form of neural filling-in underlying perceptual filling-in of a surface, there needs to be an explicit representation of the surface. If surfaces were represented entirely by the responses to their boundaries, nothing would need to fill-in. However, until recently, it was far from clear whether an explicit representation of surface brightness exists. In experimental terms, there are two major questions: (1) Do neurons somewhere in the brain respond to light in the absence of contrast? (2) If there are responses in the absence of contrast, do they correlate with physical luminance, perceived brightness, or something else?

Our first effort to answer these questions used the dynamic form of brightness induction described above in psychophysical experiments. The primary reason for choosing this stimulus was the strength of the perceptual effect. Imagine covering a visual receptive field (RF) with a gray patch of light while areas surrounding this patch are modulated from black to white. While the surround changes, the brightness of the gray patch is induced, changing from a light gray to a dark gray. But does the neuron's response change even though the physical properties in the region covering the RF are fixed? The answer is that it all depends on where one looks in the visual system.

We recorded from single cells in the retina, lateral geniculate nucleus (LGN), and primary visual cortex of anesthetized cats (Rossi et al., 1996; Rossi and Paradiso, 1999). After the RF was mapped, the dynamic induction stimulus was positioned such that a large central gray patch covered the RF. The patch was always much larger than the RF, extending 3–5 degrees beyond the RF boundary on either side. Flanks the same size as the central patch were positioned on either side. The luminance of the flanking patches was modulated from light to dark sinusoidally in time. Two principal control stimuli were used (see Fig. 4-4A, far left column). In one stimulus, the luminance of the area covering the RF was modulated rather than the flanks. This tested whether responses were better correlated with the luminance or the brightness of the central patch. The second control had a large black patch covering the RF, instead of a gray patch, while the flanks were modulated. If light from the flanks directly modulated the response of the neuron (e.g., scattered light), this should be revealed with this control stimulus. However, as there is no perceptual induction when the central patch is black, the neuron's response should not be affected by the flank modulation if the response represents brightness.

To study the responses of retinal ganglion cells, we recorded from their axons in the optic tract. It is important to keep in mind that the stimuli employed were sized such that the central patch encompassed both the center and surround of the RF; any effects of the flanks were from beyond the RF. As would be expected from the low-pass frequency response of retinal neurons, many cells were somewhat activated by a gray patch of light covering their RF. Furthermore, some cells responded in a phase-locked manner to luminance modulation within the RF. When the dynamic induction stimulus was used, cell responses were generally constant, along with the luminance of the patch covering the RF, rather than modulated. Taken together, the optic tract recordings with different stimuli indicate that the neurons are responsive to luminance in the absence of contrast, but the responses do not correlate with perceived brightness.

In many regards, the results were similar when recordings were made in LGN layers A and A1. A static gray patch in the RF often elicited a neuronal response, and the response varied as the luminance of the central patch was modulated. There were also neurons that showed modulated responses when the flank luminance was varied in time. However, the fact that the response modulation to the flanks was generally greater when the central patch covering the receptive field was black rather than gray suggests that light scattering was probably involved rather than a brightness representation. Occasionally, cells were encountered that did appear to have responses correlated with brightness. As these were similar to cells observed in striate cortex, but were much less common, we will discuss them in the context of the cortical recordings.

Many cortical neurons were found to respond only in stimulus conditions that produced perceptual changes in brightness in the area corresponding to the RF. An example of this is shown in Figure 4-4A. The third row of this figure shows the response of a neuron to the presentation of a constant gray field flanked on either side by luminance-varying fields of equal size. The RF was 4 degrees wide and was centered on the central gray area, which was 14 degrees across. The response of the neuron was phase-locked to the frequency of the luminance mod-

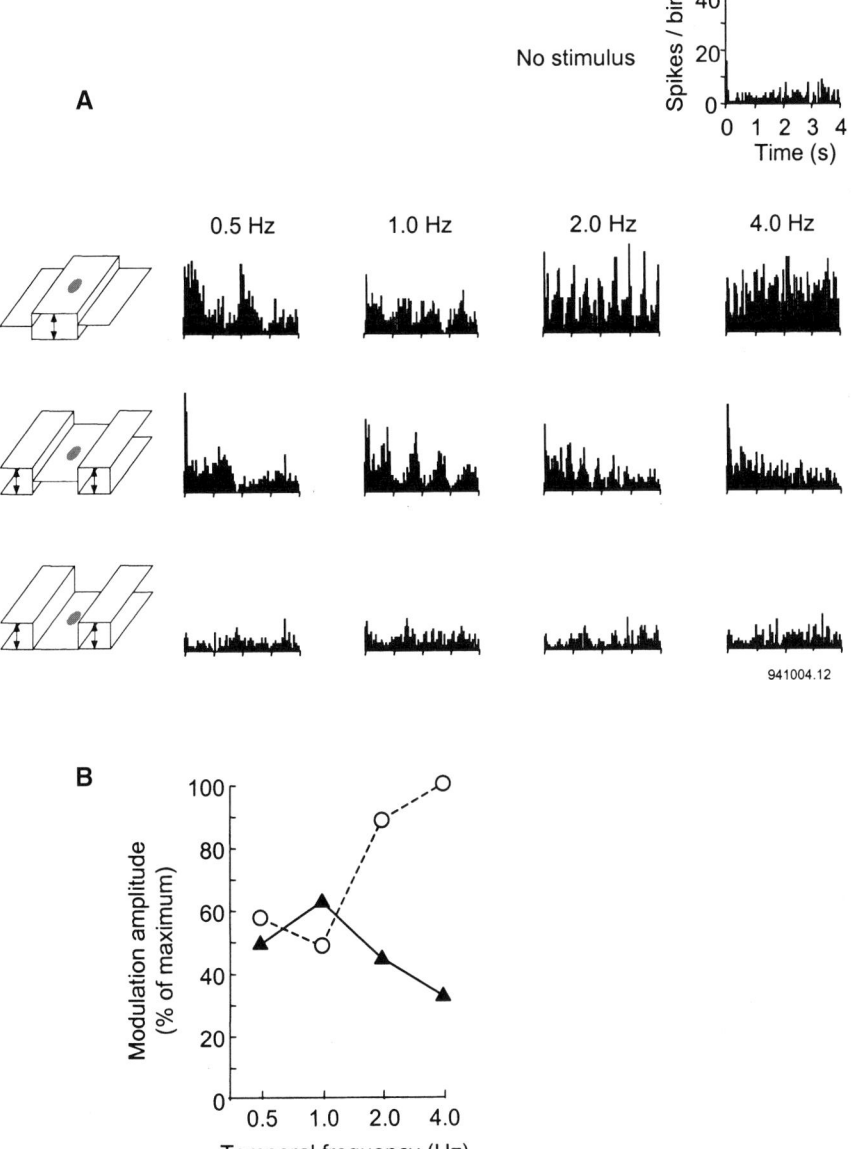

**Figure 4-4.** Brightness induction in primary visual cortex. (A) Temporal frequency of luminance modulation affects the response to induction (row 3) and control (rows 2 and 4) stimuli differently. Responses to luminance modulation rates of 0.5, 1.0, 2.0, and 4.0 Hz are shown. (B) The amplitude of response modulation plotted as a function of temporal frequency for the striate neuron shown in (A). Solid triangles represent the response to the induction stimulus and open circles to luminance modulation covering the receptive field (RF). The modulation amplitude is expressed as the percentage of the maximum response.

ulation in the stimulus flanks. There was no such response when the central portion of the stimulus was black (fourth row). This is an important distinction because there is perceptual induction of brightness changes in the stimulus with the gray center (third row) but not in the stimulus with the black center (fourth row). In our sample of 160 striate neurons, 120 (75%) had responses that were modulated and phase-locked to the luminance changes outside the RF.

A comparison of the responses in the different conditions suggests that the firing of the neuron in Figure 4-4A (and others) was more closely correlated with the brightness in the area covering the RF than with the luminance of any particular portion of the stimulus. This was seen in the strong response modulation when the stimulus center was gray (a condition that yields perceptual induction) compared to the weak response modulation when the center was black (a condition that does not cause induction). A correlation with brightness is also found when one compares the responses to luminance modulation within the RF and luminance modulation in the flanks. When light covering the receptive field was modulated, the response was maximal when the central area was brightest (and the luminance of the modulated light was highest). When the flanks were modulated, the response was again greatest when the central area was brightest, but in this case the luminance of the modulated flanks was lowest. The response was clearly not determined by the overall amount of light present in the stimulus.

Beyond noting that flank modulation outside the RF influenced the response of many striate neurons, we used additional analyses to examine the extent of the response correlation with brightness. One concern was that some neurons exhibited significant response modulation when the stimulus center was black or gray. The response of these neurons might be partly associated with brightness, but this could not be proven in the presence of what appeared to be scattering. We chose the conservative criterion that neurons were considered for further analysis only if the modulation amplitude in the induction condition was more than twice that in the center black condition. This left 49 (31% of the total 160) neurons that had responses not easily accounted for by scattering, suggesting that the responses to modulation of the stimulus flanks involved neural interactions from beyond the classical RF. We did not find a systematic relationship between classical RF properties (orientation selectivity, spatial tuning, simple vs. complex) and the magnitude of the response to the brightness induction stimuli. These neurons were located in all layers 2–6, and they were of both simple and complex types. For these 49 neurons, the phase of the temporal response and the response across temporal frequencies were analyzed for possible correlations with brightness perception.

As described in the previous section, one of the hallmarks of the dynamic brightness induction effect is that brightness changes are perceived only at low modulation rates in comparison to the rates of direct luminance modulation that elicit brightness variations. In other words, at higher modulation rates, there is a significant difference in the degree of perceived brightness modulation with real and induced brightness. Physiologically, we found differences in the amplitudes of response modulation in the induction and center modulation conditions. In the induction condition, the response of the neuron in Figure 4-4A was largest at low temporal frequencies and *decreased* as the rate of flank modulation was increased above 1.0 Hz (third row). However, when the luminance of the central area was modulated, the response amplitude progressively *increased* with increasing temporal frequency (second row). A significant difference in the induction and center modulation conditions is clearly evident in the averaged data (Fig. 4-4B).

Another characteristic of dynamic induction is that the perceived temporal phase of the brightness variations is in approximate antiphase to the luminance variations in the flanks. Of course, if the luminance of the area covering the receptive field is modulated, brightness and luminance changes covary (i.e., they are in phase). Therefore, perceptually, brightness changes are 180 degrees out of phase between the induction condition and the center modulation condition. For the neurons with responses not attributable to light scattering, the response phase differences between the induction and luminance modulation conditions were diverse, but the great majority were near either 0 degrees or 180 degrees.

The responses of neurons in striate cortex correlate with perceived brightness in four ways: the neural responses were modulated at the frequency of the surrounding luminance modulation; the response modulation occurred in conditions that elicited brightness induction but not in similar conditions that did not produce induction; in the induction conditions, the response modulation greatly decreased as the temporal frequency increased; there was a complete phase shift between induction and center modulation conditions. However, cells that appeared to follow brightness based on one criterion did not always do so according to other criteria. In the population sampled, roughly 10% of the neurons showed responses that correlated with brightness in every test run. Another 20% followed brightness but did not show a 180 degree phase shift in the induction condition. We take the estimate of 10%–30% of V1 neurons having brightness-correlated responses as conservative for two reasons. First, we did not count cells that we otherwise would have counted if the response in the center-black condition was even 50% of the response in the induction condition. Second, we did not systematically vary stimulus size. Conceivably, we would have seen more brightness correlations if we had searched for optimal stimuli.

Applying the criteria used in the cortical analysis, 2 of the 75 LGN neurons had responses correlated with brightness and none did in the optic tract. It remains to be determined whether brightness-correlated responses develop between the LGN and striate cortex or whether the occasional LGN responses result from cortical feedback.

## *Lightness Perception, Lightness Constancy, and Lateral Interactions in Visual Cortex*

The induction studies described above suggest that at least for a subgroup of neurons in striate cortex, there is an explicit representation of surface qualities such as brightness. The logical hypothesis to explain the induction physiology results is that outside cortical RFs, there are areas that modulate the response to a stimulus in the RF. While there have been many studies of interactions from outside striate RFs, virtually all have used lines or gratings as stimuli (i.e., contrast within the RF). However, when a uniform surface covers the RF, interactions from areas beyond the RF are not reliably the same as those that would be found with line or grating stimuli (MacEvoy and Paradiso, 1998). From one cell to another, there is considerable diversity in the modulatory effects that light outside the RF has on the response to a surface covering the RF. The most common effect is surround suppression. The prevalence of surround suppression, and its large spatial range, offer an explanation for the induction effect noted above. The modulatory areas outside the RF cannot drive the cortical neuron alone (i.e., there is no response when the area covering the RF is black), but when the cell is excited by a central stimulus, such as the gray patch, the flanks can alter the response. The *in phase* and *out of phase* responses recorded with luminance modulation of the patch covering the RF versus the flanks can be accounted for by areas beyond the RF that are either facilitatory or inhibitory.

The net effect of surround interactions on neurons in striate cortex is to make them largely lightness constant. Mimicking perceptual experiments on lightness constancy, the RF of a neuron was encompassed by a single patch of a monochromatic Mondrian stimulus (MacEvoy and Paradiso, 2001). Each patch in the Mondrian stimulus was assigned a reflectance value as if it were a piece of paper (Fig. 4-5A).

In *illumination* conditions, changes in illumination were simulated by adjusting the luminance of every patch in a manner consistent with its fixed reflectance. Across conditions, the luminance values of various patches changed by different amounts, but all contrast ratios between patches were constant, just as they would be for patches of paper under varying illumination. The Mondrian stimulus was presented for 5 seconds at each of five randomly intermixed illumination intensities. Psychophysical studies using similar stimuli have shown that human observers perceive the lightness of the patches to be constant when the simulated illumination is changed (see Arend and Spehar, 1993). In control con-

**Figure 4-5.** Lightness constancy in cat V1 neurons. (A) Changes in illumination were simulated on a computer monitor by assigning reflectances to patches on the display, one patch covering a neuron's receptive field (RF). Luminance changes of the RF patch and other patches could be made in a manner either consistent or inconsistent with overall changes in illumination. (B) Data from one cell show a response correlated with both luminance and lightness when only the luminance of the RF patch is changed (dotted line). When the entire Mondrian is changed in a manner consistent with overall increases in illumination, the response is relatively fixed (solid line). This response correlates with the stable lightness of the RF patch but not with the luminance of the patch. (C) Distribution of slopes from plots of response rates versus RF patch luminance. When only the luminance of the RF patch changes, V1 neurons on average show a positive correlation between response rate and RF patch luminance (solid bars; mean indicated by arrow at 0.11). When the Mondrian is varied in a manner consistent with changes in overall illumination, the average V1 response is unchanged (hatched bars; mean indicated by arrow at $-0.01$).

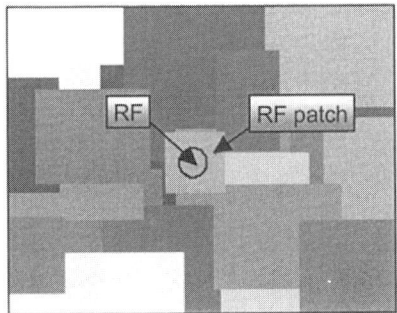

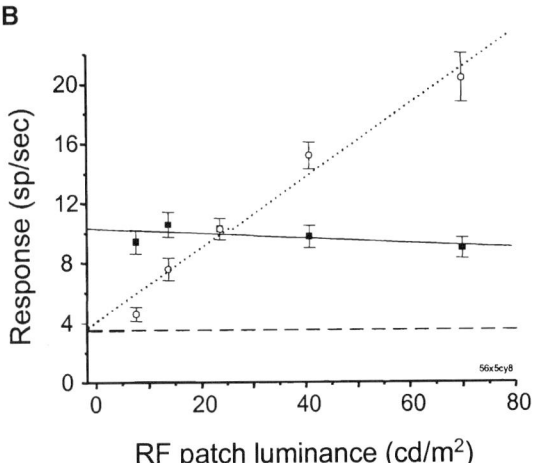

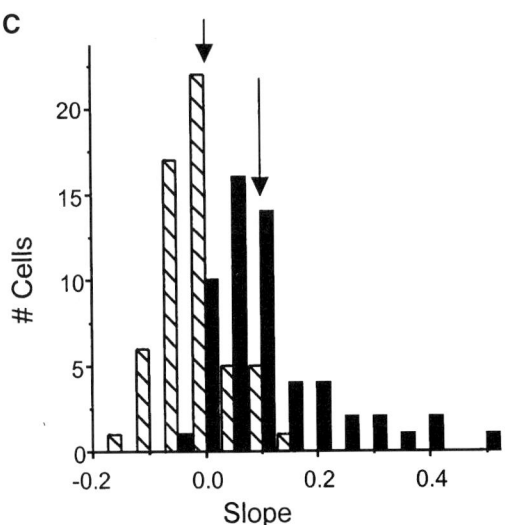

ditions, the RF patch was varied across exactly the same luminance settings as in the illumination conditions. However, the rest of the patches in the Mondrian stimulus were fixed at the mean values used in the illumination conditions. Consequently, the average contrast of the RF patch on the Mondrian stimulus reversed sign as RF patch luminance increased. The luminance settings in the control conditions were inconsistent with overall changes in illumination.

By analyzing the responses of neurons across the illumination and control conditions, we compared the way responses varied when changes in the luminance of the RF patch could or could not be accounted for by changes in overall illumination. Figure 4-5B shows the average firing rate of a neuron across the illumination and control conditions. In the control conditions, the neuron's response progressively increased as the luminance of the RF patch increased even though the contrast within the RF was fixed. In these control conditions, the lightness of the RF patch was correlated with its luminance. In the illumination conditions, the responses to identical stimuli within the RF were quite different: The responses were considerably more similar across the same range of intensities. Figure 4-5C shows the distribution of slopes in the illumination and control conditions for all 57 neurons completely characterized. The average slope in the control conditions was 0.11 compared to $-0.01$ in the illumination conditions.

Thus, in the control conditions, the average response was correlated with the luminance of the patches in the RF and with the lightness of the patches. In the illumination conditions, the average response was also correlated with lightness, but in this case the response was lightness constant, as was the stimulus perceptually. On average, in the illumination conditions, luminance changes beyond the RF counterbalanced the effect of luminance changes within it. These data extend the induction results by showing that the correlation observed between single cells and brightness applies to striate cortex on average, both in situations that are and are not lightness constant perceptually. This is all the more significant because of the behavioral importance of lightness constancy. It has been argued that lightness and color would be of little use if they were not largely immune to changes in illumination.

## *Spreading Activation in Primary Visual Cortex*

The physiological and psychophysical results discussed to this point are consistent in that large-scale spatial interactions appear to be involved in the construction of a lightness representation for surfaces. Neural interactions give rise to single-cell responses in striate cortex that exhibit both brightness induction and lightness constancy. These results support the hypothesis that there is an explicit rather than an inferred representation of surfaces. But does this representation involve filling-in? While the answers to this question are not yet definitively established, there are several physiological demonstrations of spreading activity in visual cortex. Optical imaging studies of the cortical point-spread function have shown that a focal visual stimulus evoked a wave of propagating activity in V1 that extended radially for 10 mm (Grinvald et al., 1994; Das and Gilbert, 1995).

More recently, Bringuier et al. (1999) have demonstrated large integration fields in primary visual cortex of the cat by measuring intracellular postsynaptic potentials. They found that the latency of these postsynaptic potentials increased with the distance of the stimulus away from the center of the integration field. These subthreshold measures indicate that stimulation of an isolated area in visual cortex results in spreading activation that extends far beyond the RF.

A possible consequence of spreading activation has been observed in the latency of action potentials in striate cortex of the alert macaque monkey (Rossi et al., 2001). In this study, it was found that over 40% of striate neurons responded to a surround texture stimulus presented 1 degree beyond the border of the RF in the absence of direct RF stimulation (see Fig. 4-6A). To determine the spatial extent over which a surround stimulus alone could evoke a response, we systematically varied the distance of the inner border of the surround texture from the RF. Figure 4-6B illustrates the response of a single neuron, having a 1 degree RF, to the surround stimulus presented at different distances from the RF. This figure demonstrates that the surround stimulus elicited a significant response even when the boundary of the surround was 2 degrees from the RF's center (i.e., clearly outside the RF). Moreover, the response latency increased as the surround stimulus was presented farther from the RF. The systematic increase in response latency with stimulus distance is shown for this neuron in Figure 4-6C. Figure 4-6D illustrates the same relationship for our sample of 82 neurons that had RFs 1 degree in diameter or smaller. This figure shows that there was an abrupt increase in the response latency when the surround was more than 0.5 degree from the RF's center. Response latencies continued to increase to a maximum of 105 msec as the distance between the surround and the RF center increased to 2.5 degrees, beyond which the response latency was approximately constant. It is conceivable that our observations of long-latency, extra-RF responses with surround textures represent a suprathreshold manifestation of the spreading activity described above.

As already discussed, the neuronal response to induced changes in brightness has a slow time course, evidenced by the low pass characteristics of the temporal tuning (see Fig. 4-4B). This observation has been extended in a recent study that examined the response properties of striate neurons to the static presentation of an induction stimulus (Kinoshita and Komatsu, 2001). This study showed that the later portion of the response (100–200 ms after stimulus onset) was best correlated with the surround luminance, rather than the luminance of the area corresponding to the RF. This long latency response to the surround is consistent with the low temporal cutoff frequency observed perceptually and physiologically with dynamic brightness induction.

## Summary and Conclusions

It is clear from the physiological studies of brightness induction and brightness constancy that there is an explicit representation of brightness information reflected in the firing rate of some neurons at the earliest stages of cortical pro-

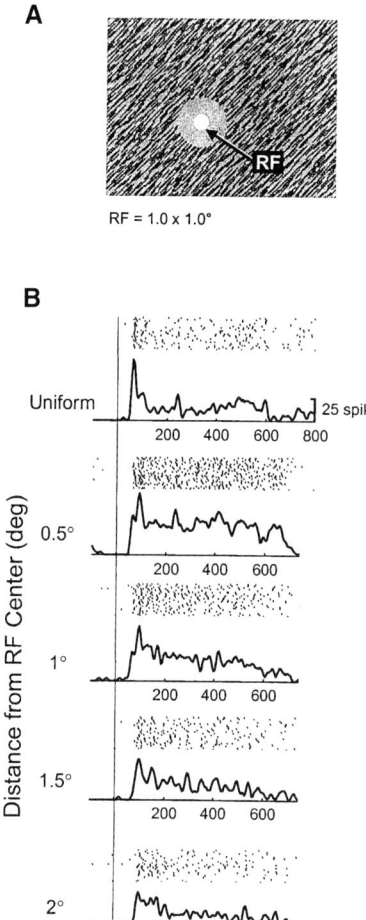
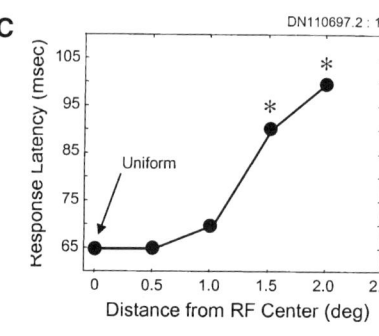
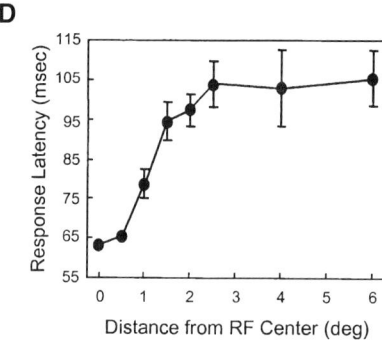

**Figure 4-6.** Spreading activity in macaque V1. (A) Spatial configuration of the surround texture relative to the receptive field (RF), represented by the white disk. The circular figure defined by the texture was centered on the RF. The luminance of the circular figure formed by the texture was identical to the luminance of the display during the intertrial interval, so that the luminance in the region of the RF remained constant during the presentation of the surround texture and the intertrial interval. The size of the RF, as measured with small bar stimuli, was 1.0 × 1.0 degrees. The luminance contrast of the texture elements was 48%. (B) Response of a single V1 neuron to the uniform texture and to surround textures presented 0.5 to 2.0 degrees from the center of the RF. The response to each stimulus is shown both as rasters (top of each panel), in which each dot is a single action potential and successive lines are different trials, and as average spike density functions (bottom of each panel). The stimulus duration was 500 ms beginning at time zero, indicated by the vertical line extending through each panel. For this neuron, no significant response could be elicited to surround textures presented more than 3 degrees from the center of the RF. (C) The response latency of the same neuron plotted as a function of the distance of the texture from the RF center. An asterisk (*) indicates that the latency of the response to the surround stimulus was significantly greater than the latency of the response to the uniform texture (one-tailed $t$-test, $p < .01$). (D) Average onset latency as a function of figure diameter. Data shown are for single-unit and multiunit V1 sites with RF sizes 1 degree across or smaller that exhibited significant responses to the surround texture when presented alone. Error bars represent standard errors of the mean.

cessing. Converging evidence from both perceptual and physiological studies of brightness indicates that the underlying neural mechanisms serving brightness perception are relatively slow, requiring time to integrate information from large areas of the visual field in order to determine the brightness of a given area. It should be noted that these neurons do not represent a subpopulation of specialized *brightness cells*. The same neurons are also sensitive to other stimulus properties such as spatial frequency and orientation. Rather, our results suggest that the neurons in striate cortex are capable of multiplexing information about contours and stimulus properties that are better correlated with the perceptual attributes of surfaces. One would like to know if the observations of spreading activity in visual cortex are related to perceptual filling-in of surface properties. Unfortunately, at present, there is no direct physiological evidence that links perceptual filling-in to the propagation of signals in visual cortex.

*Acknowledgments*

The authors wish to thank their collaborators in the research discussed: Robert Desimone, Sigrid Hahn, WooJin Kim, Sean MacEvoy, Cynthia Rittenhouse, and Leslie Ungerleider.

## References

Arend LE and Spehar B (1993) Lightness, brightness, and brightness contrast. 1. Illuminance variation. *Percept Psychophys* 54:446–456.

Bringuier V, Chavane F, Glaeser L, and Fregnac Y (1999) Horizontal propagation of visual activity in the synaptic integration field of area 17 neurons. *Science* 283:695–699.

Cohen MA and Grossberg S (1985) Neural dynamics of brightness perception: Features, boundaries, diffusion, and resonance. *Percept Psychophys* 36:428–456.

Das A and Gilbert CD (1995) Long-range horizontal connections and their role in cortical reorganization revealed by optical recording of cat primary visual cortex. *Nature* 375:780–784

De Valois RL, Webster MA, De Valois KK, and Lingelbach B (1986) Temporal properties of brightness and color induction. *Vision Res* 26:887–897.

Diamond AL (1955) Foveal simultaneous contrast as a function of inducing area. *J Exp Psych* 50:144–152.

Gerrits HJM, de Haan B, and Vendrik AJH (1966) Simultaneous contrast, filling-in process and information processing in man's visual system. *Exp Brain Res* 11:411–430.

Gerrits HJM and Vendrik AJH (1970) Simultaneous contrast, filling-in process and information processing in man's visual system. *Exp Brain Res* 11:411–430.

Grinvald A, Lieke EE, Frostig RD, and Hildesheim R (1994) Cortical point-spread function and long-range lateral interactions revealed by real-time optical imaging of macaque monkey primary visual cortex. *J Neurosci* 14:2545–2568.

Heinemann E (1955) Simultaneous brightness induction as a function of inducing- and test-field luminances. *J Exp Psych* 50:89–96.

Heinemann E (1972) Simultaneous brightness induction. In: Jameson D and Hurvich LM (eds), *Handbook of Sensory Physiology VII: Visual Psychophysics*. New York: Springer Verlag, pp. 146–169.

Hess C and Pretori H (1894) Messende Untersuchungen über die Gesetzmässigkeit des simultanen Helligkeitcontrastes. *Albert von Graefe's Archiv Ophthalmol* 40:1–24.

Kinoshita M and Komatsu H (2001) Neural representation of the luminance and brightness of a uniform surface in the macaque primary visual cortex. *J Neurophysiol* 86:2559–2570.

Komatsu H, Murakami I, and Kinoshita M (1996) Surface representation in the visual system. *Cogn Brain Res* 5:97–104.

Krauskopf J (1963) Effect of retinal image stabilization on the appearance of heterochromatic targets. *J Opt Soc Am* 53:741–744.

Larimer KS and Piantanida T (1988) The impact of boundaries on color: Stabilized image studies. *Soc Photo-Opt Instrument Eng* 901:241–247.

MacEvoy SP, Kim W, and Paradiso MA (1998) Integration of surface information in primary visual cortex. *Nat Neurosci* 1:616–620.

MacEvoy SP and Paradiso MA (2001) Lightness constancy in primary visual cortex. *Proc Natl Acad Sci USA* 98:8827–8831.

Paradiso MA and Hahn S (1996) Filling-in percepts produced by luminance modulation. *Vision Res* 36:2657–2663.

Paradiso MA and Nakayama K (1991) Brightness perception and filling-in. *Vision Res* 31:1221–1236.

Riggs LA, Ratliff F, Cornsweet JC, and Cornsweet TN (1953) The disappearance of steadily fixated visual test objects. *J Opt Soc Am* 43:495–501.

Rossi AF, Desimone R, and Ungerleider LG. (2001) Contextual modulation in primary visual cortex of macaques. *J Neurosci* 21:1698–1709.

Rossi AF and Paradiso MA (1996) Temporal limits of brightness induction and mechanisms of brightness perception. *Vision Res* 36:1391–1398.

Rossi AF and Paradiso MA (1999) Neural correlates of perceived brightness in the retina, LGN, and striate cortex. *J Neurosci* 19:6145–6156.

Rossi AF, Rittenhouse CD, and Paradiso MA (1996) The representation of brightness in primary visual cortex. *Science* 273:1104–1107.

Wallach H (1948) Brightness constancy and the nature of achromatic colors. *J Exp Psych* 38:310–324.

Walls GL (1954) The filling-in process. *Am J Optom Arch Am Acad Optom* 31:329–341.

Yarbus AL (1967) *Eye Movements and Vision.* New York: Plenum.

# 5

# Mechanisms of Surface Completion:
## Perceptual Filling-In of Texture

### LOTHAR SPILLMANN AND PETER DE WEERD

*Perceptual filling-in* refers to the interpolation of information across regions of visual space where that information is physically absent. Is there evidence in favor of active spreading of surface features during perceptual filling-in? Psychophysical studies of texture filling-in suggest that there is. The data indicate that a fast and active interpolation process contributes not only to the perceptual filling-in of figures by their backgrounds during fixation, but also to filling-in across scotomas and to filling-in during normal surface perception. During perceptual filling-in, these interpolation mechanisms appear to interact with various mechanisms of figure–ground segregation. These mechanisms include low-level representations of boundaries, as well as higher-level factors such as perceptual salience of the figure and directed attention. Neurophysiological and anatomical findings will be presented that show strong support for active interpolation of neuronal activity during filling-in, as well as for the interaction between interpolation and segregation mechanisms. When retinal or subcortical injury causes deafferentation of visual cortical neurons, interpolation mechanisms in retinotopic areas that contribute to the completion of surfaces during normal perception, may induce a remapping of visual space onto cortex. Taken together, the data refute recent proposals that question the existence of isomorphic neural correlates of perceptual filling-in.

## Mechanisms of Texture Filling-In

### *Phenomena of Texture Filling-In: Interactions Between Boundary Representations and Interpolation Processes*

Texture fading is one of the more recent and more complex examples of a series of fading phenomena whose scientific study dates back to Troxler (1804). Troxler showed that with strict fixation, a small perimetric stimulus presented in the periphery of the visual field rapidly faded into the background and vanished from view. This phenomenon, known as *Troxler's effect* (Pirenne, 1962), was attributed to local adaptation (Adrian, 1928; Clarke, 1961; Aulhorn and Harms, 1972) and filling-in (Walls, 1954). More recently, figures shown on a textured background, away from a fixation spot (Fig. 5-1), have been demonstrated to become filled-in with the texture during prolonged fixation (e.g., Ramachandran and Gregory, 1991; Spillmann and Kurtenbach, 1992; De Weerd et al., 1995, 1998). Strict fixation is required for the target to disappear from view, and any eye movements make it reappear (see Gerrits et al., 1984).

Whereas in Troxler's (1804) original study a single stationary target appeared to fade into a uniform background, later investigators showed that moving and flickering stimuli were also prone to Troxler's effect (Spillmann et al., 1984). For example, a slowly rotating disk sector will first appear to come to a standstill before fading into the background (Hunzelmann and Spillmann, 1984; Harris et al., 1990). Likewise, a flickering light source will appear to stop flickering and then disappear (Schieting and Spillmann, 1987; Anstis, 1996). Similarly, Anstis (1989) showed that a figure filled with coherently drifting dots (first-order motion) on a dynamic visual noise background faded from view within seconds of fixation.

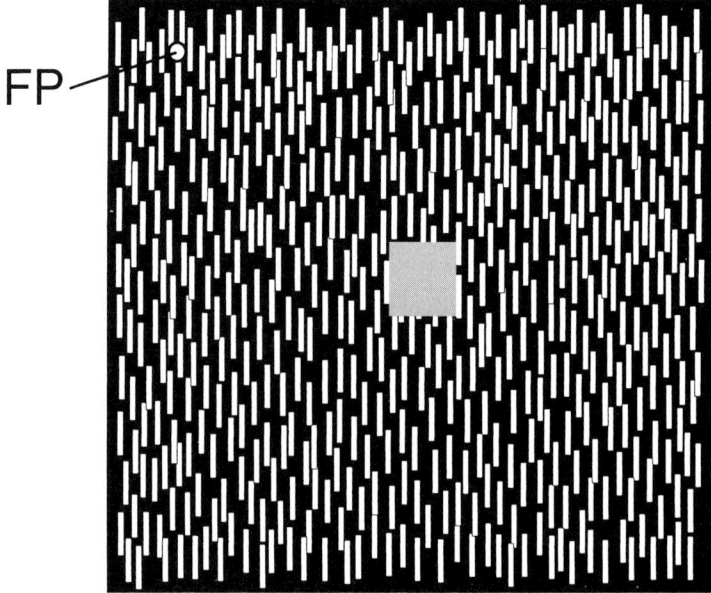

**Figure 5-1.** Neural mechanism for filling-in of an artificial scotoma. Stimulus pattern used in psychophysical experiments with humans and neurophysiological experiments with monkeys. During continued fixation at a fixation point (FP), humans report that the gray square perceptually fills in with the surrounding texture. (*Source:* Adapted from De Weerd et al., 1995)

A common factor in all these examples is that veridical information about the stimulus is lost in favor of surface uniformity. Typically, what appears as a figure merges into the background under conditions of prolonged fixation.

The filling-in of a peripherally presented figure by its background during prolonged fixation is similar in some respects to the perceptual completion of simple line figures or patterns across the blind spot, or across scotomas caused by retinal, subcortical, or cortical lesions (for a review see Durgin et al., 1995; Ramachandran, 1995). The filling-in of texture across a (migraine) scotoma was reported as early as 60 years ago, when Lashley (1941, pp. 338–339) wrote: "Talking with a friend, I glanced just to the right of his face, whereon his head disappeared. His shoulders and necktie were still visible, but the vertical stripes in the wallpaper behind him seemed to extend right down to the necktie. Quick mapping revealed an area of total blindness covering about 30 degrees, just off the macula."

The above examples illustrate that two types of texture filling-in should be distinguished: texture filling-in across a scotoma and filling-in of a figure by the surrounding texture induced by prolonged fixation. The question to be asked then is: Are the two phenomena subserved by the same or similar mechanisms, and could such mechanisms also be relevant for normal perception? In both filling-in across scotomas and filling-in of figures during fixation, information is interpolated across a region in the visual field where that information is physically absent. An obvious difference between the two phenomena is their time course. Filling-in across scotomas is instantaneous, but filling-in of a figure by its ground during prolonged fixation takes time. This suggests that in the latter type of filling-in, there is a factor that delays the filling-in process, which may play no role during filling-in of scotomas.

A common factor invoked in explanations of phenomena exhibiting delayed filling-in is adaptation. Specifically, for delayed filling-in of figures by their backgrounds during fixation, Gerrits et al. (1966) proposed that filling-in occurs because of the adaptation of inhibitory neural effects generated by border representations, which during normal perception prevent surface features from spreading beyond surface boundaries (Neumann and Mingolla, 2001; see also Chapters 2 and 8). The better the fixation, the faster adaptation will take place and the earlier the onset of filling-in is expected. The finding that artificial retinal stabilization of a stimulus dramatically reduces the time for filling-in by the background (Ditchburn and Ginsborg, 1952; Riggs et al., 1953; Yarbus, 1967) fits with the idea that the adaptation of mechanisms representing boundaries adds significantly to the time required for the filling-in of a figure by its background (Gerrits et al., 1984) during prolonged fixation.

In this chapter, we propose that delayed filling-in of a figure by its ground during fixation and quasi-instantaneous filling-in across a scotoma both represent interactions between interpolation processes and boundary representations. In the former case, perceptual filling-in occurs following slow adaptation of boundary representation mechanisms, after which fast interpolation of background information across the region previously occupied by the figure takes place. In the latter case, since a real scotoma contained within a large surface does not correspond to any boundaries in the image, the spread of surface information across the scotoma is quasi-instantaneous and is contained by surface boundaries present outside the scotoma. The fast spread of surface information across a scotoma, or between existing surface boundaries, may be an important factor in normal surface perception. The following section focuses on the role of boundary representations in filling-in.

## *The Role of Boundary Representations*

Texture spreading in the Ehrenstein figure provides an excellent example of interactions between boundary representations and surface interpolation. This figure, in its simplest version, consists of four black radial lines arranged at right angles, and in collinear opposition, around a central gap. In the resulting illusion, a bright illusory disk delineated by a sharp illusory contour is perceived to be superimposed on the gap. When a colored cross is used to bridge the gap (van Tuijl, 1975; for a review see Bressan et al., 1997), a disk-shaped veil of neon color spreading is produced in the Ehrenstein figure. This veil has recently been shown to elicit a cortical afterimage, presumably from adaptation of the neural circuits representing the perceptually filled-in surface (Shimojo et al., 2001). Similarly, when a cross consisting of two hatched or stippled lines is inserted into the gap, texture spreading is perceived within the bounds of the illusory circle (Watanabe and Cavanagh, 1991).

These illusions illustrate that interpolation processes are contained within boundary representations. Hence, the delayed filling-in of a gray patch by its textured background during prolonged fixation suggests a slow adaptation of the figure's boundary representations, after which fast filling-in can take place (Ramachandran, 1992). Several authors (e.g., Ramachandran and Gregory, 1991; De Weerd et al., 1995) have referred to the gray patch in the texture as an *artificial scotoma*[7] (a term coined by Gerrits and Timmerman, 1969). The quasi-instantaneous nature of filling-in within the illusory boundaries in the Ehrenstein figure fits with the idea that filling-in plays a role in the perception of surfaces during normal perception.

The idea that adaptation of boundary representations is an important predictor of the time required for filling-in was tested by De Weerd et al. (1998). They measured the time to filling-in of a gray square on a black background filled with small white vertical bars that moved dynamically, as in visual noise on a detuned television set (Fig. 5-1). Various square sizes and eccentricities were used. Based on estimates of cortical magnification in lower-order human visual cortex (Sereno et al., 1995), they found that the time to filling-in of a square was linearly related to the total contour length of the square's projection onto the visual cortex, rather than to its retinal image size. Computational studies suggest that longer boundary representations require more time to adapt (Grossberg, 1987a, 1987b; Francis et al., 1994; Grossberg, 1994), supporting the idea that adaptation of boundary representations determines fading time. Because the length of the cortical boundary representation of the figure was correlated with its cortical projection area, the cortical projection area itself could have been important as well, and further experiments are required to determine the effects of each factor alone. However, the time required for filling-in of stimuli corresponding to rectangular cortical projections did not correlate with the shortest distance across the cortical projection, which is what would be expected if the time required for filling-in corresponded to a slow, seconds-long interpolation process rather than to the adaptation of boundary representations.

Because cortical magnification curves are similar in the different retinotopic areas, except for a scaling factor to account for differences in size among those areas (Sereno et al., 1995), it was impossible to determine which of the retinotopic areas would be critically involved in texture fading and filling-in. However, the data did suggest that filling-in of dynamic texture is not carried out by higher-order regions in the temporal cortex where the magnification factor is independent of eccentricity (Sereno et al., 1995).

The data taken together support the idea that perceptual filling-in of a figure by its background during fixation results from a *two-stage process*. First, there is a slow adaptation of mechanisms that normally keep the figure segregated from its background (cancellation). Both the adaptation of more localized boundary representations and the adaptation of more global, high-level figure–ground segregation processes may contribute to a failure of segregation. Second, following breakdown of segregation, there is a fast interpolation process by which the region previously occupied by the figure becomes invaded by the background (substitution).

In the following sections, we will highlight several aspects of the filling-in phenomenon that have been at the center of recent debate. To begin, psychophysical experiments will be described that investigate the hypothesis that there exist fast interpolation processes that *actively* spread surface features within bounded surfaces. Thereafter, psychophysical experiments will be discussed that indicate that interactions between these interpolation processes and boundary representations are modulated by effects of salience and directed attention.

## *Evidence for the Existence of Fast Interpolation Processes*

The idea that fast interpolation processes could form the basis of filling-in across both artificial and real scotomas, such as the blind spot, has generated passionate debate. There have been two principal competing hypotheses in the literature (Pessoa et al., 1998). The first hypothesis suggests that filling-in results from *tagging* an entire region using information from its surround. This hypothesis is related to Dennett's (1991) proposal that active filling-in does not exist: The brain would not fill-in information across scotomas, but would simply ignore the absence of information by symbolically labeling the region devoid of information with the information label present in the surround (*more of the same*). Following this logic, neural activity related to filling-in might be found in high-level areas representing surfaces, object parts, or objects, where such symbolic operations might take place, but there should be no isomorphic representation of filling-in in lower-order retinotopic areas. In other words, filling-in of a region in the visual field would not be mimicked by the spread of neural activity into the representation of that region in retinotopically organized cortex (for a discussion see Churchland and Ramachandran, 1996).

A second proposal is the active spreading hypothesis. According to this hypothesis, information from the edge of a figure propagates into the enclosed region to fill-in the void (Gerrits et al., 1966; Gerrits and Vendrik, 1970; De Weerd et al., 1995). Pessoa and Neumann (1998) recently discussed filling-in in terms of regularization theory (i.e., a tendency of the visual system to produce a uniform distribution even in the face of sparse input). According to this theory, active lateral spreading occurs not only during filling-in of scotomas and filling-in of a figure during prolonged fixation, but also during normal surface perception.

Paradiso and Nakayama (1991) obtained psychophysical evidence for active, fast spreading of brightness. The authors examined the time course of filling-in for a white disk briefly presented on a black background to one eye, followed by various kinds of smaller masks (a horseshoe, a ring) presented to the contralateral eye. They found that the masks interfered with the perception of brightness in the central disk. The authors concluded that the lines acted as a barrier to the spread of brightness from the edge toward the center, thereby preventing the disk from becoming uniformly filled-in (see Chapter 4). Through systematic manipulation of the time difference between disk and mask (stimulus onset asynchrony), they computed a speed of 110 to 150 deg/sec for brightness propagation (see also Paradiso and Hahn, 1996; Rossi and Paradiso, 1996). Importantly, the longest time difference at which masking was effective increased with surface size, suggesting that progressive lateral interactions are involved in mediating brightness. Motoyoshi (1999) performed an experiment similar to that of Paradiso and Nakayama (1991) with texture. He found that a small annular mask flashed to one eye, after the presentation of a large oriented line texture to the other eye, strongly suppressed the perception of texture within the annular mask (Fig. 5-2). By analogy with brightness filling-in, he attributed this suppression to the interruption of texture spreading from the edge to the center of the stimulus pattern. Motoyoshi arrived at a speed of propagation comparable to that for brightness.

Interestingly, the detection of a pop-out stimulus, such as a single line oriented orthogonally to the surrounding lines, was not affected by the mask, even though it was embedded in the texture surrounded by the mask (see also Caputo, 1996, 1998). This finding suggests that pop-out operations take place before filling-in. It is known that pop-out occurs preattentively (Bergen and Julesz, 1983; Nothdurft, 1991, 1993) or requires little attention (Joseph et al., 1997). These preattentive processes may play a role in the detection and representation of boundaries in the image. The idea that boundary segmentation precedes interpolation is consistent with the proposal that spreading activation is contained within existing boundary representations.

These psychophysical studies argue against the idea that active spreading does not exist. Specifically, the fact that active spreading of a feature across a surface

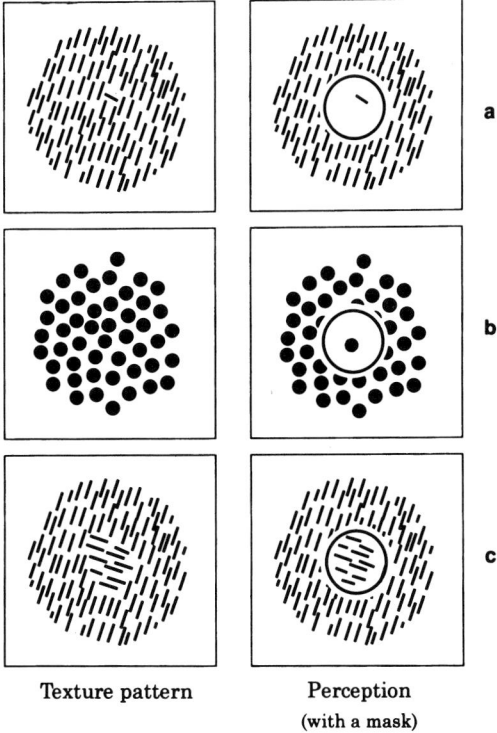

**Figure 5-2.** Suppression of texture filling-in. A thin ring mask briefly presented to one eye will suppress the perception of texture presented to the other eye (a, b). Whereas lines of identical orientation will be masked, a single pop-out line or orthogonal texture within the enclosed area will resist suppression and remain visible (a, c) (*Source:* Motoyoshi, 1999, with permission)

or scotoma, though fast, requires time, in a way that is correlated with the distance over which spreading must take place, argues against the idea that filling-in is a *symbolic* operation. The need for an active filling-in process can also be understood in terms of a basic property of visual neurons. Visual neurons are specialized in the detection of contrast and respond poorly when homogeneous stimuli cover their receptive field (RF). For example, cells in early visual areas respond vigorously to changes in luminance contrast (bars, edges), but respond weakly to homogeneous levels of luminance (surfaces). If there were no active filling-in processes to spread different brightness levels at either side of edges over the surface areas bounded by these edges, then the world might look like a skeleton of boundaries delineating hollow surfaces rather than a world of solid surfaces and objects. The same reasoning holds for surface features other than luminance, such as texture. A neuron's response to a given local element in its RF is inhibited by similar elements surrounding it outside the RF (e.g., Van

Essen et al., 1991). As a consequence, the response of striate and extrastriate neurons to large-scale texture is relatively weak, as is the case for large-scale luminance stimuli. The existence of texture filling-in is compatible with the idea that the coding of individual texture elements by neurons with small RFs is insufficient to generate a large, uniform surface representation. Hence, spreading activity emanating from the boundaries of a surface defined by texture contrast (Lamme, 1995; Sillito et al., 1995) is critical for the perception of extended textured surfaces.

Would a spread of activation in a retinotopic map preserve higher-order statistics of the texture, something that is not an issue in cases of simple brightness or color filling-in? The psychophysical evidence suggests that texture filling-in does not preserve all of the texture's statistics. When observers report filling-in of a gray region by a texture of surrounding alphanumeric characters (Ramachandran and Gregory, 1991), they perceive the texture but cannot read the filled-in characters. Similarly, fading of a region of jumbled L's surrounded by regularly arranged crosses (Bergen, 1991) leads to perceived regularization of the figure area (in rows and columns), but without a clear perception of whether the L's change to crosses (Fig. 5–3). Thus, only the more elementary aspects of the texture are preserved during filling-in (see also Gyoba, 1997).

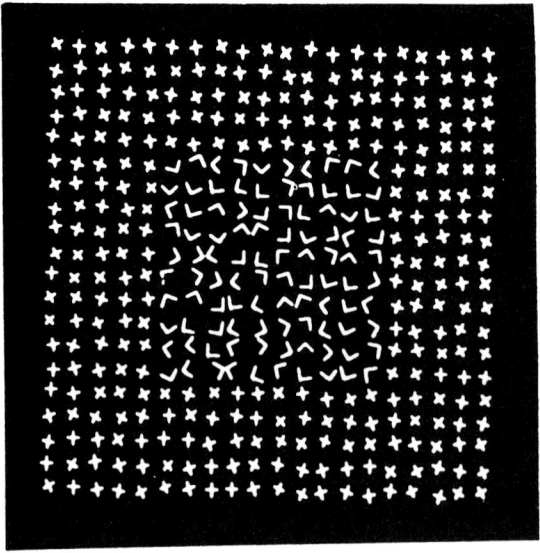

**Figure 5-3.** Fading of perceived texture segmentation. Crosses in various orientations surround a pop-out square of randomly oriented L's whose positions are shuffled relative to one another. If one fixates at a corner, the conspicuous disorder of the L-shaped elements will rapidly give way to greater regularity, and after a few seconds the target square will appear to become embedded in the background (*Source:* Bergen and Julesz, 1983. Reprinted with permission from *Nature*, Macmillan Magazines Limited)

This section provides psychophysical evidence in favor of an active interpolation mechanism during (texture) filling-in across scotomas, during filling-in of figures by their background, and during normal surface perception. In the previous section, we presented evidence suggesting that the time required for filling-in of a figure by its background depends on the adaptation of a signal generated by boundary representations, which normally prevents surface features from spreading beyond surface boundaries. We indicated in that section that the time required for filling-in may also depend on factors other than mechanisms of boundary representation. These factors include perceptual salience and attention.

## The Role of Perceptual Salience for Figure–Ground Segregation and Perceptual Filling-In

An experiment by De Weerd et al. (1998) indicated an influence upon filling-in of the perceptual salience of the figure as a whole relative to the background. They found that for a given square size, filling-in by the texture background (Fig. 5-1) took more time when an equiluminant square was red than when it was gray. The authors suggested that the stronger perceptual salience of the red square delayed the failure of figure–ground segregation and perceptual filling-in by the background texture.

To elucidate the relationship between filling-in and salience, Stürzel and Spillmann (2001) conducted a psychophysical study using figures defined by three different types of texture contrast, with their border lengths (circumferences) held constant (Fig. 5-4, top). In the first stimulus, the figure was composed of an array of short, vertically oriented bars surrounded by a background of similar bars with a different orientation (orientation contrast). Abutting edges between figure and ground were avoided because preliminary data showed that this was an extra factor influencing salience. In the second stimulus, the figure was a single polygon with the number of corners ranging from 3 to 10 surrounded by equally large circles (shape contrast). In the third stimulus, the figure consisted of a cluster of dots arranged in a disorderly manner and surrounded by dots forming a regular lattice (order or regularity contrast).

For each of these three classes of stimuli, the salience of the figure was changed by varying the strength of the (physical) texture contrast between figure and ground. As a measure of perceptual salience, magnitude estimates and reaction times were obtained, in addition to the time required to perceive filling-in (time to first disappearance). For each stimulus, increasing the strength of the (physical) texture contrast increased the perceptual salience of the stimulus; in accordance, it also increased the time required for fading. Results for the three kinds of stimuli agreed reasonably well. This is shown in Figure 5–4 (bottom), which plots fading time for all three types of texture contrast as a function of perceptual salience (magnitude estimation). A near-linear relationship was found between salience and textural contrast. It thus appears that it is the perceptual salience of the figure, rather than a particular physical texture contrast, that pre-

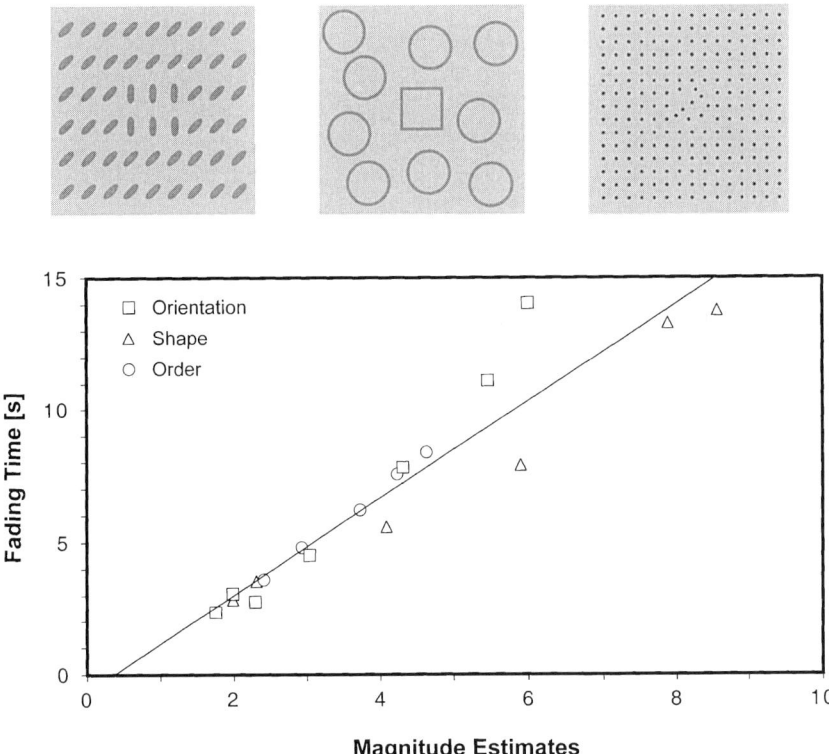

**Figure 5-4.** Fading and filling-in of texture contrast patterns. Top: Schematic representation of texture stimuli chosen to study time to disappearance in relation to textural salience. Target size 2 × 2 degrees, fixation 10 degrees lateral. Bottom: Fading time for orientation contrast, shape contrast, and order contrast are plotted as a function of rated strength by magnitude estimation (*Source:* Adapted from Stürzel and Spillmann, 2001).

dicts the time required for filling-in (see also Welchman and Harris, 2001). The data support the idea that the time before filling-in of a figure by its ground is, at least in part, determined by the adaptation of processes representing global factors, such as salience, that contribute to the segregation of figure and ground.

## *The Role of Directed Attention for Figure–Ground Segregation and Perceptual Filling-In*

Lou (1999) reported that one or more of a set of three colored disks (e.g., green) to which attention was directed faded more rapidly than three simultaneously presented disks of a different color (e.g., red) that were not attended to. The shapes were presented equidistantly from a central fixation spot on a gray background. Smith and De Weerd (2001) replicated this somewhat paradoxical result using figures presented on a large, dynamic texture background. They obtained the same result when the two sets of figures differed in shape rather than color. In addition, the same effects were obtained by using just two figures, one of which was attended and the other unattended. Thus, it appears that the facilitatory effect of attention on fading and filling-in can be generalized to a variety of stimuli. Why would a figure to which attention is directed (in a top-down manner) fill in sooner with the surrounding background than an identical figure at a matched eccentricity to which attention is not directed?

Many physiological studies in monkey extrastriate cortex show that when a target and distracters are presented inside a neuron's RF, attention to the target strongly diminishes the influence of the distracters on the activity of that neuron (Moran and Desimone, 1985; Chelazzi et al., 1993; Treue and Maunsell, 1996; for a review see Desimone and Duncan, 1995). If attention is focused on a target (the figure) and the background is considered a distracter, then the influence of the background on the response of a neuron whose RF encompasses parts of the figure and its background should diminish. This diminution might be considered equivalent to a reduction in the size of the textured surround of a gray square. It has been shown that the addition of texture around a figure more than a few degrees away from the figure *delays* the onset of filling-in (Welchman and Harris, 1999). Directing attention to the region of the figure thus may eliminate the influences from parts of the background far removed from the figure, thereby reducing the time required for filling-in.

It should be pointed out that De Weerd et al. (1998) found that the addition of texture far away from the figure did not influence the time required for filling-in. In contrast to Welchman and Harris (1999), De Weerd et al. (1998) randomized the eccentricity and size of the figure in their experiment, on a trial-by-trials basis, whereas Welchman and Harris (1999) presented identical stimuli for a number of consecutive trials before moving to the next experimental condition, which likely was more effective in picking up effects of remote background. Since Lou's (1999) and Smith and De Weerd's (2001) studies were carried out in a non-randomized fashion as well, Welchman and Harris's (1999) study is directly relevant for the interpretation of the attention effects in these two studies.

It is possible that attention directed to the region of the figure includes background elements in the immediate vicinity of the figure's boundaries. This attentional enhancement of background elements just outside the boundaries may increase the background's effectiveness in *penetrating* failing boundary representations. This idea is supported by Ramachandran (1992), who found that when a black line and a white line intersecting each other are presented across the blind spot, only the attended line is filled-in. Grouping of similar elements or features around the figure by attention may rely on mechanisms such as synchronization (Engel et al., 1991) or selective enhancement of neural activity (Roelfsema and Singer, 1998). Thus, the tendency to bind similar attended elements in the immediate surroundings of the figure together may tip the balance between the drive to interpolate and the drive to segregate in favor of interpolation, thereby reducing the time required for perceptual filling-in.

The data suggest that, at least during prolonged fixation, sustained top-down attention to a peripherally presented stimulus does not enhance its segregation from the background. In contrast, the facilitation of filling-in by attention indicates a more speedy failure of figure–ground segregation. Furthermore, when attention is captured (bottom-up attention) by a figure that is made more salient than others (see previous section), the data suggest that the increase in the time required for filling-in caused by the enhanced segregation of the figure from its ground is much larger than any decrease that might be induced by top-down attention. Thus, secondary top-down attention effects on figure–ground segregation resulting from attention capture are not an explanation for the delay of filling-in when a figure's salience is high.

## An Anatomical and Physiological Basis for Texture Filling-In

### Physiological Evidence for Delayed Filling-In Across an Artificial Scotoma

Psychophysical studies have provided evidence for an active interpolation process, and they suggest that this active interpolation takes place in retinotopically organized areas. While these data are suggestive, direct demonstrations of interpolation processes would require the measurement of neural activity in the cortical representation of the figure while it is filled-in perceptually by the background. Such a demonstration would directly challenge the objections that have been formulated against an isomorphic neural correlate of perceptual filling-in in retinotopically organized areas (Dennett, 1991).

De Weerd et al. (1995) recorded from single V2 and V3 neurons in the macaque, whose RFs were centered on a gray figure (a square) presented on a dynamic texture background (see Fig. 5-1). The dynamic texture was made up of short white line elements randomly moving on a black ground. The monkey was trained to maintain fixation while activity was recorded from neurons whose RFs were contained within the square, which was presented away from fixation. For the larger squares used the RFs were contained entirely within the gray square, but for the smaller squares the dynamic texture impinged upon the RF of the neuron from which recordings were made. The neurons responded with a brief transient response at stimulus onset, followed by a steep fall-off of activity and a subsequent slow increase in the discharge rate. This *climbing activity* reached the level of *control activity* measured with the same dynamic texture, but with the square (and thus the RF) physically filled with texture (Fig. 5-5). The time required for the climbing activity to converge with the control activity corresponded to the time required for human observers to perceive filling-in of the square by its background. Thus, around the time that the cells in V2 and V3 of the monkey could not distinguish between a texture with a square and the same texture without a square, human subjects reported perceptual filling-in. The authors therefore suggested that the climbing activity was a correlate of perceptual filling-in.

De Weerd et al. (1995) further suggested that the initial onset transient was driven by an excitatory input from regions close to the edge of the classical RF and that the subsequent fall-off of the signal was due to inhibition from the sur-

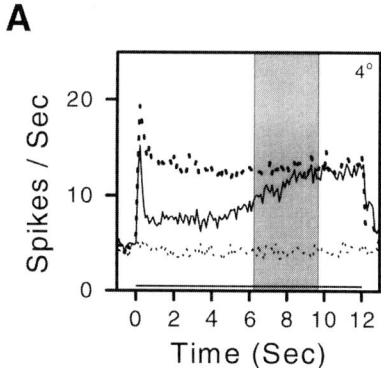

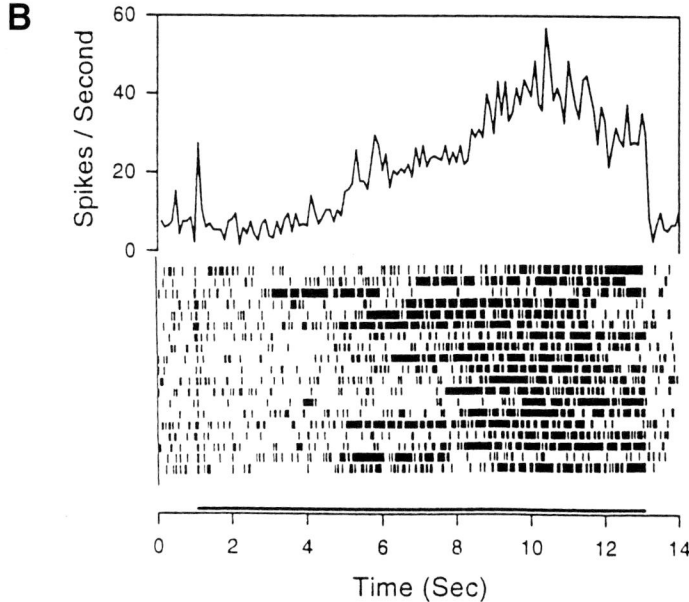

**Figure 5-5.** Neuronal response to a gray square on a dynamic texture (see Fig. 5-1). (A) Average histogram from 78 V2 and V3 cells recorded in two monkeys when a gray square (4 degrees) covered the receptive field (RF) (solid line), when the square was absent and replaced with texture in the RF (thick dotted line), and when no stimulus was present at all (baseline). The horizontal line at the bottom indicates the duration of stimulus presentation. The shaded region illustrates the range of times at which human subjects started to experience filling-in. (*Source:* De Weerd et al., 1995, with permission) (B) Individual neuron's response. The RF of the cell was centered over the square and straddled its edges. The cumulative histogram (top panel) shows a brief response at stimulus onset followed by gradual climbing activity. Individual response traces (bottom), with tick marks indicating spikes, show sharp transitions between periods of low activity and periods of high activity (which may correspond to periods of filling-in). Tick marks in response traces blend together during periods of high activity.

round. As the inhibition adapted over time, excitatory inputs from the surround started to drive the cell, producing climbing activity and its perceptual correlate, fading and filling-in. The decrease of the inhibitory signal may reflect the degradation of figure–ground segregation. De Weerd et al. (1995) provided direct evidence for this inhibitory signal: For the largest squares, activity decreased below spontaneous firing rates during initial presentation of the square over the RF. The strength of that inhibition was a good predictor of the strength of climbing activity measured with smaller squares in the same neuron (see Chapter 15, Fig. 15-1).

The slow time course of climbing activity that develops over several seconds does not correspond to the much faster sudden disappearance of the figure. To understand the relationship between climbing activity in average histograms and filling-in, it is useful to inspect single-trial activity traces. Particularly informative in this respect are cells that showed strong activity when the square (and thus the RF) was filled-in physically with texture. The large difference in activity between conditions with and without texture inside the RF presumably made those neurons more likely to also display strong activity during perceived filling-in of texture into their RFs. In these cells, a gray square presented in their RFs led to low baseline activity for several seconds, followed by a discrete period of activity marked by sudden onset and offset. In some trials, several discrete periods of activity could be discerned, each lasting for several seconds. The sudden onset and offset of activity in individual trials is in agreement with the fact that perceptual filling-in (in human observers) occurred rapidly, was not permanent, and could occur repeatedly within the same trial. These finds might result from imperfect fixation. Thus, the slow increase of climbing activity in average histograms likely mirrors the variability in the onset of climbing activity and filling-in among individual trials. After normalization of activity, the average histograms could be interpreted as a representation of the probability that a given neuron would signal filling-in at a given time after stimulus onset. Hence, the data are in agreement with the idea that perceptual filling-in occurs in two steps: a slow one (measured in seconds), during which figure–ground segregation deteriorates and ultimately fails (cancellation), and a fast one (measured in milliseconds), during which background information spreads from the edge onto the target area (substitution).

The study by De Weerd et al. (1995) relied on a careful comparison of neuronal activity in V2 and V3 cells with human reports of perceptual filling-in obtained under identical stimulus conditions. However, comparing perceptual filling-in and its presumed neural correlate within an individual observer would greatly enhance the claim that both are related. Recently, a component of visually evoked cortical potentials has been reported that correlates with the perception of texture filling-in (Romani et al., 1999).

*Physiological Evidence for Fast Filling-In Across a Real Scotoma*
Interpolation across real scotomas is quasi-instantaneous, because there are no neural mechanisms that segregate such scotomas from the rest of the visual field, and thus no adaptation of segregation mechanisms is necessary prior to interpo-

lation. In a particularly compelling example of fast interpolation, Fiorani et al. (1992) obtained responses from the blind spot region of area V1 of the monkey when stimulating two regions on either side of the optic disk 15 degrees apart (see Chapter 9). These distances are several times the length of conventional RFs, implying a functional (and structural) convergence much larger than is commonly expected. Although the blind spot is present from birth and thus represents a special case of a scotoma, these physiological findings suggest that our unawareness of it may be based on a filling-in process (interpolation) that uses mechanisms similar to the intracortical connections underlying filling-in across other kinds of scotomas and across normally perceived surfaces. In monkeys, filling-in has been demonstrated behaviorally for the blind spot (Komatsu and Murakami, 1994) and a retinal scotoma (Murakami et al., 1997), as well as an artificial scotoma (see Chapters 10 and 15).

Based on the above evidence, one might conclude that filling-in across the blind spot takes place in V1, and that filling-in across artificial scotomas takes place in V2 and V3. Alternatively, it is possible that filling-in of elementary features such as luminance can be observed at various cortical stages including V1, while filling-in of more complex surface features such as texture may depend upon extrastriate cortex.

*Horizontal Connections, Lateral Spread of Neural Activity, and Figure–Ground Segregation*
Although it cannot be excluded that reciprocal connections between cortical areas (e.g., Van Essen, 1985; Distler et al., 1993) play a role in perceptual filling-in, especially given the effects of cognitive factors such as attention, the lateral spreading of activity during filling-in suggests strong contributions of horizontal connections between pyramidal cells in visual cortex. The evidence for horizontal connections within the cortex is abundant. There is evidence in the monkey (McGuire et al., 1991; Gilbert and Wiesel, 1992) and cat (Lund et al., 1993) that pyramidal axons extend up to about 7 mm, capable of transmitting information from the edge of a figure to the enclosed inner section. There is anatomical and physiological evidence for both excitatory and inhibitory influences (Maffei and Fiorentini, 1976; Nelson and Frost, 1978, 1985; Lamme, 1995; Sillito et al., 1995; Sillito and Jones, 1996; Levitt and Lund, 1997). Lateral spread of activation has also been demonstrated using optical recording techniques (Grinvald et al., 1994; Das and Gilbert, 1995b). These studies show signal propagation on a time scale of milliseconds compatible with the speed of fast perceptual filling-in.

Horizontal long-range interactions of this kind may form the basis for perceptual filling-in during normal surface perception and for filling-in across retinal and central scotomas (Eysel, 1997; Eysel and Schweigart, 1999). They may also lead to a better understanding of the large-scale spreading of graininess and twinkle after adaptation to a gray target on a dynamic visual noise background (Spillmann and Kurtenbach, 1992; Ramachandran et al., 1993; Hardage and Tyler, 1995; Tyler and Hardage, 1998) and of the cooperative processes involved in the formation of smooth surfaces and sharp edges in random dot stereograms or kinematograms (Frisby, 1979; van de Grind et al., 1983; for a review see Spillmann and Werner, 1996). The involvement of horizontal connections in perceptual filling-in is also supported by the finding that there are limits to the size of a figure that can be filled-in during maintained fixation (e.g., about 6 degrees in De Weerd et al., 1998).

Horizontal connections have also been implied in a variety of physiologically measured contextual effects, which are induced from regions outside the classical RF (for a review see Allman et al., 1985) and which contribute to figure–ground segregation. Knierim and Van Essen (1992) and Kastner et al. (1999) measured responses from V1 neurons to a line element in their RFs when that line was surrounded either by identical elements outside the RF or by differently oriented elements. Response suppression was maximal with identical elements in the surround. These findings indicate that V1 is involved in the detection of pop-out elements, and suggest a role of V1 in figure–ground segregation when the boundaries are defined by a clear difference (texture contrast) in one or more stimulus dimensions. For example, Zipser et al. (1996) found that V1 neurons were able to code texture-defined and other types of figure boundaries several degrees away from their classical RFs. Hence, horizontal connections may be crucially involved both in figure–ground segregation and in the spread of activity from the background that occurs when figure–ground segregation fails. In this sense, it may be said that pop-out (figure–ground segregation) and fading (interpolation) constitute opposite ends of the same perceptual continuum (Derrington, 1996).

*Long-Term Effects of Real Scotomas:*
*Remapping of Visual Space in Cortex*
We have focused so far upon the short-term effects (within seconds) induced by the presentation of artificial scotomas over the RFs of visual neurons. However, what are the long-term effects of the deafferentation of visual cortical neurons that follow permanent damage at the receptor level (real scotomas)? This question has been investigated in the visual system by inducing small retinal lesions using laser burns. The finding that V1 neurons that have been deafferented may begin to fire again has been interpreted in terms of RF reorganization due to long-range interactions (Gilbert and Wiesel, 1992). In anesthetized cats, Pettet and Gilbert (1992) found that within minutes of focal lesioning in corresponding parts of both retinas, silenced neurons whose RFs were just inside the lesion boundary could be reactivated by probe stimuli presented outside the edge of the scotoma. A likely explanation is the recruitment of collaterals mediating (previously ineffective) excitatory inputs from nearby afferents through disinhibition of preexisting synapses. This kind of remapping resulted in the increase of a neuron's RF size associated with a shift in its location toward the edge of the lesion, so that many such neurons collectively covered the area of the scotoma (Gilbert and Wiesel, 1992; Pettet and Gilbert, 1992; Das and Gilbert, 1995a). No remapping was observed after lesioning in one eye only (Kaas et al., 1990; Chino et al., 1992, 1995).

Pettet and Gilbert (1992) and Gilbert (1992) described analogous effects when using an artificial scotoma. The artificial scotoma consisted of a uniform area superimposed on a dynamic textured background and covering the RF of the V1 neuron from which recordings were made. Under these conditions, continued mapping of the RF with small moving bars revealed an expansion by up to a factor of 5 within minutes. This expansion suggests that following the functional deafferentation of part of the retinotopic map, the cortical representation of the scotoma decreased (shrinkage hypothesis), while the representation of the surrounding area expanded.

An alternative view is that the increases in responsivity of V1 neurons with RFs contained within an artificial or real scotoma are caused by changes in contrast gain (Ohzawa et al., 1985; DeAngelis et al., 1995). That idea, however, does not easily account for the psychophysical findings generated under stimulus conditions similar to those that are hypothesized to induce RF expansion of V1 neurons. Indeed, Kapadia et al. (1994) demonstrated that objects lying near the borders of the scotoma appeared to be pulled toward the visual field defect. Similarly, a patient with a homonymous paracentral scotoma was reported to perceive an object (e.g., the shoulder of his doctor) projecting into his scotoma as narrower than the same object on the other side (Safran et al., 1999). Also, of two equally long lines, the one crossing the scotoma looked shorter. In agreement with the idea of shrinkage of the representation of the scotoma, Reich et al. (1997) found evidence for the underestimation of the size of objects presented across artificial scotomas. On the other hand, Tripathy et al. (1995) found no shrinkage across the blind spot. Given that the blind spot is present from birth, a failure to find shrinkage may be related to the development of compensatory mechanisms.

While it is clear that the relatively slow time course of RF expansion in area V1 described by Gilbert and colleagues (Gilbert and Wiesel, 1992; Pettet and Gilbert, 1992) does not easily lend itself to an explanation of perceptual filling-in, the resulting remapping of visual space onto cortical area V1 points to a capability of reorganization that may be important after injury and during particular kinds of skill learning (Chapters 13 and 15). It is possible that the activity in areas V2 and V3 found by De Weerd et al. (1998) facilitates RF expansion and remapping in lower-order cortex. This top-down influence is an idea analogous to some models of skill learning, which propose a *reverse hierarchy* by feedback, in which plasticity in higher-order cortex precedes and modulates plasticity in lower-order cortex (see Chapter 15).

*Clinical Relevance*
Filling-in is regularly observed in, and has consequences for, the clinical assessment of retinal scotomas in eye patients. Safran and Landis (1996) report that visual field defects from retinal pathology or laser treatment tend to fill-in with information from the surround, prompting patients to ignore or underestimate their defects. For example, patients suffering from diabetic retinopathy may have up to 1500 scotomas of 0.5 to 2 degrees in diameter each in their peripheral retinas (summing to a large areal deficit), yet they do not spontaneously report any holes in their visual fields. Similar observations are known from hemianopic patients after damage to the visual pathways (see Chapter 11).

One way of making scotomas visible to the patient is by noise–field campimetry. On a dynamic noise background, scotomas appear to have less flicker and are perceived as brighter or darker than surrounding areas (Aulhorn and Köst, 1989). As a rule, visualization depends on lesion site and age. Whereas optic nerve lesions (e.g., in glaucoma) may be visualized for years, long-standing scotomas due to postgeniculate lesions usually cannot be detected by this method (Kolb et al., 1995). This is particularly true for scotomas due to lesions of the optic radiation (Schiefer et al., 1998). A modified technique (component perimetry) has been developed to overcome this problem (Bachmann and Fahle, 2000).

Another procedure to make patients aware of their field defect is through the use of the Amsler grid, which consists of thin orthogonal lines (Achard et al., 1995). Here again, filling-in of scotomas leads to underestimation of the size of the visual defect so that, for example, patients with age-related macular degeneration report a much smaller scotoma than measured on the tangent screen (Fig. 5-6A). Furthermore, there seems to be competition between the neuronal mechanisms mediating perception of the diagonal line and the grid (Fig. 5-6B). A survey shows that half of the scotomas are not detected at all, presumably as a result of perceptual completion. Even scotomas of up to 6 degrees may go unnoticed.

Fading and filling-in may also obscure the slowly advancing blindness occurring in glaucoma (Cibis, 1964) and the ring scotomas in retinitis pigmentosa, which often remain undetected until late in the disease. This failure to "see" one's

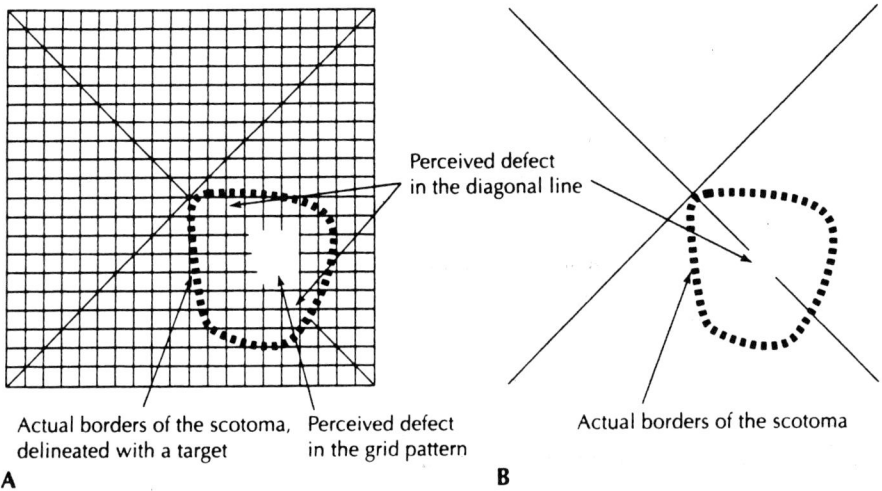

**Figure 5-6.** Difference between perceived and measured size of scotoma. (A) Patient's homonymous paracentral scotoma assessed with the Amsler grid compared to the same scotoma measured with a small perimetric test spot (dotted border). (B) The diagonal line shown in isolation is partially completed within the scotoma, but not when shown in conjunction with the Amsler grid (*Source:* Safran and Landis, 1996, with permission)

own scotoma is likely due to the fact that, because of the permanence of these real scotomas, they may induce significant reorganization in the lateral geniculate nucleus and visual cortex, possibly through sprouting and increased axon arborization (Eysel et al., 1981; Darian-Smith and Gilbert, 1994).

## Conclusion

With prolonged fixation, targets defined by texture contrast rapidly fade and disappear into the background in a way similar to that of targets defined by brightness, color, and motion. Psychophysical and neurophysiological evidence suggests a two-stage mechanism for the filling-in of figures by their background: Gradual breakdown of the segregation of a figure from its ground is followed by fast filling-in of background features through the region formerly occupied by the figure. These segregation processes comprise both lower-level mechanisms of boundary representation and higher-level attentive and cognitive factors. Based on studies discussed in this chapter, we propose that the interpolation processes active during the filling-in of figures by their grounds are similar to the interpolation processes occurring through scotomas and through surface regions in the visual field. Later in this book, a link will be proposed between fast interpolation processes during perceptual filling-in and slower RF expansions observed after deafferentation of visual cortical neurons (Chapter 10), which may lead to a remapping of visual space onto retinotopic cortical areas (Chapter 15).

*Acknowledgments*
This work was supported by DFG Grants LS 67/5–2 and 8–1 (to LS) and in part by NIH Grant 5 R01 MH61972–02 to PDW. The authors are indebted to Drs. J.S. Werner, S.P. Tripathy, U. Schiefer, and S. Kastner for valuable comments and to W. Ehrenstein, G. Grah, L. Maloney, E. Peterhans, and B. Heider for carefully reading a draft of the manuscript.

## Note

1. The term *artificial scotoma* may be misleading and must be interpreted in the proper context. In the context of a theory of filling-in based on interactions between filling-in processes and boundary representations, a uniform area on a differently colored or textured background becomes a real scotoma only after figure–ground segregation fails. Before that, the uniform patch is a figure on a ground.

## References

Achard OA, Safran AB, Duret FC, and Ragama E (1995) Role of the completion phenomenon in the evaluation of Amsler grid results. *Am J Ophthalmol* 120:322–329.
Adrian ED (1928) *The Basis of Sensations. The Action of the Sense Organs.* London: Christophers.

Allman J, Miezin F, and McGuinness, E (1985) Stimulus specific responses from beyond the classical RF: Neurophysiological mechanisms for local–global comparisons in visual neurons. *Annu Rev Neurosci* 8:407–430.

Anstis S (1989) Kinetic edges become displaced, segregated and invisible. In: Lam, DMK and Gilbert CD (eds), *Neural Mechanisms of Visual Perception*. Houston: Gulf Publishing Company, pp 247–260.

Anstis S (1996) Adaptation to peripheral flicker. *Vision Res* 36:3479–3485.

Aulhorn E and Harms H (1972) Local adaptation. In: Jameson D and Hurvich LM (eds), *Visual Psychophysics, Handbook of Sensory Physiology*, Vol. VII/4, Berlin: Springer, pp 128–129.

Aulhorn E and Köst G (1989) Noise–field campimetry: A new perimetric method (snow campimetry). In: Heijl A (ed), *Perimetry Update 1988/1989*. Proceedings of the VIIIth International Perimetry Society Meeting. Amsterdam: Kugler and Ghedini, pp 331–336.

Bachmann G and Fahle M (2000) Component perimetry: A fast method to detect visual field defects caused by brain lesions. *IOVS* 41:2870–2886.

Bergen JR (1991) Theories of visual texture perception. In: Regan DM (ed), *Vision and Visual Dysfunction*, Vol. 10, *Spatial Vision*. New York: Macmillan, pp 114–134.

Bergen JR and Julesz B (1983) Parallel versus serial processing in rapid pattern discrimination. *Nature* 303:696–698.

Bressan P, Mingolla E, Spillmann L, and Watanabe T (1997) Neon color spreading: A review. *Perception* 26:1353–1366.

Caputo G (1996) The role of the background: Texture segregation and figure–ground segmentation. *Vision Res* 36:2815–2826.

Caputo G (1998) Texture brightness filling-in. *Vision Res* 38:841–851.

Chelazzi L, Miller EK, Duncan J, and Desimone R (1993) A neural basis for visual search in the inferior temporal cortex. *Nature* 363:345–347.

Chino YM, Kaas JH, Smith EL III, Langston AL, and Cheng H (1992) Rapid reorganization of cortical maps in adult cats following restricted deafferentation in the retina. *Vision Res* 32:789–796.

Chino YM, Smith EL III, Kaas JH, Langston AL, and Cheng H (1995) Receptive-field properties of deafferented visual cortical neurons after topographic map reorganization in adult cats. *J Neurosci* 15:2417–2433.

Churchland PS and Ramachandran VS (1996) Filling-in: Why Dennett is wrong. In: Akins K (ed), *Perception*. New York: Oxford University Press, pp 132–157.

Cibis PA (1964) Lokaladaptation. *Ber Dtsch Ophthal Ges* 66:193–202.

Clarke FJJ (1961) Visual recovery following local adaptation of the peripheral retina (Troxler's effect). *Opt Acta* 8:121–135.

Darian-Smith C and Gilbert CD (1994) Axonal sprouting accompanies functional reorganization in adult cat striate cortex. *Nature* 368:737–740.

Das A and Gilbert CD (1995a) RF expansion in adult visual cortex is linked to dynamic changes in strength of cortical connections. *J Neurophysiol* 74:779–792.

Das A and Gilbert CD (1995b) Long-range horizontal connections and their role in cortical reorganization revealed by optical recording of cat primary cortex. *Nature* 375:780–784.

DeAngelis GC, Anzai A, Ohzawa I, and Freeman RD (1995) RF structure in the visual cortex: Does selective stimulation induce plasticity? *Proc Natl Acad Sci USA* 92:9682–9686.

Dennett DC (1991) *Consciousness Explained*. Boston: Little, Brown and Company.

Derrington A (1996) Vision: Filling in and pop out. *Curr Biol* 6:141–143.

Desimone R and Duncan J (1995) Neural mechanisms of selective visual attention. *Annu Rev Neurosci* 18:193–222.

De Weerd P, Desimone R, and Ungerleider LG (1998) Perceptual filling-in: A parametric study. *Vision Res* 38:2721–2734.

De Weerd P, Gattass R, Desimone R, and Ungerleider LG (1995) Responses of cells in monkey visual cortex during perceptual filling-in of an artificial scotoma. *Nature* 377:731–734.

Distler C, Boussaoud D, Desimone R, and Ungerleider LG (1993) Cortical connections of inferior temporal area TEO in macaque monkeys. *J Comp Neurol* 334:125–150.

Ditchburn RW and Ginsborg BL (1952) Vision with a stabilized retinal image. *Nature* 170:36–37.

Durgin FH, Tripathy SP, and Levi DM (1995) On the filling-in of the visual blind spot: Some rules of thumb. *Perception* 24:827–840.

Engel AK, König P, and Singer W (1991) Direct physiological evidence for scene segmentation by temporal coding. *Proc Natl Acad Sci USA* 88:9136–9140.

Eysel UT (1997) Perilesional cortical dysfunction and reorganization. In: Freund H-J, Sabel BA, and Witte OW (eds), *Brain Plasticity (Advances in Neurology 73)*. Philadelphia: Lippincott-Raven Publishers, pp 195–206.

Eysel UT, Gonzales-Aguilar F, and Mayer U (1981) Time-dependent decrease in the extent of visual deafferentation in the lateral geniculate nucleus of adult cats with small retinal lesions. *Exp Brain Res* 41:256–263.

Eysel UT and Schweigart G (1999) Increased RF size in the surround of chronic lesions in the adult cat visual cortex. *Cereb Cortex* 9:101–109.

Fiorani M, Rosa MGP, Gattass R, and Rocha-Miranda CE (1992) Dynamic surrounds of RFs in primate striate cortex: A physiological basis for perceptual completion? *Proc Natl Acad Sci USA* 89:8547–8551.

Francis G, Grossberg S, and Mingolla E (1994) Cortical dynamics of feature binding and reset: Control of visual persistence. *Vision Res* 34:1089–1104.

Frisby JP (1979) *Seeing: Illusion, Brain and Mind.* Oxford: Oxford University Press.

Gerrits HJM, deHaan B, and Vendrik AJH (1966) Experiments with retinal stabilized images. Relations between the observations and neural data. *Vision Res* 6:427–440.

Gerrits HJM, Stassen HPW, and van Erning LJThO (1984) The role of drifts and saccades for the preservation of brightness perception. In: Spillmann L and Wooten BR (eds), *Sensory Experience, Adaptation, and Perception.* Hillsdale, NJ: Lawrence Erlbaum Associates, pp 439–459.

Gerrits HJM and Timmerman GJMEN (1969) The filling-in process in patients with retinal scotomas. *Vision Res* 9:439–442.

Gerrits HJM, Stassen HPW, and van Erning LJT (1984) The role of drifts and saccades for the preservation of brightness perception. In: Spillmann L and Wooten BR (eds), *Sensory Experience, Adaptation, and Perception.* Hillsdale, NJ: Lawrence Erlbaum Associates, pp 439–459.

Gerrits HJM, van Erning LJThO, and Eijkman EGJ (1988) Afterimages: A collective term for percepts of different origin. *Exp Brain Res* 72:279–286.

Gerrits HJM and Vendrik, AJH (1970) Simultaneous contrast, filling-in process and information processing in man's visual system. *Exp Brain Res* 11:411–430.

Gilbert CD (1992) Horizontal integration and cortical dynamics. *Neuron* 9:1–13.

Gilbert CD and Wiesel TN (1992) RF dynamics in adult primary visual cortex. *Nature* 356:150–152.

Grinvald A, Lieke EE, Frostig RD, and Hildesheim R (1994) Cortical point-spread function and long-range interactions revealed by real-time optical imaging of macaque monkey primary visual cortex. *J Neurosci* 14:2545–2548.

Grossberg S (1987a) Cortical dynamics of three-dimensional form, color, and brightness perception: I. Monocular theory. *Percept Psychophys* 41:87–116.

Grossberg S (1987b) Cortical dynamics of three-dimensional form, color, and brightness perception: II. Binocular theory. *Percept Psychophys* 41:117–158.

Grossberg S (1994) 3-D vision and figure–ground separation by visual cortex. *Percept Psychophys* 55:48–120.

Gyoba J (1997) Loss of a forest: Perceptual fading and filling-in of static texture patterns. *Perception* 26:1317–1320.

Hardage L and Tyler CW (1995) Induced twinkle aftereffect as a probe of dynamic visual processing mechanisms. *Vision Res* 35:757–766.

Harris JP, Calvert JE, and Snelgar SR (1990) Adaptation to peripheral flicker: Relationship to contrast thresholds. *Vision Res* 30:381–386.

Hunzelmann N and Spillmann L (1984) Movement adaptation in the peripheral retina. *Vision Res* 24:1765–1769.

Joseph JS, Chun MM, and Nakayama K (1997) Attentional requirements in a "preattentive" feature search task. *Nature* 387:805–807.

Kaas JH, Krubitzer LA, Chino YM, Langston AL, Polley EH, and Blair N (1990) Reorganization of retinotopic cortical maps in adult mammals after lesions of the retina. *Science* 248:229–231.

Kapadia MK, Gilbert CD, and Westheimer G (1994) A quantitative measure for quantitative short-term cortical plasticity in human vision. *J Neurosci* 14:451–457.

Kastner S, Nothdurft HC, and Pigarev IN (1999) Neuronal responses to orientation and motion contrast in cat striate cortex. *Vis Neurosci* 16:961–980.

Knierim JJ and van Essen DC (1992) Neuronal responses to static texture patterns in area V1 of the alert macaque monkey. *J Neurophysiol* 67:961–980.

Kolb M, Petersen D, Schiefer U, Kolb R, and Skalej M (1995) Scotoma perception in white-noise–field campimetry and postchiasmal visual pathway lesions. *German J Ophthalmol* 4:228–233.

Komatsu H and Murakami I (1994) Behavioral evidence of filling-in at the blind spot of the monkey. *Vis Neurosci* 11:1103–1113.

Lamme V (1995) The neurophysiology of figure–ground segregation in primary visual cortex. *J Neurosci* 15:1605–1615.

Lashley KS (1941) Patterns of cerebral integration indicated by the scotomas of migraine. *Arch Neurol Psychiatry* 46:331–339.

Levitt JB and Lund JS (1997) Contrast dependence of contextual effects in primate visual cortex. *Nature* 387:73–76.

Lou L (1999) Selective peripheral fading: Evidence for inhibitory sensory effect of attention. *Perception* 28:519–526.

Lund JS, Yoshioka T, and Levitt JB (1993) Comparison of intrinsic connectivity in different areas of macaque monkey cerebral cortex. *Cereb Cortex* 3:148–162.

Maffei L and Fiorentini A (1976) The unresponsive regions of visual cortical RFs. *Vision Res* 16:1131–1139.

McGuire BA, Gilbert CD, Rivlin PK, and Wiesel TN (1991) Targets of horizontal connections in macaque primary visual cortex. *J Comp Neurol* 305:370–392.

Moran J and Desimone R (1985) Selective attention gates visual processing in the extrastriate cortex. *Science* 299:782–784.

Motoyoshi I (1999) Texture filling-in and texture segregation revealed by transient masking. *Vision Res* 39:1285–1291.

Murakami I, Komatsu H, and Kinoshita M (1997) Perceptual filling-in at the scotoma following a monocular retinal lesion in the monkey. *Vis Neurosci* 14:89–101.

Nelson JI and Frost B (1978) Orientation selective inhibition from beyond the classical RF. *Brain Res* 139:359–365.

Nelson JI and Frost B (1985) Intracortical facilitation among co-oriented co-axially aligned simple cells in cat striate cortex. *Exp Brain Res* 6:54–51.

Neumann H and Mingolla E (2001) Computational neural models of spatial integration in perceptual grouping. In: Shipley TF and Kellman PJ (eds), *From Fragments to Objects—Segmentation and Grouping in Vision.* Amsterdam: Elsevier Science Publishers, pp 353–400.

Nothdurft HC (1991) Texture segmentation and pop-out from orientation contrast. *Vision Res* 31:1073–1078.

Nothdurft HC (1993) The role of features in preattentive vision: Comparison of orientation, motion and color cues. *Vision Res* 33:1937–1958.

Ohzawa I, Sclar G, and Freeman RD (1985) Contrast gain control in the cats's visual system. *J Neurophysiol* 54:651–676.

Paradiso MA and Hahn S (1996) Filling-in percepts produced by luminance modulation. *Vision Res* 36:2657–2663.

Paradiso MA and Nakayama K (1991) Brightness perception and filling-in. *Vision Res* 31:1221–1236.

Pessoa L and Neumann H (1998) Why does the brain fill-in? *Trends Cogn Sci* 2:422–424.

Pessoa L, Thompson E, and Noë A (1998) Finding out about filling-in: A guide to perceptual completion for visual science and the philosopy of perception. *Behav Brain Sci* 21:723–748.

Pettet MW and Gilbert CD (1992) Dynamic changes in receptive-field size in cat primary visual cortex. *Proc Natl Acad Sci USA* 89:8366–8370.

Pirenne MH (1962) Light adaptation. I. The Troxler phenomenon. In: Davson H (ed), *The Eye*, Vol. 2. New York and London: Academic Press, pp 197–199.

Ramachandran VS (1992) Blind spots. *Sci Am* 266:85–91.

Ramachandran VS (1995) Perceptual correlates of neural plasticity in the adult human brain. In: Papathomas TV and Chubb C (eds), *Early Vision and Beyond.* Cambridge, Mass.: MIT Press, pp 227–247.

Ramachandran VS and Gregory RL (1991) Perceptual filling-in of artificially induced scotomas in human vision. *Nature* 350:699–702.

Ramachandran VS, Gregory RL, and Aiken W (1993) Perceptual fading of visual texture borders. *Vision Res* 33:717–721.

Reich LN, Nguyen TT, and Levi DH (1997) Artificial scotomas and spatial localization (abstract). *IOVS* 38:2970.

Riggs LA, Ratliff F, Cornsweet JC, and Cornsweet TN (1953) The disappearance of steadily fixated visual test objects. *J Opt Soc Am* 43:495–501.

Roelfsema PR and Singer W (1998) Detecting connectedness. *Cereb Cortex* 8:385–396.

Romani A, Caputo G, Callieco R, Schintone E, and Cosi V (1999) Edge detection and surface filling-in as shown by texture visual evoked potentials. *Clin Neurophysiol* 110:86–91.

Rossi AF and Paradiso MA (1996) Temporal limits of brightness induction and mechanisms of brightness perception. *Vision Res* 36:1391–1398.

Safran AB, Achmard O, Duret F, and Landis T (1999) The "thin man" phenomenon: A sign of cortical plasticity following inferior homonymous paracentral scotomas. *Br J Ophthalmol* 83:137–142.

Safran AB and Landis T (1996) Plasticity in the adult visual cortex: Implications for the diagnosis of visual field defects and visual rehabilitation. *Curr Opin Ophthalmol* 7:53–64.

Schiefer U, Skalej M, Kolb M, Dietrich TJ, Kolb R, Braun C, and Petersen D (1998) Lesion location influences perception of homonymous scotomata during flickering random dot pattern stimulation. *Vision Res* 38:1303–1312.

Schieting S and Spillmann L (1987) Flicker adaptation in the peripheral retina. *Vision Res* 27:277–284.

Sereno MI, Dale AM, Reppas JB, Kwong KK, Belliveau JW, Brady TJ, Rosen BR, and Tootell RB (1995) Borders of multiple visual areas in humans revealed by functional magnetic resonance imaging. *Science* 268:889–893.

Shimojo S, Kamitani Y, and Nishida S (2001) Afterimage of perceptually filled-in surface. *Science* 293:1677–1680.

Sillito AM, Grieve KL, Jones HE, Cudeiro J, and Davis J (1995) Visual cortical mechanisms detecting focal orientation discontinuities. *Nature* 378:492–495.

Sillito AM and Jones HE (1996) Context-dependent interactions and visual processing in V1. *J Physiol* 90:205–209.

Smith E and De Weerd P (2001) Interactions between attention and perceptual filling-in. *Cogn Neurosci Abstr* 2001:149.

Spillmann L and Kurtenbach A (1992) Dynamic noise backgrounds facilitate target fading. *Vision Res* 32:1941–1946.

Spillmann L, Neumeyer C, and Hunzelmann N (1984) Adaptation an ruhende, bewegte und flimmernde Reize. In: Herzau V (ed), *Pathophysiologie des Sehens. Grundlagenforschung und Klinik der visuellen Sensorik (Aulhorn-Festschrift). Klin Monatsbl Augenheilkde* (Suppl) 98:68–78.

Spillmann L and Werner JS (1996) Long-range interactions in visual perception. *Trends Neurosci* 19:428–434.

Stürzel F and Spillmann L (2001) Texture fading correlates with stimulus salience. *Vision Res* 41:2969–2977.

Treue S and Maunsell JHR (1996) Attentional modulation of visual motion processing in cortical areas MT and MST. *Nature* 382:539–541.

Tripathy SP, Levi DM, Ogmen H, and Harden C (1995) Perceived length across the physiological blind spot. *Vis Neurosci* 12:385–402.

Troxler D (1804) Ueber das Verschwinden gegebener Gegenstände innerhalb unseres Gesichtskreises. In: Himly K and Schmidt JA (eds), *Ophthalmische Bibliothek II.2.* Jena: F Frommann, pp 1–119.

Tyler CW and Hardage L (1998) Long-range twinkle induction: An achromatic rebound effect in the magnocellular processing system? *Perception* 27:203–214.

van de Grind WA, Doorn AJ, and Koenderink JJ (1983) Detection of coherent movement in peripherally viewed random dot patterns. *J Opt Soc Am* 73:1674–1683.

Van Essen DC (1985) Functional organization of primate visual cortex. In: Jones EG and Peters AA (eds), *Cerebral Cortex*, Vol. 3. New York: Plenum Press, pp 259–329.

Van Essen DC, Felleman DJ, DeYoe EA, and Knierim JJ (1991) Probing the primate visual cortex: Pathways and perspectives. In: Valberg A and Lee BB (eds), *From Pigments to Perception—Advances in Understanding Visual Processess.* New York and London: Plenum Press, pp 227–237.

van Tuijl HFJM (1975) A new visual illusion: Neonlike color spreading and complementary color induction between subjective contours. *Acta Psychol* 39:441–445.

Walls GL (1954) The filling-in process. *Am J Optom Arch Am Acad Optom* 31:329–341.

Watanabe T and Cavanagh P (1991) Texture and motion spreading, the aperture problem, and transparency. *Percept Psychophys* 50:459–464.

Welchman AE and Harris JM (1999) Disappearing tricks: How the area of surrounding texture affects perceptual fading (abstract). *Perception* 28:S104d.

Welchman AE and Harris JM (2001) Filling-in the details on perceptual fading. *Vision Res* 41:2107–2117.

Yarbus AL (1967) *Eye Movements in Vision* (Haigh B trans). New York: Plenum Press.

Zipser K, Lamme VA, and Schiller PH (1996) Contextual modulation in primary visual cortex. *J Neurosci* 15:7376–7389.

# 6

## Searching for the Neural Mechanism of Color Filling-In

### RÜDIGER VON DER HEYDT, HOWARD S. FRIEDMAN, AND HONG ZHOU

In this chapter we will discuss a perceptual phenomenon in which visual stimuli seem to assume the color and brightness of the surrounding region and thereby vanish from perception. We will first review the basic findings and theories in order to clarify the origin of the ideas that guided recent neurophysiological studies. We will then review those recent studies that tried to solve the puzzle of filling-in by means of single-cell recording in monkeys.

There are four conditions under which color filling-in has been observed. One is the filling-in of the blind spot in monocular viewing. If seen against a surface of uniform color, the part of the visual field corresponding to the blind spot appears in the color of that surface, although obviously no color signals are generated at the blind spot. Second, patients with a scotoma (which may be caused by a lesion of the retina or visual pathways) report filling-in of the region corresponding to the scotoma. The third condition is artificial stabilization of the retinal image. Image stabilization can be achieved, for example, by mounting a small projector with a suction cap on the eye (Iarbus, 1957; Gerrits et al., 1966; Yarbus, 1967). The stabilized stimulus appears to fade gradually and to assume the color of the surrounding region. The fourth condition is known as *Troxler's effect*. During steady fixation, visual scenes gradually lose contrast until some objects disappear from perception (Troxler, 1804, cited in Fiorentini et al., 1989). Disappearance, however, generally means filling-in since the final appearance of the stimulus depends on the color of the background (Spillmann et al., 1984; Livingstone and Hubel, 1987). Thus, it is clear that this phenomenon cannot be fully explained by local processes such as adaptation, but also involves filling-in. The events observed under steady fixation (Zhang and von der Heydt, 1995; Friedman et al., 1999) are similar to those that occur under artificial image stabilization (Krauskopf, 1963; Gerrits et al., 1966; Yarbus, 1967; Ditchburn, 1973) but are generally more variable, presumably because of the irregularity of residual eye movements.

Thus, perceptual filling-in of color can occur in parts of the visual field for which no retinal signals exist (across the blind spot and other scotomas), but it can also occur over intact retinal regions under conditions of image stabilization. In the former case, filling-in occurs immediately or very rapidly, whereas in the latter case, it takes appreciable time, usually several seconds.

It has been hypothesized that all of the above observations share a common neural mechanism that is basic to the perception of color and brightness of surface in general (Walls, 1954; Gerrits and Vendrik, 1970; Cohen and Grossberg, 1984; Paradiso and Nakayama, 1991; see also Pessoa et al., 1998). Specific theories of filling-in postulate that perception is based on an image representation held in a two-dimensional array of neurons, in which color signals spread in all directions except across borders formed by contour activity (Gerrits and Vendrik, 1970; Cohen and Grossberg, 1984; Arrington, 1994). The process is thought to be analogous to physical diffusion, with contours acting as diffusion barriers for the color and brightness signals. As a result, these signals tend to fill the regions between the contours evenly, like water filling in the space between dikes. Since this theory assumes pointwise representation of visual information (the activity of each element of the array represents either color or contour strength for one location in the visual field), we will call it the *isomorphic filling-in theory*. Although the above studies differ widely in various aspects, we think it is fair to regard them as exemplifications of the same theory.

The isomorphic filling-in theory originated with the observations made in patients with visual scotomas and the striking phenomena discovered in retinal image stabilization (Ditchburn and Ginsborg, 1952; Riggs et al., 1953; Krauskopf, 1963; Gerrits et al., 1966; Yarbus, 1967). A detailed neural theory emerged when Gerrits and colleagues compared these observations with single-cell recordings from the cat optic tract, lateral geniculate nucleus (LGN), and striate cortex published by other authors at the time. It may be worthwhile to recapitulate here the basic arguments, as summarized in Gerrits and Vendrik (1970).

The neural representation of a stimulus, such as a bright uniform disk, was found to differ from the perception of that stimulus in two ways: First, the neurons generally responded to the onset of the stimulus with a brief transient elevation of the firing rate, whereas perception of brightness and color is constant over time. Second, the spatial distribution of neural activity was uneven—high for the border regions and low for the inner area of the disk—whereas the disk appears uniform in perception. In addition, with image stabilization, the color of the disk was perceived for several seconds before it appeared to be filled-in, but the transient elevation of the firing rate lasted for less than 0.1 second. Therefore, Gerrits and coworkers concluded that the moment of perceptual filling-in was not related to the decay of neural activity at those levels. Instead, they postulated a neural representation, called the *higher center*, in which the short afferent bursts are integrated and stored with a relatively long time constant. The additivity of integration at this level was demonstrated by applying luminance increments and decrements to a stabilized stimulus. The role of the contrast borders in forming diffusion barriers was shown by demonstrating that a large bright disk that had faded would reappear completely upon small displacements, even though the displacements modulated the illumination of receptors near the borders, but not of receptors near the center of the disk. When a stabilized bright bar that had faded was subsequently moved along its long axis, it created the perception of brightness spreading from behind the leading edge and darkness spreading from behind the trailing edge, while most of the lateral borders remained invisible (Yarbus, 1967, Fig. 46; Gerrits and Vendrik, 1970, Fig. 3). Thus, it seemed as if brightness and darkness signals were generated at the moving contrast borders, and as if the spreading of these signals was limited only by the moving borders, whereas the stationary borders were permeable.

The observation of delayed filling-in is an important point. It has been argued that the observation of perceived uniformity does not necessarily require the assumption of a filling-in process. Spatial filling-in might simply reflect the fact that different physical patterns of luminance distribution can be physiologically equivalent (Ratliff, 1978; see Fiorentini et al., 1989, for further references). For example, Cornsweet's luminance pattern is perceived as a uniform disk because both produce essentially the same patterns of neural activity. The same explanation would hold for filling-in of blind spot and scotomas. However, the experience of a color change occurring during physically constant stimulation suggests that filling-in is a physiological process and not just a convention of coding.

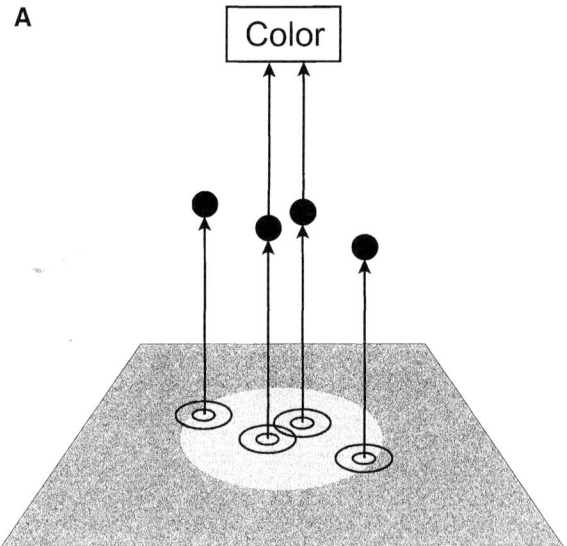

**Figure 6-1.** Three theories about the neural representation of surface color. (A) The naive concept assumes that the color of the disk is represented by the cells whose receptive fields are distributed over the surface of the disk. (B) The color filling-in theory assumes that the color signals generated by receptive fields at the borders of the disk propagate to cells representing the interior of the disk. (C) The symbolic color representation theory assumes that the signals from edge-selective receptive fields on the borders of the disk are integrated at a higher level to produce a signal that represents the color of the disk.

# Searching for the Neural Mechanism of Color Filling-In

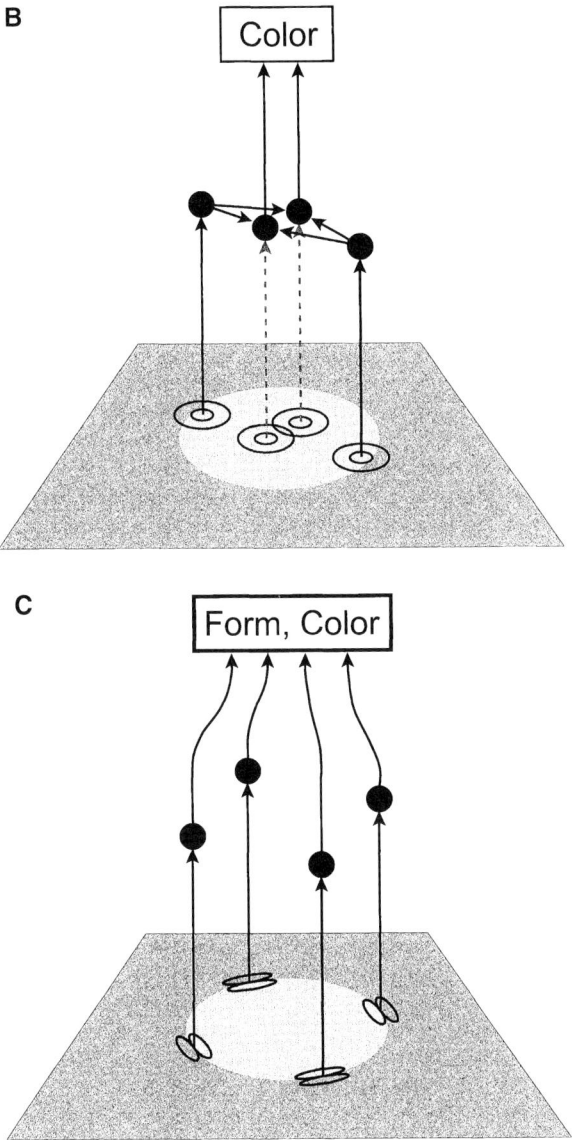

**Figure 6-1.** (*Continued*)

In Figures 6-1A–C we have summarized the arguments described above in cartoon form. It appears natural to assume that perception of the color of a surface is given by the activity of the cells whose receptive fields point at the surface (Fig. 6-1A). However, this is clearly not the case, as shown by a variety of filling-in phenomena (e.g., color is perceived at the blind spot in the absence of receptive fields; yellow and blue are perceived in the center of the fovea, which lacks S-cones). According to the isomorphic filling-in theory (Fig. 6-1B), color is also represented by the activity of cells whose receptive fields point at the surface, but it is assumed that these cells receive additional activation through horizontal connections that keeps their activity level high despite mechanisms of lateral inhibition that tend to suppress surface activity and despite the transient nature of the afferent signals. The dashed arrows in Figure 6-1B indicate the unreliable afferent signals. The lateral activation comes from receptive fields at contrast borders. These signals are strong, because receptive fields are exposed to contrast, and reliable, because the border produces continuous light modulation even during fixation due to small residual eye movements. The lateral connections also activate the cells representing the blind spot region which have receptive fields only in one eye, keeping up their activity when that eye is occluded. Figure 6-1C illustrates an alternative hypothesis to explain filling-in. This hypothesis assumes that image information is transformed at the cortical level into an oriented feature representation from which form and color are derived at a subsequent stage. This could be a stage of preliminary grouping based on rather mechanistic bottom-up processing or an *object file* generated by means of attentional feature binding. In this model, color is represented not in an isomorphic manner, but as an attribute of an object or proto-object (tentative association of features by low-level mechanisms). This theory also explains the perceptual observations, but in a completely different way: Blind spots and scotomas generate no border signals because there are no cortical cells whose receptive fields straddle their borders. Therefore, they do not give rise to object representations. However, if a large disk is presented over a scotoma, it generates the proper contrast border signals from which the shape and color of the disk are derived. Retinal stabilization of a stimulus causes adaptation of border signals, leading to its perceptual disappearance. What is perceived, then, is the color of the "underlying" object whose representation is based on signals of more distant borders which are not stabilized. Small eye movements will revive the adapted border signals, regenerating the object representation. Since this theory postulates a change at a symbolic level of representation (e.g., cessation of activity in a group of cells representing an object), we call it the *symbolic filling-in theory*.

Limitation of space precludes the discussion of all the phenomena of filling-in that have been reported, but the arguments sketched so far may convince the reader that virtually every finding can be explained easily and parsimoniously by the isomorphic as well as the symbolic theory. Despite many attempts to decide the case by psychophysical experiments, the mechanisms of color filling-in are still unknown.

## Literature Review

We shall review recent attempts to clarify the basis of color filling-in by means of single-cell recording. The earlier attempts to relate perception to neural activity by Gerrits and coworkers, as reviewed above, are unsatisfactory in two respects. First, human perception was compared with neurophysiological data from cats, whose visual system differs markedly from ours, particularly in regard to color vision. For better comparison with human perception, we need to study the neural activity in a primate species. Second, the arguments were indirect, via the spatiotemporal characteristics of neural processing (as measured, for example, with flashing spots of light). Much more convincing evidence could be obtained by recording the activity of neurons directly under the conditions in which filling-in occurs.

### Immediate Filling-in

Even though the visual system of macaque monkeys is known to be similar to that of humans, we need proof that monkeys also experience color filling-in. Komatsu and colleagues have recently demonstrated this for filling-in through the blind spot and through retinal scotomas (Komatsu and Murakami, 1994; Murakami et al., 1997). Monkeys were taught to discriminate between disks and rings. When a ring was then presented over the blind spot so that its inner contour fell on the blind region, the animals responded as if a disk were presented.

Komatsu and colleagues also analyzed the activity of cells of the blind spot representation in striate cortex (area V1) and found cells, in layers 4–6, that responded to large stimuli covering the blind spot (Komatsu et al., 2000). Most of these cells had particularly large classical receptive fields, with a residual field in the eye of the blind spot, and therefore responded to small stimuli near the blind spot (that is, stimuli that do not produce perceptual filling-in). However, some cells had only small classical receptive fields in the seeing eye inside the region corresponding to the blind spot. These cells did not respond to small stimuli near the blind spot but did respond if a large stimulus covered it, which is exactly the condition that produces perceptual filling-in. Thus, there seem to be connections that can transmit color and brightness information into the blind region. The exact nature of this pathway is not yet clear; convergence of afferent signals, horizontal intracortical connections (as suggested in Fig. 6-1B), or feedback projections from extrastriate areas could all play a role.

### Delayed Filling-in

The experiments discussed so far dealt with filling-in of scotomas and did not examine the role of contours as diffusion barriers for color signals, which is an important feature of the isomorphic filling-in theory. Only after the cessation of contour activity under stabilized vision can color signals spread across the contours and fill the enclosed area. Whereas the spread of signals must be relatively fast because even large stimuli appear uniform shortly after stimulus onset (Paradiso and Nakayama, 1991; Arrington, 1994), the breakdown of the dikes of contour activity under stabilization apparently takes some time (Gerrits and Vendrik, 1970). Thus, the critical question is: Does the neural activity change at the time of delayed filling-in?

To answer that question, we first need to know if monkeys perceive color filling-in under steady fixation like humans. Zhang (1995) and Friedman et al. (1999) developed a method for measuring perceptual filling-in that can be applied to humans as well as monkeys. They used a disk–ring stimulus in which the disk–ring border was of moderate contrast and blurred, whereas the outer border of the ring was of high contrast and sharp (Fig. 6-2, right). The result was that the disk tended to disappear after a few seconds under steady fixation, whereas the outer contour of the ring was perceived much longer, and the area of the disk appeared to be filled in with the color of the ring (Krauskopf, 1967). We used the complementary colors red and green for the disk and ring, and assigned these colors alternatively to the disk and ring so as to keep local color adaptation constant over the test sessions (complementary colors add up to neutral). Color saturation was set at 30% of the maximum that was attainable on a cathode ray tube color monitor. Despite being desaturated, the hues could be clearly perceived. The subjects had to fixate their gaze on a fixation target 2.5 degrees from the center of the disk. Fixation was controlled by having subjects respond to an orientation

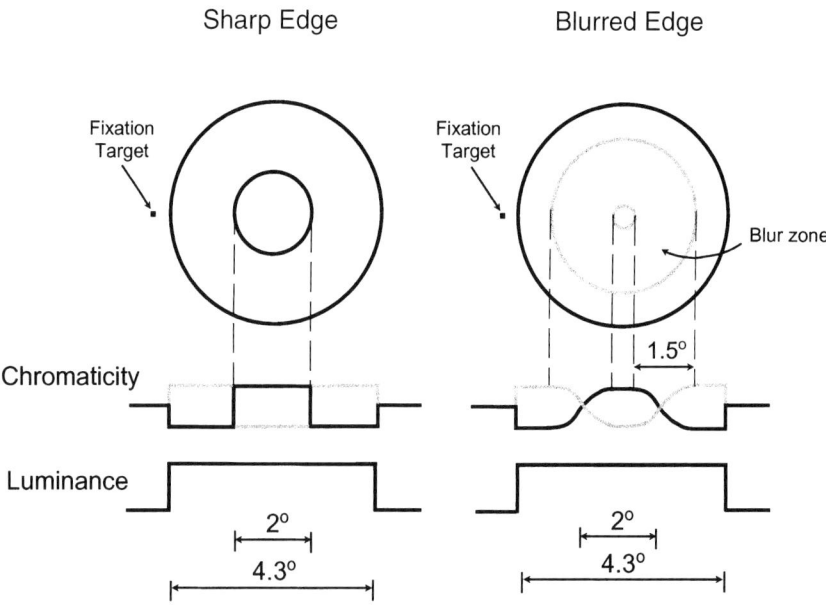

**Figure 6-2.** The visual stimuli used to study color filling-in. The shapes of the stimuli are shown at the top, and the chromaticity and luminance profiles at the bottom. The stimuli were disk–ring configurations in which the border between the disk and ring could be sharp (left) or blurred (right). Either kind of stimulus was presented statically, and moving, the disk subscribing a circular path of 8 arc minute radius at 1 Hz. The dimensions apply to the psychophysical experiments in which desaturated red and green colors were used. Similar configuration were used for the neural recordings, but colors were chosen according to the color selectivity of each cell. (*Source:* Modified from Friedman et al., 1999)

change of a small fixation target that occurred randomly in some trials and could be detected only in foveal vision. The monkeys were rewarded if they responded within 0.4 second after the target change. If they missed this interval, they were not rewarded and were punished by delaying the beginning of the next trial. Eye position was monitored with an infrared pupil tracking system, and larger eye movements were also punished by reward withholding and delay.

Monkeys cannot be instructed to respond to a visual illusion. However, they can be trained to signal reliably a physical color change in the stimulus that resembles the illusion of filling-in. We expected that when a monkey was well trained, it would then respond also in randomly inserted test trials in which there was no physical change, but instead an illusory change of color. This strategy works only if the subject confuses the illusory change with a physical change. Thus, if a monkey does not respond in those test trials, it may be either because the animal does not perceive filling-in or because the physical changes do not mimic the perceptual filling-in well enough. However, if a monkey responds consistently in the absence of a physical change under certain conditions, this would be strong evidence that it experiences illusory filling-in under these conditions.

Using the method described above, we have compared filling-in in humans and monkeys (Friedman et al., 1999). Two classes of stimuli were randomly intermixed: *control stimuli* in which the physical color of the disk was gradually changed to that of the ring and *test stimuli* in which the physical colors remained constant (Fig. 6-3). The transition time for the control stimuli varied from trial to trial. The human subjects were instructed to respond when the disk merged with the ring, forming a large, uniform disk. The monkeys were first trained for several months with only control trials in which they were rewarded if they indicated the moment when the disk merged with the ring. In the beginning, a fast color transition occurred at a randomized time in each trial. Later, the time constant of color change was also randomized and gradually extended, so that a response was required as early as 1.5 seconds after stimulus onset in some trials and as late as 7 seconds in others. The animals were then tested with a mixture of control trials (92%) and test trials (8%). In test trials they were rewarded randomly. To see if the subjects performed the task as intended, the disk was presented in four different modes: static or moving (circular oscillation), and with a sharp or blurred border. Since sharp borders and movement are both known to reduce the probability of perceiving filling-in, we expected that the frequency of responses would be affected accordingly.

The results of this experiment showed that for monkeys as well as for human subjects, blurred disks were more likely to produce a filling-in response than were sharp disks, and static disks were more likely to produce this response than moving disks. Figure 6-4 shows the probability of filling-in responses for the static-blurred condition as a function of time after stimulus onset. Filling-in responses began to occur after 3–4 seconds; by the end of 6 seconds the probability reached 22%–80%, depending on the subject. While the rate of the increase varied among subjects, the time course was remarkably similar between humans and monkeys. It can be seen that responses before 3 seconds were extremely rare. This is in

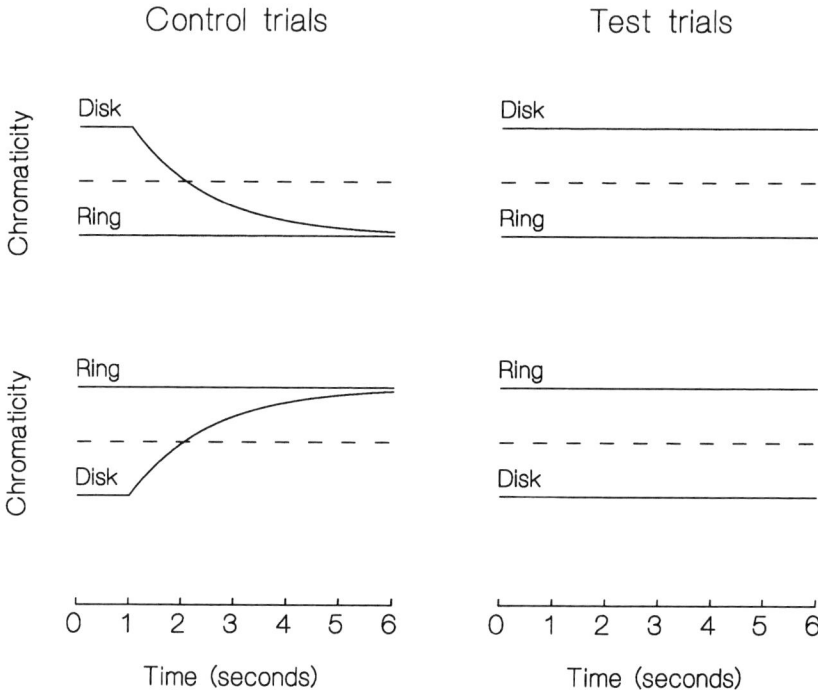

**Figure 6-3.** Test trials and control trials. In test trials, disk and ring colors were constant. In control trials, the color of the disk was first constant for a variable interval and then exponentially approached the ring color, with a variable time constant. (*Source:* Modified from Friedman et al., 1999)

contrast to the control trials (92% of all trials), in which 25% of the responses occurred before 3 seconds, indicating that the monkeys responded when they perceived the change, not when they expected it. Thus, the dependence on the stimulus condition and the distribution of response times are strong evidence that monkeys perceive color filling-in under steady fixation, just as humans do.

## Some Basic Facts About Cortical Coding of Colored Figures

Before we discuss the neurophysiological processes during delayed filling-in, we have to clarify a few points about the cortical representation of colored figures. First of all, Gerrits' assumption that uniform illumination of receptive fields produces only weak excitation of cells in the visual pathways does not hold for chromatic stimuli in the monkey. The most common type of cell in the monkey LGN, the color-opponent center-surround cell (type I; Wiesel and Hubel, 1966), responds well to uniform illumination. These cells respond maximally if the receptive field is centered on the surface of a chromatic figure (De Valois and Pease, 1971). It is only at the cortical level that color surface responses are reduced

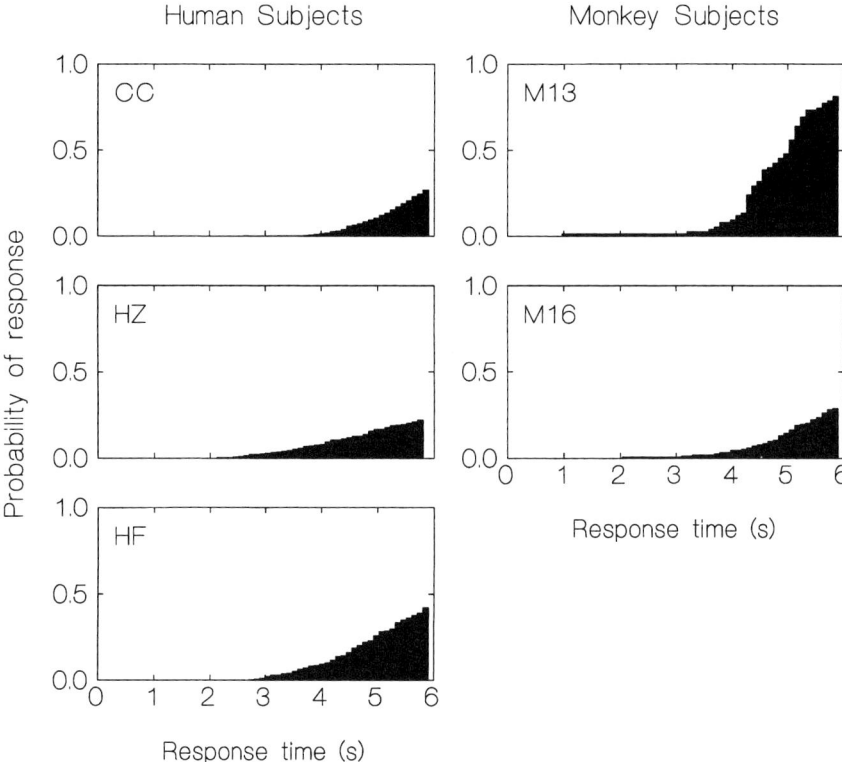

**Figure 6-4.** The probability of filling-in responses for the blurred disk–ring stimulus as a function of time after stimulus onset. The stimulus colors were constant, red and green. Distributions are shown for three human subjects and two monkeys. (*Source:* Modified from Friedman et al., 1999)

(Hubel and Wiesel, 1968; Thorell et al., 1984). Recordings from alert behaving monkeys (von der Heydt et al., 1996; Friedman et al., 2002) show that, in layers 2–3 of V1, 85% of cells respond almost exclusively to contrast borders (*edge cells*: surface response <25% of edge response), while only 15% can be activated by larger uniform stimuli centered on the receptive field (*surface cells*).[1] The proportions in area V2 are quite similar. Thus, although the relative amount of surface activity is greatly reduced in the cortex compared to the LGN, surface signals still exist.

The second point is that, contrary to common belief, color selectivity is as common among orientation-selective cells as it is among unoriented cells (Michael, 1978a, 1978b; Thorell et al., 1984; Levitt et al., 1994; Leventhal et al., 1995; von der Heydt et al. 1996). Since the vast majority of cells in the superficial layers of V1 and in V2 are orientation selective, this means that far more color information is present in oriented than in unoriented signals (Friedman et al., 2002). Furthermore, many of these cells not only provide color information, but are also selective for contrast polarity at the border. For example, a cell may respond to a gray-red border of a certain orientation, but not to a red-gray border of the same orientation.

Thus, the physiological facts, as presently known, are compatible with both the isomorphic and symbolic theories (Figs. 6-1B and 6-1C). It is possible that afferent surface signals are suppressed at the cortical level, as Gerrits and Vendrik (1970) suggested, and that the sporadic surface responses observed in the cortex are the result of the filling-in process (Fig. 6-1B). On the other hand, many oriented border contrast signals also exist from which surface color could be derived (Fig. 6-1C).

## *Surface and Border Signals During Perceptual Filling-In*

The crucial question is how surface and border signals behave during perceptual fading and filling-in. Consider a display like the one in Figure 6-2, with two different colors, such as red in the center and green in the surrounding ring. If the isomorphic filling-in theory is right, then cells representing the center should signal "red" after stimulus onset and then change to signal "green" when the display changes perceptually to a large, uniform disc. For the border signals, both theories predict a decline during fading: In the isomorphic theory, the cessation of border signals makes the disk borders permeable for color signals; in the symbolic theory, it causes the disk representation to vanish.

We have recorded the activity of cells in visual cortex while the monkey was performing the filling-in task (Friedman, 1998; see also Zhou et al., 2000, for general methods). Surface cells (as defined above) were tested with the uniform center of the disk placed over the receptive field, edge cells with the disk–ring border placed on the receptive field at the optimum orientation. Figures 6-5 to 6-7 show the time courses of activity for four different stimulus conditions (differences within stimulus conditions between trials in which the animal did and did not signal filling-in will be discussed later on).

Figure 6-5 shows the responses of a surface cell of area V1. The firing rate of the neuron is plotted as a function of time after stimulus onset. Each data point represents the mean firing rate during 0.5 second; error bars show standard errors of the means. Filled symbols and solid lines represent responses for disks of the "good" color (for this cell, red); open symbols and dashed lines represent responses for disks of the "bad" color (green). The left side shows the activity during control trials in which the color of the disk was physically changed to that of the ring; the right side shows the activity during test trials in which the display was constant. The top panels are for blurred disks, the bottom panels for disks with sharp contours.

It can be seen that the firing rate in the test trials remained fairly constant, high for the optimum color and low for the complementary color, during 6 seconds of fixation. Note also that the neural responses did not decay faster in the blurred than in the sharp border condition. By contrast, when the disk was filled in physically, the responses changed accordingly (left panels of Fig. 6-5). The

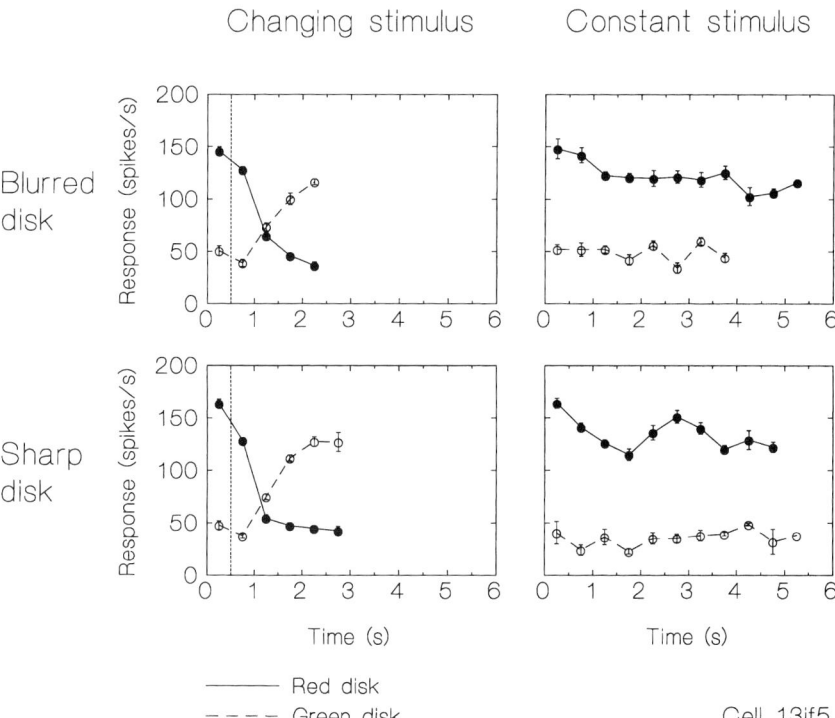

**Figure 6-5.** The responses of a V1 cell to disk–ring stimuli centered over its receptive field in control trials (left) and test trials (right). Filled symbols, initial disk color optimal (red); open symbols, initial disk color complementary (green). Error bars represent standard errors of the means. Only one of four control conditions with different timing is shown: 0.5 second constancy with subsequent exponential change of 1 second time constant; the vertical line indicates onset of change. When the disk color changed physically, the firing rate changed correspondingly (left), but during the perceptual color changes experienced with the blurred disk, it remained nearly constant (top right).

firing rate followed the changing chromaticity rather faithfully. The two curves for good-to-bad and bad-to-good color changes cross each other.

A variety of color-selective cells were tested. While red was the preferred color for the cell of Figure 6-5, very similar results were obtained for green-selective cells. Using eight pairs of equiluminant colors and nine pairs of colors that differed in luminance, including grays, we selected, for each cell, the pair that produced the greatest response difference. For Figures 6-6 and 6-7 we calculated, for each cell, the difference between the responses to the two complementary color stimuli (solid and dashed curves of Fig. 6-5). (We assume here that color information is encoded in the balance of activity between pairs of cells

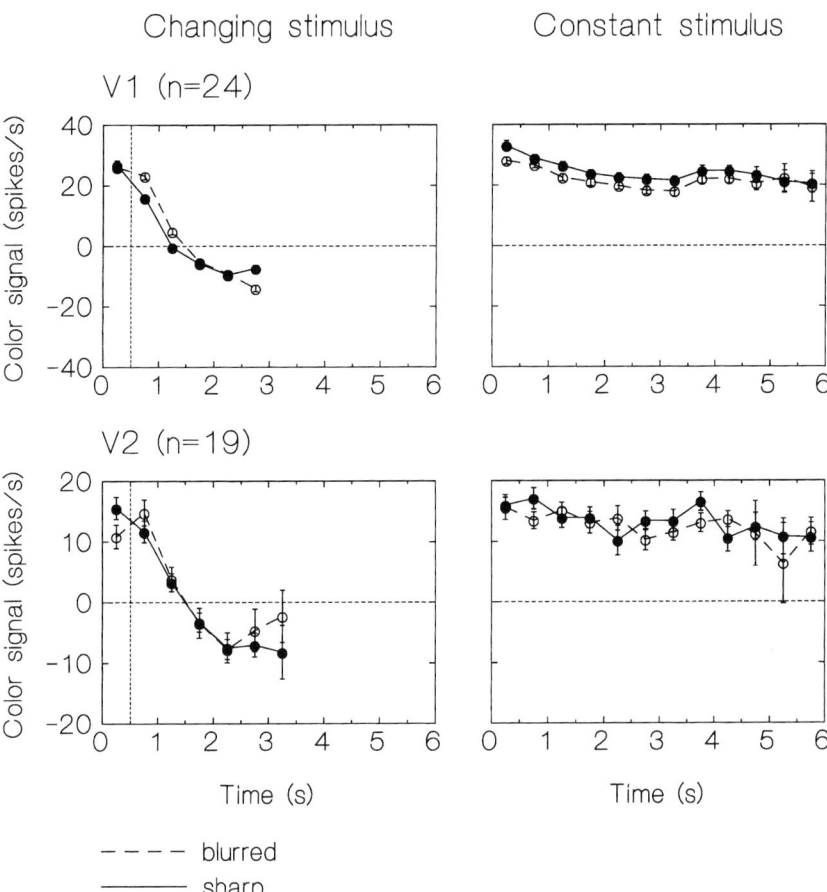

**Figure 6-6.** The averaged color signals of the surface cells studied in V1 and V2 (V1 cells mostly from layers 2–3). The difference between the optimal and complementary color trials is plotted as a function of time after stimulus onset. Filled and open symbols represent sharp and blurred border conditions. Error bars represent standard error of the mean. As in Figure 6-5, the averaged surface signals followed the physical color changes but remained nearly constant during perceptual changes. Note that stimuli with blurred and sharp borders produced very similar signals, whereas filling-in was perceived significantly more often with blurred than with sharp borders.

with opposite color preference but otherwise identical receptive fields. We infer the responses of the two cells from the responses of one cell to the two opposite colors.)

In Figure 6-6 we plotted the mean color signals of the surface cells tested in areas V1 and V2, weighting each cell by its color modulation index (the differ-

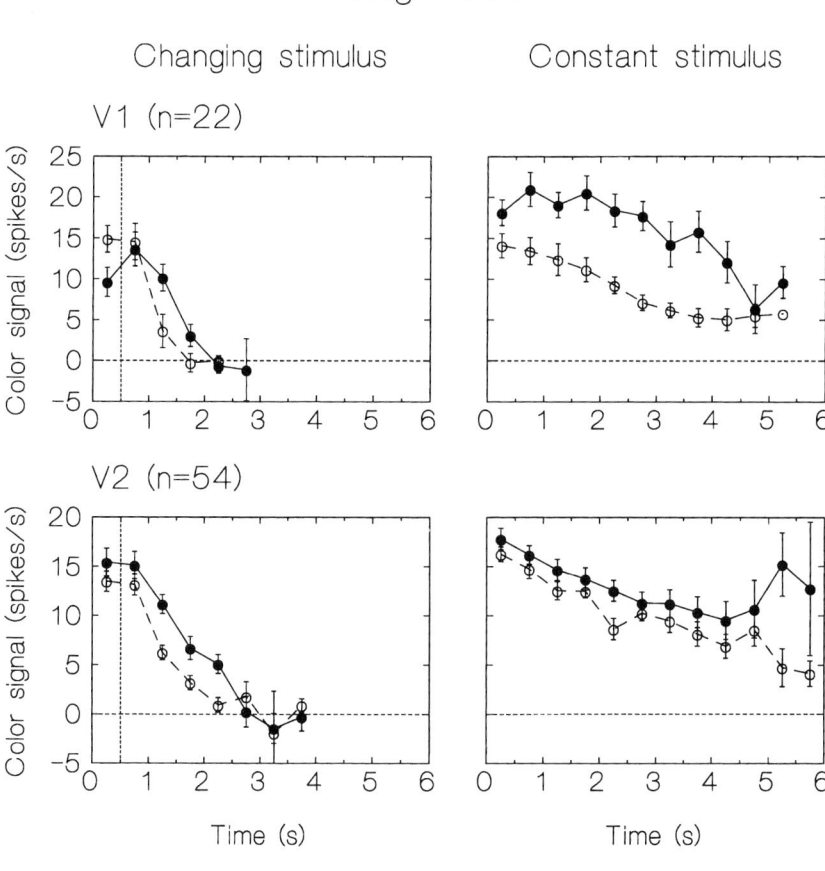

**Figure 6-7.** The averaged color signals of the edge cells of areas V1 and V2 (V1 cells mostly from layers 2–3). The border between the disk and ring was placed in the receptive field at an optimal orientation. The difference between the responses to the borders of optimal color contrast and the reversed contrast is plotted as a function of time. Other conventions are as for Figure 6-6. When the disk color changed physically, the edge signals followed the stimulus contrast, approaching zero within 3 seconds. When the colors were constant, the edge signals also decayed, but more slowly. The edge signals were significantly smaller for blurred disks than for sharp disks.

ence between the responses to the optimal color and the complementary color divided by the sum of the two). As in Figure 6-5, the left panels represent the changing color condition, the right panels the constant color condition. Responses to sharp border stimuli are plotted with filled symbols and solid line, responses to blurred border stimuli with open symbols and dashed lines. The results from areas V1 (where cells were recorded mainly from layers 2 and 3) and V2 are quite similar. It can be seen that the color surface signals crossed from positive to negative in trials in which the disk changed from one color to its complement. However, when the stimulus colors did not change, the responses remained fairly constant. The finding of sustained color signals over 6 seconds is in contrast to the behavioral filling-in responses, which indicated that in many trials the perceived color had changed to the complementary color by 6 seconds (80% of the trials in M13, 25% in M16, Fig. 6-4). Furthermore, the responses for the blurred and sharp border conditions were almost identical, in contrast to the behavioral filling-in responses, which were more frequent for the blurred border than for the sharp border.

As mentioned, the great majority of color-sensitive cells are edge selective. We studied the responses of these cells to the border between disk and ring in our filling-in paradigm. Figure 6-7 shows the time course of the color edge signals. As for the surface condition, we calculated the difference between the responses for the two color conditions, that is, the difference between the responses to the edges of the preferred and nonpreferred polarities. Again, cells were weighted by their color modulation index calculated as above, but from the responses to edges of opposite contrast polarities.

The predictions for border signals are different from those for surface signals. While the color of the disk changes to the complementary color, the contrast at the border between disk and ring decays to zero. As can be seen in Figure 6-7, the color edge signals decreased to zero in the control trials, reflecting the contrast decay (left). However, the signals decreased also, more slowly, in the test trials in which the contrast was constant (right). This decay was faster for the blurred than for the sharp border condition (dashed line versus solid line).

We also looked at the difference within stimulus conditions between trials in which the monkeys signaled filling-in and those in which they did not. We expected to see an earlier drop of activity in trials with a filling-in response. We found that the firing rate of the edge responses was slightly lower in these trials, while there was no difference in the slope of decay—neither in the surface responses nor in the edge responses. However, the behavioral data from the single-cell recording sessions were less clear than the data from the psychophysical experiments (Friedman et al., 1999), presumably because during the recording sessions the animal had to switch back and forth between the difficult filling-in task and the simpler fixation task that was used to explore and map receptive fields, and also because stimulus location and color varied according to the receptive fields of the neurons studied.

## *Relating Neural Signals and Behavioral Response*

In this section we discuss the question of how the time course of neural color signals should be related to the psychophysical data on filling-in. To illustrate the problem, we consider a simple model. The logic is as follows: We assume that (1) perception of the disk color is based on the activity of a group of color-selective cells, (2) a continuous signal S, such as a membrane potential, is derived by pooling and smoothing the spike trains, and (3) a filling-in response is generated when S reaches a critical limit. Whatever hypothesis we make about S, the same critical limit must account for the illusion as well as the perception of physical filling-in.

In the case of the isomorphic theory, S is derived from the surface signals. The disk appears to be filled in when its color signal equals that from the ring. We can determine the value of the disk color signal at this moment from the trials with physical color change: In the case of a sharp-edged disk whose color changed with a 1 second time constant, the monkeys responded about 3 seconds after stimulus onset. From the plots of the neural signals of V2, for example, we see that the mean color surface signal had reached about $-8$ spikes/second at this time (filled circles in Figure 6-6, bottom left panel). Thus, $-8$ spikes/sec is the level of the color surface signal at which the disk blends in with the ring when the color changes physically, and this must also be the critical limit for illusory filling-in. In Figure 6-8A we have replotted the surface response data for the blurred constant stimuli (open circles in Figure 6-6, bottom right panel) and fitted a regression line to the data points. This line describes the slow decay of the color signal of the disk. The horizontal dotted line indicates the critical limit. (The sloping dashed line and the curve at the bottom are explained below.)

In the case of the symbolic theory, S is derived from edge cells and the critical limit should be zero because uniformity of color was the response criterion in the task. Indeed, the mean response of V2 edge cells at the time when filling-in was perceived for the physical color change (3 seconds) was close to zero (Fig. 6-7, lower left panel). In Figure 6-8B we have replotted the mean response data of the V2 edge cells for the blurred constant stimuli with their regression line. This line intersects zero at about 8 seconds.

Because signal S varies from trial to trial, it can hit zero sooner or later than the mean signal. The signal characteristics of S depend on the variability of the single-cell responses, the number of cells pooled, their possible correlation, and the time constant of temporal integration. We do not know these parameters. However, since the probability of filling-in responses in the behavioral experiments started to rise at 3–4 seconds (Fig. 6-4), the standard deviation (SD) of S should be such that a line 2 SD below the regression line would intersect the limit at about 4 seconds. The dashed lines in Figure 6-8B mark the $\pm 2$ SD band assuming an SD of 4 spikes/sec. This is the only free parameter in the model. The curve shows the approximate shape of the resulting probability distribution of model responses. It is comparable to the behavioral distributions of Figure 6-4.[2] In the case of the color surface signal, we would have to assume a much larger SD, on the order of 16 spikes/sec, to obtain filling-in responses by 4 seconds (dashed line in Fig. 6-8A). However, because of the slow decay of the mean signal strength (the linear extrapolation reaches the limit only 25 seconds after stimulus onset), the probability of responses would rise extremely slowly. This is not at all what the behavioral responses show.[3] The mismatch would be even greater for the color surface signals of V1, which are still more sustained than those of

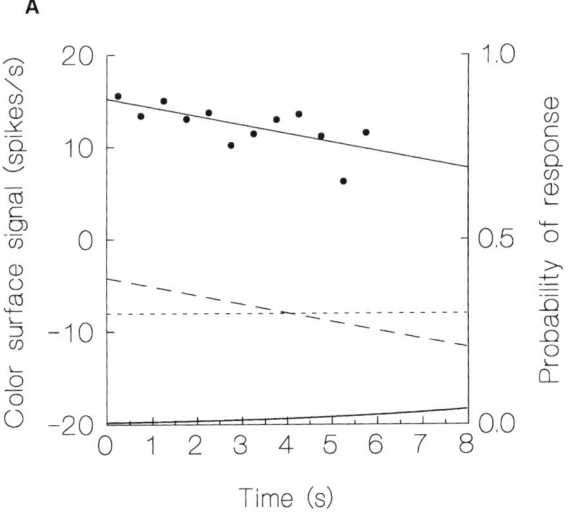

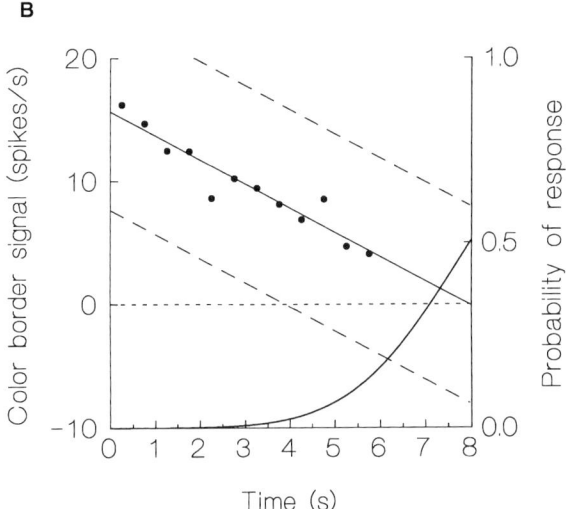

**Figure 6-8.** Model calculation relating neural signals to behavioral data. Predictions of the probability of behavioral filling-in responses are derived from (A) the surface signals and (B) the edge signals of V2. Dots with regression lines represent the averaged color signals of V2 cells (left scale) as a function of time after stimulus onset. The curve at the bottom indicates the predicted cumulative probability of filling-in (right scale). See text for further explanation.

V2. Preliminary results from area V4 indicate that the color surface signals there are also sustained and do not change at the time of perceptual filling-in.

## Discussion

Information about the color and brightness of a surface is represented in two ways in the visual cortex: by the activity of neurons whose receptive fields point at the surface and by the responses of neurons whose receptive fields straddle the border of the surface.

Our recordings from the visual cortex of monkeys during perceptual filling-in failed to show the corresponding change of the surface activity. We conclude that the physiological evidence is incompatible with the isomorphic filling-in theory which assumes that color signals spread from the borders into uniform regions (Fig. 6-1B). We believe that our results do not depend on the particular choice of colors. We have used pairs of complementary colors for the disk and ring (and switched them between trials to keep color adaptation constant). However, informal observations showed that similar filling-in would be obtained with other colors, for example, a gray patch surrounded by a colored ring or vice versa. We are aware that the comparison of neural signals with perception, even in the same animal, is fraught with problems. In our experiments, the stimulus parameters used for psychophysics and neural recording were not exactly the same. For example, the colors were varied in the physiological experiments, whereas only red and green were used for the psychophysical study, fixation of gaze might have varied, and so on. However, even with these uncertainties in mind, it seems impossible to reconcile the sustained character of the color surface signals with the signal change postulated by the isomorphic filling-in theory.

The physiological data are compatible with the symbolic theory of filling-in which only postulates a decay of border signals (Fig. 6-1C). In this theory, the perceived color of the blurred disk would be represented by the pooled color edge signals of the disk. Under reasonable assumptions about the variability of the pooled signal, the distribution of behavioral filling-in responses can be modeled. Thus, the gradual decay of border signals might explain the delayed perception of filling-in under conditions of image stabilization including Troxler's effect. Referring to Figure 6-1C, we assume that the border signals sustain representations of two objects: a light disk on top of a dark square. The disk is perceived as long as the color edge selective cells are activated by the border of the disk. When their activity ceases, the disk representation disappears and a uniform square is perceived whose color is given by the cells that are activated by the borders of the square. In this theory, the cessation of all border activity inside a region is the condition for perceiving the region as uniform. We do not assume that uniformity is merely the default assumption; rather, we think that circuits exist that detect the absence of edge responses.

The proposition that object color is computed from border signals raises some interesting questions about the nature of the color edge signals and the way they are combined. The process of combination obviously requires information about which border signals have to be included and which not. In general, this problem is more complex than in the case of a circular disk. Indeed, many psychophysical studies have shown that factors that determine the perception of spatial layout and contours also affect the perception of color and brightness. Examples are the brightness effect of illusory contours, perception of transparent colors, and brightness illusions in displays of three-dimensional shapes (see, for example, Kanizsa, 1979; Nakayama et al., 1990; Adelson, 1993). We conjecture that all these phenomena can be explained naturally by assuming that color and brightness are derived from orientation-selective edge responses.

Of particular importance is the phenomenon of *border ownership*, the tendency to perceive borders as belonging to one of the adjacent regions, as if the borders were occluding contours of objects in space (Koffka, 1935). We have recently shown that border ownership coding emerges early in the visual cortex. Edge-selective cells in areas V2 and V4 were found to carry information about the side of the surface to which an edge belongs (Zhou et al., 2000; von der Heydt et al., 2002). In effect, each contrast border is represented by two groups of cells. For an isolated border, both groups are active, but if there are cues that indicate that a border is due to spatial occlusion, one group is activated while the other is suppressed. Such cells can be thought of as having receptive fields with a pointer that indicates the side of the surface to which the border belongs. In this representation, the color of a surface could be computed by selectively integrating the activity of those cells whose pointers converge toward the center of the surface. Future research might reveal this hypothetical stage of integration in the cortex.

The fact that the time course of the edge signals seems to explain naturally the delay and the rise of the probability of filling-in (Fig. 6-8B) suggests that filling-in is not entirely a process of the hypothetical stage of symbolic coding, but is initiated at the level of local feature representation. This is in agreement with psychophysical results showing that filling-in depends on stimulus properties such as movement, contrast, size, and blur (Spillmann et al., 1984; Zhang and von der Heydt, 1995).

Our finding that the color signals of surface cells did not reverse according to the perceptual color reversal indicates that these signals are not the result of a filling-in process as sketched in Figure 6-1B, but simply reflect a property of the color signals from the retina. The finding of sustained activity in response to constant illumination of the receptive field contradicts the widespread opinion that responses in the visual pathways are generally transient (Walls, 1954; Gerrits and Vendrik, 1970). Sustained activity was the rule not only for color, but also for luminance contrast stimuli.

Given the behavioral evidence for a perceptual color reversal, the finding of sustained color surface signals is puzzling. It means that a perceptual color change, say from red to green, can occur despite continued strong "red" signals from surface cells in V1 and V2. Although surface cells are only a small minority in these areas, the fact that such cells are found in V2 as well as V1 indicates that they do not merely represent a transitory stage of processing (Friedman et al., 2002). Perhaps these signals are not directly involved in representing object color, but serve to monitor illumination changes as required for color constancy.

Our results in the color/brightness domain are formally comparable to those of De Weerd et al. (1995), who found filling-in of neural texture responses in areas V2 and V3. The emergence of texture activity in neurons with receptive fields inside an untextured region of the stimulus in that study contrasts with the persistent absence of responses to disks of the non-preferred color of neurons in our study (Fig. 6-6). However, we have to keep in mind that the analogy is purely formal. Other observations also indicate that filling-in of texture is different from filling-in of color. For example, color filling-in produces an afterimage that depends on the adapting color, whereas the aftereffect of texture filling-in is not related to the texture of the preceding stimulation (Hardage and Tyler, 1995).

In conclusion, by comparing visual cortical neuron activity with behavioral responses in monkeys, we find that the illusory perception of filling-in under steady fixation can be related to a gradual decay of color border signals. We find no evidence for surface filling-in at the level of neuronal signals. These findings suggest that the visual system computes surface color from orientation-selective border responses.

*Acknowledgments*

We wish to thank Ofelia Garalde for technical assistance and Todd Macuda for stylistic improvements. Supported by NIH Grant EY02966 and Human Frontier Science Program RG31. HSF was supported by the Whitaker Foundation.

## Notes

1. *Surface cell* is short for *surface-responsive cell* and does not imply a special role in surface representation.

2. The exact shape of the distribution depends on the power spectrum of S (cf. Gerstein and Mandelbrot, 1964). For example, if S varies rapidly, it would generally hit the critical limit before the mean. If it varies slowly, this would occur in about half of the trials. The curve in Figure 6-8B corresponds to a slowly varying Gaussian signal.

3. We assumed that the limit is constant, that is, that the color signal of the ring remains constant while the color signal of the disk changes, in keeping with the filling-in hypothesis. If the ring color signal also changes, but in the opposite direction, the resulting probability of filling-in would rise faster but would still reach only 5% after 6 seconds, compared to an average of 42% observed behavioral responses.

## References

Adelson EH (1993) Perceptual organization and the judgment of brightness. *Science* 262:2042–2044.

Arrington KF (1994) The temporal dynamics of brightness filling-in. *Vision Res* 34:3371–3387.

Cohen MA and Grossberg S (1984) Neural dynamics of brightness perception: Features, boundaries, diffusion, and resonance. *Percept Psychophys* 36:428–456.

De Valois RL and Pease PL (1971) Contours and contrast: Responses of macaque lateral geniculate cells to color and luminance figures. *Science* 171:694–696.

De Weerd P, Gattass R, Desimone R, and Ungerleider LG (1995) Responses of cells in monkey visual cortex during perceptual filling-in of an artificial scotoma. *Nature* 377:731–734.

Ditchburn RW (1973) *Eye Movements and Visual Perception.* Oxford: Clarendon Press.

Ditchburn RW and Ginsborg BL (1952) Vision with a stabilized retinal image. *Nature* 170:36–37.

Fiorentini A, Baumgartner G, Magnussen S, Schiller PH, and Thomas JP (1989) The perception of brightness and darkness: Relations to neuronal receptive fields. In: Spillmann L and Werner JS (eds), *Visual Perception: The Neurophysiological Foundations.* San Diego: Academic Press, pp 129–161.

Friedman H (1998) Neural Mechanisms of Object Color Representation in Areas V1, V2 and V4 of Macaque Visual Cortex. PhD Thesis, Johns Hopkins University, Baltimore: Maryland.

Friedman HS, Zhou H, and von der Heydt R (1999) Color filling-in under steady fixation: Behavioral demonstration in monkeys and humans. *Perception* 28:1383–1395.

Friedman HS, Zhou H, and von der Heydt R (2002) The coding of uniform color figures in monkey visual cortex. *J Physiol* (in press).

Gerrits HJM, de Haan B, and Vendrik AJH (1966) Experiments with retinal stabilized images. Relations between the observations and neural data. *Vision Res* 6:427–440.

Gerrits HJM and Vendrik AJH (1970) Simultaneous contrast, filling-in process and information processing in man's visual system. *Exp Brain Res* 11:411–430.

Gerstein GL and Mandelbrot B (1964) Random walk models for the spike activity of a single neuron. *Biophys J* 4:41–68.

Hardage L and Tyler CW (1995) Induced twinkle aftereffect as a probe of dynamic visual processing mechanisms. *Vision Res* 35:757–766.

Hubel DH and Wiesel TN (1968) Receptive fields and functional architecture of monkey striate cortex. *J Physiol (Lond)* 195:215–243.

Iarbus AL (1957) A new method of studying the activity of various parts of the retina. *Biophysics* 2:165–167.

Kanizsa G (1979) *Organization in Vision: Essays on Gestalt Perception.* New York: Praeger Publishers.

Koffka K (1935) *Principles of Gestalt Psychology.* New York: Harcourt, Brace and World.

Komatsu H, Kinoshita M, and Murakami I (2000) Neural responses in the retinotopic representation of the blind spot in the macaque V1 to stimuli for perceptual filling-in. *J Neurosci* 20:9310–9319.

Komatsu H and Murakami I (1994) Behavioral evidence of filling-in at the blind spot of the monkey. *Vis Neurosci* 11:1103–1113.

Krauskopf J (1963) Effect of retinal image stabilization on the appearance of heterochromatic targets. *J Opt Soc Am* 53:741–743.

Krauskopf J (1967) Heterochromatic stabilized images: A classroom demonstration. *Am J Psychol* 80:634–637.

Leventhal AG, Thompson KG, Liu D, Zhou Y, and Ault SJ (1995) Concomitant sensitivity to orientation, direction, and color of cells in layers 2, 3, and 4 of monkey striate cortex. *J Neurosci* 15:1808–1818.

Levitt JB, Kiper DC, and Movshon JA (1994) Receptive fields and functional architecture of macaque V2. *J Neurophysiol* 71:2517–2542.

Livingstone MS and Hubel DH (1987) Psychophysical evidence for separate channels for the perception of form, color, movement, and depth. *J Neurosci* 7:3416–3468.

Michael CR (1978a) Color vision mechanisms in monkey striate cortex: Simple cells with dual opponent-color receptive fields. *J Neurophysiol* 41:1233–1249.

Michael CR (1978b) Color-sensitive complex cells in monkey striate cortex. *J Neurophysiol* 41:1250–1266.

Murakami I, Komatsu H, and Kinoshita M (1997) Perceptual filling-in at the scotoma following a monocular retinal lesion in the monkey. *Vis Neurosci* 14:89–101.

Nakayama K, Shimojo S, and Ramachandran VS (1990) Transparency: Relation to depth, subjective contours, luminance and neon color spreading. *Perception* 19:497–513.

Paradiso MA and Nakayama K (1991) Brightness perception and filling-in. *Vision Res* 31:1221–1236.

Pessoa L, Thompson E, and Noe A (1998) Finding out about filling-in: A guide to perceptual completion for visual science and the philosophy of perception. *Behav Brain Sci* 21:723–748.

Ratliff F (1978) A discourse on edges. In: Armington JC, Krauskopf J, and Wooten BR (eds), *Visual Psychophysics and Physiology.* New York: Academic Press, pp 299–314.

Riggs LA, Ratliff F, Cornsweet JC, and Cornsweet TN (1953) The disappearance of steadily fixated visual test objects. *J Opt Soc Am* 43:495–501.

Spillmann L, Neumeyer C, and Hunzelmann N (1984) Adaptation an ruhende, bewegte und flimmernde Reize. *Klin Monatsbl Augenheilkunde Beiheft* 98:68–78.

Thorell LG, De Valois RL, and Albrecht DG (1984) Spatial mapping of monkey V1 cells with pure color and luminance stimuli. *Vision Res* 24:751–769.

von der Heydt R, Zhou H, and Friedman H (1996) The coding of extended colored figures in monkey visual cortex. *Soc Neurosci Abstr* 22:951.

von der Heydt R, Zhou H, and Friedman HS (2002) Neural coding of border ownership: Implications for the theory of figure–ground perception. In: Behrmann M, Kimchi R, and Olson CR (eds), *Perceptual Organization in Vision: Behavioral and Neural Perspectives.* Hillsdale, NJ: Lawrence Erlbaum Associates (in press).

Walls GL (1954) The filling-in process. *Am J Optom* 31:329–341.

Wiesel TN and Hubel DH (1966) Spatial and chromatic interactions in the lateral geniculate body of the rhesus monkey. *J Neurophysiol* 29:1115–1156.

Yarbus AL (1967) *Eye Movements and Vision.* New York: Plenum Press.

Zhang X (1995) Objective measurement of perceptual filling-in. Master's thesis, Johns Hopkins University, Baltimore.

Zhang X and von der Heydt R (1995) Determinants of filling-in. *Invest Ophthalmol Vis Sci* 36:S469.

Zhou H, Friedman HS, and von der Heydt R (2000) Coding of border ownership in monkey visual cortex. *J Neurosci* 20:6594–6611.

# 7

# Effects of Modal versus Amodal Completion Upon Visual Attention:
A Function for Filling-In?

## GREG DAVIS AND JON DRIVER

As the various contributions in this book illustrate, the term *filling-in* has been used to refer to a variety of perceptual phenomena (see also Petry and Meyer, 1987; Pessoa et al., 1998, for reviews). While these phenomena may have some common features, they also differ in several salient respects. Accordingly, we begin by clarifying the particular sense in which we shall refer to filling-in. First, it is important to distinguish *perceptual* filling-in, from *neural* filling-in (Pessoa et al., 1998). We are concerned here with perceptual filling-in, without speculating on whether or not this may reflect particular forms of neural filling-in, such as spread of neural firing across topological banks of feature detectors and so on. Second, while the conclusions we draw may apply to other cases, we shall focus specifically upon perceptual filling-in of color and brightness. Third, in addressing the possible functions of such perceptual filling-in in this chapter, we shall be concerned with cases where regions of visual space become filled-in with *illusory* color and brightness. We argue that a close comparison of modal and amodal completion may be particularly revealing about the possible functions of such illusory filling-in.

Many recent studies on the general issue of filling-in have instead examined processing at blind spot regions in our visual field, which arise monocularly due to a small area in each retina where no receptors exist (e.g., Durgin et al., 1995; Chapter 9, this volume). The case of the retinal blind spot has provided a classic arena for many disputes about the nature of filling-in. Indeed, there has even been debate about whether or not the blind spot region does in fact get perceptually filled-in phenomenally with the color and brightness of surrounding regions despite the monocular absence of input. While some authors (e.g., Ramachandran and Gregory, 1991) accept that such phenomenal filling-in of color and brightness does occur, other authors have pointed out that instead, the absence of monocular input there might simply be ignored (e.g., Dennett, 1991). A third alternative might be that the unstimulated region is *sewn up*, such that its spatial extent is not represented perceptually (e.g., Durgin et al., 1995; Chapter 9, this volume).

The enduring controversy over even the basic phenomenology of filling-in at blind spot regions illustrates that, while the blind spot has been the focus of much useful work, it may not be an optimal candidate for studying filling-in. Blind spots arise in the peripheral visual field, where acuity is limited, so that some aspects of phenomenal perception are consequently hard to resolve. The ensuing lack of agreement over even the basic phenomenology of the blind spot region has hindered research in this area, and we argue here that other cases may provide less controversial examples for studying processes associated with phenomenal filling-in. In particular, phenomenally compelling examples of filling-in are associated with *modal-completion* processes that can be induced even for foveated regions of the visual scene, where the phenomenology at least is uncontroversial.

A well-known example can be experienced by viewing the pattern in Figure 7-1A. A central square transparent surface is perceived, appearing grayish in color throughout its extent. However, only the corner elements (where the square appears to overlap the circular elements) are actually printed. The rest of the phenomenal gray surface is illusory, with the grayness seen there providing a compelling example of phenomenal filling-in. This is one example of modal completion (Michotte et al., 1964), whereby several spatially separated fragments of the visual image are perceived to form parts of a single illusory visual surface. Critically, in such cases of modal completion, the intervening regions between the fragments become filled-in with illusory color determined by the flanking inducers.

The main question we address in this chapter is whether such filling-in of brightness and color, in cases of modal completion, is associated with any *functional* consequences beyond the production of the phenomenal illusion. What we mean by this may be illustrated by contrasting our approach with that of Kellman and Shipley (1992, p. 194), who suggested that while filling-in of brightness and color may affect the conscious phenomenology of perception for filled-in regions, this change in appearance is "superficial," having no significant impact on other perceptual or cognitive processes. Our position likewise contrasts with that of the British physicist Sir David Brewster (1832) in his classic discussion of filling-in for the blind spot case. He suggested that filling-in arose only to prevent "God's creation" being "imperfect" (due to lack of input at the retinal blind spot). In contrast with such rather nonfunctional views of filling-in, we are interested precisely in whether (for the specific case of modal completion) filling-in may have some useful function beyond the aesthetics of phenomenology for the observer (or, indeed, for any Creator!). As we discuss below, our recent research has suggested that filling-in for cases of modal completion may have some nontrivial functional consequences in addition to the impact on phenomenology.

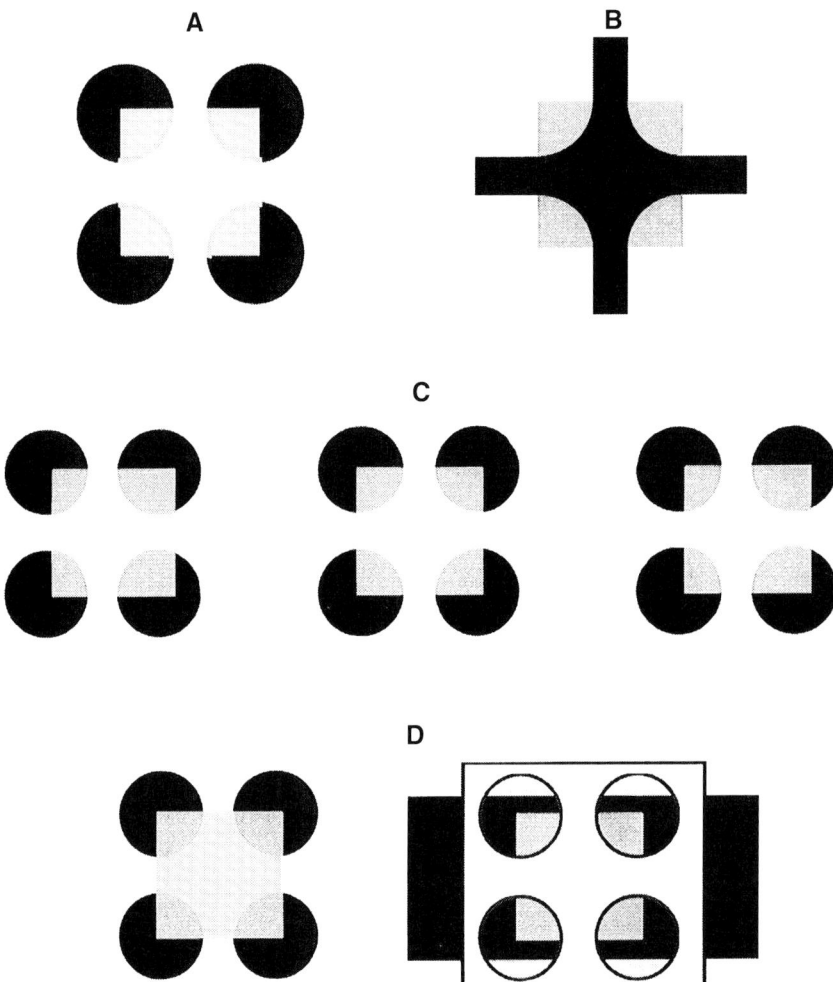

**Figure 7-1.** (A) Kanizsa rectangle pattern. Modal completion of the gray sectors yields perception of an illusory transparent gray square. (B) Pattern in which four gray sectors similar to those in (A) now undergo amodal completion behind an apparent occluder. (C) Patterns that can yield modal or amodal completion, depending upon the depth relations of the gray and black elements. If the left and central images are fused with uncrossed fusion (try this by focusing on an imaginary distant point between the two patterns), modal completion of the gray sectors will result in the front plane (appearance cartooned for nonfusers at the left of D). Alternatively if the central and right images are fused, the gray sectors are amodally completed in the back plane (appearance cartooned at the right of D). In the modal case, the gray sectors are perceived to form a transparent square overlapping four circles, with illusory gray perceived in the central region. In the amodal case, the sectors are perceived to form a partially occluded object, the visible parts of which appear as if viewed through apparent holes in the page. (D) Cartooned appearance of images in (C) when fused with uncrossed fusion. The left image in (D) illustrates the percept when the central and left images in (C) are fused. The right image in (D) illustrates the percept when the central and right images in (C) are fused.

## Modal versus Amodal Completion as a Comparison That Can Isolate Filling-In

Modal completion has two striking phenomenal characteristics that can be considered separately. First, one perceives an apparently complete *shape* on the basis of separate inducing fragments (e.g., a complete rectangle appears to be formed by the inducing pacmen in Fig. 7-1A). Second, the regions intervening between the separate inducers are phenomenally *filled-in* with illusory brightness and color that is determined by the inducers. We are concerned here with any functional effects associated with just the latter filling-in phenomena. As we noted earlier, while the term *filling-in* has been used by others to refer to a diverse range of phenomena (which may sometimes encompass shape completion of fragments), here we restrict our own usage to cases where illusory surface properties (e.g., color, brightness) are perceived in the regions between inducing fragments. This narrower definition can best be illustrated by a direct comparison of *modal* completion with another similar process termed *amodal* completion (see Fig. 7-1B).

Amodal completion occurs when several spatially separated elements in the visual input are perceived to form a single partly occluded shape. Figure 7-1B provides an example of amodal completion in which four gray elements are perceived to form parts of a single larger square that appears partly occluded by a cross shape. Note the similarity of this shape completion to the modal-completion case in Figure 7-1A. In both cases, similar inducing elements undergo shape completion to form a larger Gestalt from the fragments. This similarity between modal and amodal completion is further illustrated when the pairs of images in Figure 7-1C are fused with uncrossed fusion (see Fig. 7-1 legend). When the central and left images are fused in this manner, the gray segments in the fused image are modally completed to form a transparent rectangle in front of four circles (appearance cartooned for nonfusers in Fig. 7-1D, left). However, when the central and right images are fused, the four gray segments in the fused image are instead amodally completed as a partially occluded object, the corners of which appear to be visible as though seen through holes in the page (appearance cartooned in Fig. 7-1D, right). Note that the rightmost and leftmost images in Figure 7-1C are the same: It is only their spatial positioning relative to the central image (and hence the binocular disparity they can produce) that determines whether they fuse to yield modal or amodal completion. Kellman and Shipley (1992) recently showed that many of the stimulus constraints on shape completion are equivalent for modal and amodal completion (e.g., in terms of the spacing and alignment of inducing fragments that are required to form a strong percept of a complete shape). On the basis of such evidence, Kellman and Shipley proposed that modal and amodal completion are likely to reflect identical *shape-completion* processes.

However, despite such commonalities, modal and amodal completion still differ in the critical respect that illusory surface properties (e.g., color and brightness) get filled-in phenomenally only for the completed region in the case of modal completion, not for the case of amodal completion (e.g., compare Figs. 7-1A and 7-1B). Indeed, it was precisely this difference that originally led Michotte et al. (1964) to introduce the terms *modal completion* (i.e., inducing phenomenal illusions for properties specific to the visual *modality*, e.g., color/brightness) and *amodal completion* (inducing the impression of a completed shape, but one for which no properties seem visible in the completed region, given the apparent occlusion). Of course, cases of modal and amodal completion generally differ correspondingly in the depth relations that are apparent (i.e., a completed region in the front plane for the modal but not the amodal case). However, as will be shown later, by using appropriate control stimuli, this depth difference between modal and amodal completion can be factored out, independently of the difference in whether illusory brightness and color become filled-in phenomenally. Comparing modal and amodal completion directly can thus allow one to identify differences associated with the presence versus absence of color/brightness filling-in while using stimuli that are closely comparable in other respects and that both induce shape completion.

### Functional Roles That Seem Similar for Modal and Amodal Completion

On the above argument, any functions served equally by modal and amodal completion would not relate distinctively to the presence of filling-in (as we define it), since in our terms filling-in arises only for the modal case (see also Durgin et al., 1995). Functions that are common to modal and amodal completion may relate to shape-completion processes instead of filling-in. For example, both modal and amodal completion can integrate separate inducing elements into a single object (e.g., Kellman and Shipley, 1992), with objective consequences for judgments of the component parts (e.g., Mattingley et al., 1997; Behrmann et al., 1998). The filling-in that is specific to modal completion therefore seems tangential to these particular functional consequences.

As noted earlier, modal completion arises for completed regions that are perceived to be in front of the surrounding inducers, whereas amodal completion applies to apparently occluded regions. It might therefore be suggested that the filling-in specific to modal completion might play some functional role in representing one surface as overlapping in front of another, since this applies to modal but not amodal completion. While this remains a hypothetical possibility, we note that filling-in of illusory color and brightness, or of other surface properties, does not invariably seem required in order for one surface to be perceived as overlapping in front of another. In random-dot stereograms, for example, one can readily perceive one surface as overlapping in front of its background, even when there is no perceived or actual difference in color or brightness between these surfaces. One such example can be viewed by cross-fusing the left and right cruciform patches of dots in Figure 7-2A. When fused, these displays yield the percept of a horizontal bar that overlaps in front of a vertical bar. Note that the absence of filling-in does not seem to prevent this depth stratification from being perceived (see Michotte et al., 1964, for further examples in which surfaces are perceived to overlap in front of others without filling-in).

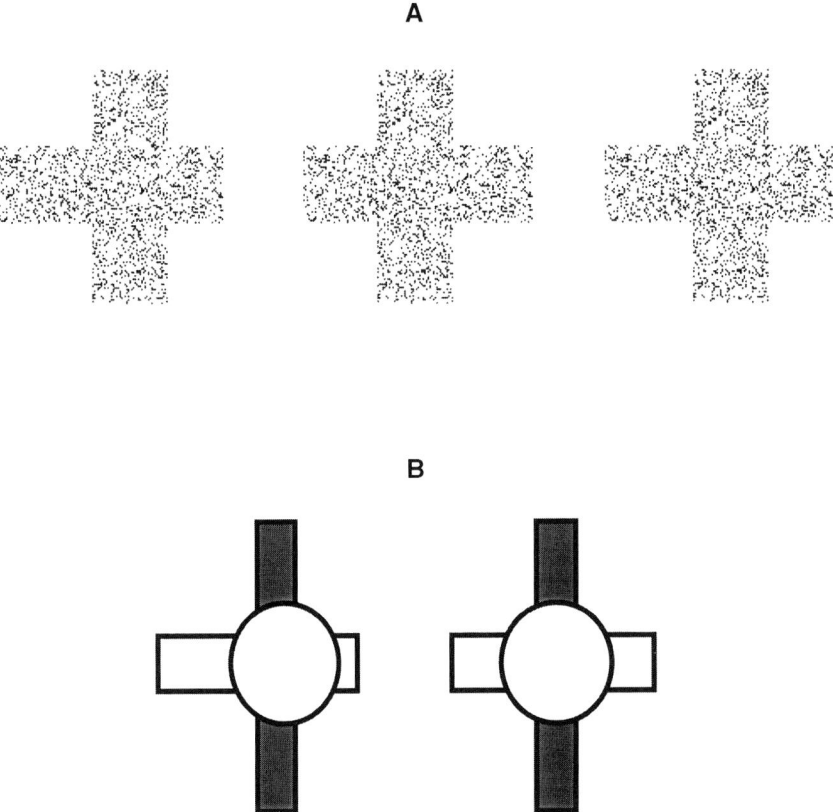

**Figure 7-2.** Two demonstrations that differences in perceived color between two overlapping surfaces are not required to see interposition in depth. (A) Fusing the left and central random-dot stereograms with uncrossed fusion (as for Figure 7-1C) yields the impression of a vertical bar in front of a horizontal bar, while fusing the central and right images in this manner causes the horizontal bar to appear nearer than the vertical bar. This perceived depth stratification at the overlap arises even though the horizontal and vertical bars have the same texture and colors. (B) Demonstration that one amodally completed surface can be perceived to overlap in front of another without the need for filling-in to arise at the region of overlap. Fusing the two images causes the clear impression of a vertical gray bar overlapping in front of a horizontal white bar, even though the region of overlap is entirely occluded from view by a circle and is thus perceived amodally (see text).

Note also that amodal completion (i.e., with no filling-in, in our terms) can arise for a surface that is perceived as overlapping in front of another. One example of this occurs when three apparent surfaces are perceived: an unoccluded surface at the front, which partially occludes a second surface at intermediate depth, which in turn partially occludes a third apparent surface in the back plane, as in Figure 7-2B, when stereo-fused (see also Kellman and Shipley, 1992). The intermediate amodally completed surface can be perceived as overlapping in front of the amodally completed surface at the back, even within the completed area (Fig. 7-2B). This provides some suggestive phenomenal evidence that filling-in of color and brightness is not required for one surface to be perceived as overlapping in front of another (though it may prove useful to corroborate this with objective measures in addition to phenomenology).

A further candidate function for the filling-in seen in modal completion might in principle relate to the processing of color and/or brightness itself. That is, the filling-in might reflect mechanisms that, in daily life, serve to extract the likely color and brightness properties of external surfaces, given the current input. These same mechanisms may produce illusory colors and brightnesses under the particular experimental conditions that induce modal completion (e.g., see Nakayama and Shimojo, 1992). Such mechanisms might in principle not apply to the completed region in the amodal case, precisely because this region appears occluded and so should have no visible color and brightness (i.e., the surface properties projected to the retina in this region should be those of the occluder instead). However, Watanabe (1995) has provided some suggestive evidence that color may be represented in the brain to some extent, even for *amodally* completed regions. He studied McCullough aftereffects, which are driven by exposure to specific combinations of color and orientation. Such an effect was found from the occluded region of amodally completed stimuli, even though no filled-in color was perceived there phenomenally.

Thus, cases of amodal and modal completion do not seem to differ in the shape-completion processes that are induced and in the functional consequences of these processes. Nor does the filling-in specific to modal completion seem required for one surface to be perceived as extending in front of another. Finally, while modal and amodal completion undoubtedly induce different color and brightness qualia, some evidence from McCollough orientation–specific color aftereffects suggests that a form of color representation may arise even for amodally completed regions in the human visual system (Watanabe, 1995). Thus, some of the most obvious candidates for a functional difference between modal and amodal completion seem less clear-cut when considered further.

In the remainder of this chapter, we focus on very different functional effects; potential differences between modal and amodal completion in terms of their relation to *visual attention*. We first review evidence from visual-search studies. These have suggested that both amodal and modal completion may arise within *parallel vision* (i.e., without serial attentive inspection of each element in a scene) and that they may do so automatically, even when against the observer's will. We then present preliminary evidence that modal and amodal completion may be differentiated in such parallel vision. Finally, we describe experiments showing that spreading of attention from inducing regions to completed regions (or vice versa) can differ significantly between otherwise comparable cases of modal versus amodal completion. This work demonstrates that the functional effects of modal and amodal completion on attention can indeed differ, in a manner that relates to the presence or absence of filling-in.

## Literature Review

### Modal and Amodal Completion in Visual-Search Tasks

In visual search, observers have to report the presence or absence of a target that is distinguishable from accompanying nontargets on the basis of one property or a combination of properties (e.g., Treisman and Gelade, 1980; Wolfe, 1998). In some cases (e.g., when the target and nontargets are of distinct colors), the time taken to determine the target's presence hardly alters as the number of nontargets in a display is augmented (yielding shallow *search slopes* when search time is plotted against number of items in a display). This effect, termed *pop-out*, can provide an index of properties that can be derived efficiently in parallel for many items in a display at once. If a particular property can either facilitate or prevent pop-out, it is held to be derived in parallel, without the need for serial attentional scrutiny

Treisman and Gelade's (1980) influential feature-integration theory suggested, in its original form, that only simple physical properties (e.g., two-dimensional [2D] orientation of edges) were extracted in parallel, but much subsequent research has shown that more complex properties can also influence target pop-out (see Wolfe, 1998). Among these more recent studies are several that have addressed whether or not modal and amodal completion can arise in parallel. In one pioneering study, He and Nakayama (1992) examined visual search for shapes that could undergo amodal completion with unrestricted viewing. Observers searched for a white L-shaped target (Figure 7-3A, left) among reversed-L nontargets (Fig. 7-3A, right). The stereoscopically induced depth of the white L and reversed-L shapes was manipulated relative to their abutting black squares. When the L and reversed-L shapes in the patterns appeared farther away than the abutting square, they could be amodally completed to yield the percept of a white square appearing partly occluded by the abutting black square. The left image in Figure 7-3B cartoons the appearance of an L-shaped pattern with unrestricted viewing under this depth arrangement. While the L shape appeared to be a complete, partly occluded square, no illusory white color is apparent in the completed region; rather, the occluded region of the perceived square (indicated by the shaded region in the figure) is perceived amodally with unrestricted viewing. However, such amodal completion could not arise when the L and reversed-L shapes appeared nearer than the black square (appearance cartooned in Fig. 7-3B, right). Moreover, the luminance configuration was inconsistent with modal completion in this depth arrangement, as explained later.

He and Nakayama (1992) reported that when the L and reversed-L shapes were nearer than the abutting squares in stereoscopic depth, the search for an L target was highly efficient and parallel, as indicated by the shallow search slopes. However, when both the L and reversed-L shapes appeared farther away than the black squares (and thus could both become amodally completed to yield partly occluded white squares), the search for the target L shape became highly inefficient, yielding steep search slopes. The latter result is consistent with amodal

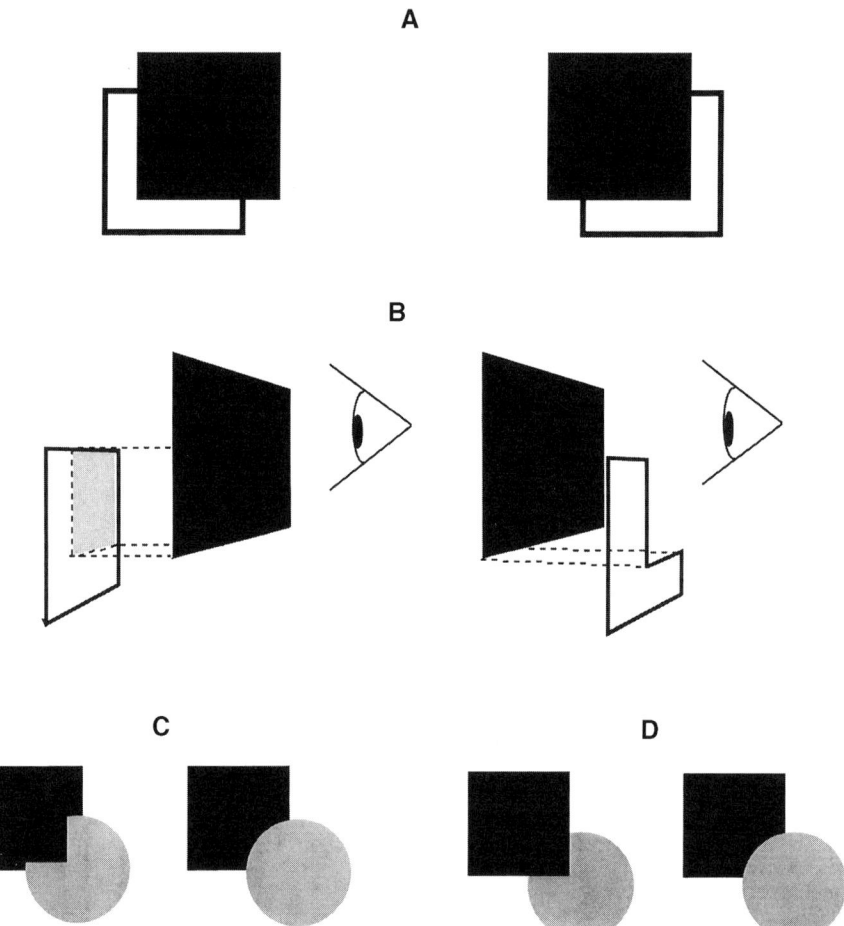

**Figure 7-3.** Example target and nontarget stimuli employed in visual-search studies of preattentive amodal completion. (A) Typical target (left) and nontarget (right) items employed by He and Nakayama (1992). (B) Cartoon of manipulation of depth relations by He and Nakayama. When the white L shape in each pattern is perceived to be farther away than the black square, with unrestricted viewing it becomes amodally completed to form a white square (left image); the amodally perceived region of the completed square is indicated by the shaded area in the figure. However, when the L shape appears nearer than the black square, it is not completed (right image). (C) Target (left) and nontarget (right) items employed by Rensink and Enns (1998) in a control study. Here the notched circle in the target can be searched for in parallel among whole-circle distractor items (right), popping out even when hidden among many of the latter. The stimuli in (D) utilize the same elements as (C), but with a change in the spatial relations between the black and gray elements such that the notched circle in the target can now be amodally completed to form a circle that appears partly occluded. With this alteration, the target cannot now be searched for in parallel, suggesting that the gray notched circle was amodally completed at preattentive stages of vision to form a whole (albeit partly occluded) circle that was then hard to distinguish from distractors like the example on the right in (D) (see text).

completion arising in parallel to make the L target and reversed-L nontargets now appear more similar to each other (i.e., both appearing as partly occluded white squares). These results therefore suggest that amodal completion can arise in parallel vision, because targets that led to efficient parallel search in the absence of amodal completion became much harder to find when amodal completion could arise in the displays. Note also that the presumed amodal completion produced its effect even though the prescribed task was to search for the "incomplete shape" (i.e., the L among reversed L's) that was physically present in the retinal image. This implies that amodal completion may arise automatically, even when its effects are highly detrimental to the prescribed task and against the intentions of the subject (see also Davis and Driver, 1998a; Driver et al., 2001). Rensink and Enns (1998) have extended and corroborated these conclusions using 2D displays that induced amodal completion via pictorial rather than stereoscopic cues to relative depth (see Fig. 7-3D).

Such results from visual search thus suggest that amodal completion can arise in parallel, within *preattentive* vision and may do so automatically. Results of searches involving modal rather than amodal completion initially suggested that a different result might apply for the modal case; but as we shall see, the eventual conclusion was that the two forms of completion behave similarly in visual search. Grabowecky and Treisman (1989) required subjects to search for Kanizsa triangles (a classic case of modal completion; Fig. 7-4A, left) induced by appropriately aligned pacman figures, among varying numbers of nontarget items made from rearrangements of similar pacmen (see Fig. 7-4A, right). They reported inefficient, apparently serial search. However, Davis and Driver (1994) subsequently argued that Grabowecky and Treisman's experiment may not have been optimal for observing parallel results for several reasons (including the sudden onset of many luminance edges that might potentially disrupt the impact of subjective edges and the possible influence of alignments between pacmen from different nontargets). Davis and Driver refined the paradigm and observed clear pop-out for pacman clusters that would be expected to induce a modally completed subjective square (Fig. 7-4B, left) among pacman clusters that should not (Fig. 7-4B, right). When arcs were added to the inducing pacmen of the target and nontargets (Fig. 7-4C, left and right, respectively) to preclude the formation of a modally complete square, pop-out no longer occurred. Additional control conditions suggested further that the pop-out effect found when modal completion could arise for the target item was not merely due to blurring at low spatial frequencies.

However, these results remained susceptible to further criticisms (e.g., see Gurnsey et al., 1996; Davis and Driver, 1998a) relating to the possibility that the search might have been based on some other property that distinguished the target (e.g., the configuration of the inducing elements themselves) rather than on the formation of a modally completed illusory square. Moreover, since the subjects' task in Davis and Driver's (1994) experiment was to look for a subjective square, the results could not in any case demonstrate that these are formed automatically (i.e., even when counter to the subjects' intentions, as in the search

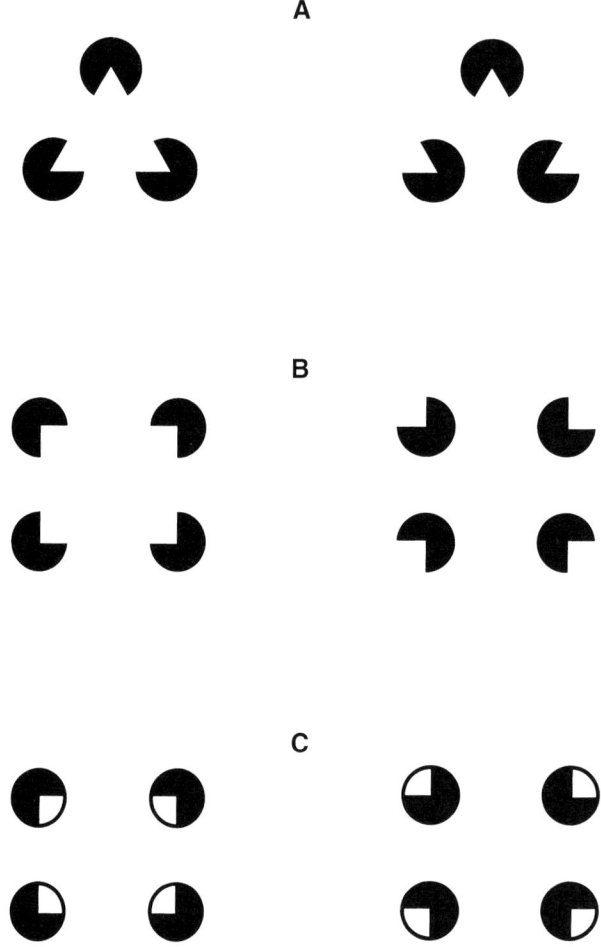

**Figure 7-4.** Example target and nontarget stimuli from visual-search studies of preattentive modal completion. (A) Target (left) and nontarget stimuli employed by Grabowecky and Treisman (1989). (B) Target (left) and nontarget stimuli employed by Davis and Driver (1994). (C) Target (left) and nontarget stimuli employed in a control experiment by Davis and Driver (1994).

experiments on amodal completion). Finally, there was at most only one modally completable stimulus in Davis and Driver's (1994) displays, so the results could not assess whether multiple stimuli can modally complete in parallel.

Davis and Driver (1998) addressed all these points in experiments that followed up the previous search studies of *amodal* completion (e.g., He and Nakayama, 1992), but now testing whether *modally* complete surfaces could serve as apparent occluders to induce amodal-completion effects in parallel vision. The logic behind the experiments was based upon that of He and Nakayama (1992) and Rensink and Enns (1998) but in addition involved modally completable stimuli. In the studies of He and Nakayama (Figs. 7-3A and 7-3B), or Rensink and Enns (Figs. 7-3C and 7-3D), *physically present* squares in the front plane had induced amodal completion to reduce search efficiency against the subjects' intentions. Davis and Driver (1998) tested whether a *modally completed* subjective square might analogously act as an occluder to induce unwanted amodal completion of an abutting notched target, just as the real squares do in Figure 7-3D.

Similarly to the search tasks employed by Rensink and Enns (1998; see Figs. 7-3C and 7-3D), observers again searched for a notched circle among complete circles. Smaller pacman stimuli were now arranged so as to produce possible subjective squares that might serve as occluders in the critical conditions (see Fig. 7-5A, left). Search slopes for the large notched circle in the target cluster, among large full circles in the nontarget clusters (e.g., Fig. 7-5A, right), were steep (indicating inefficient search) when these appeared stereoscopically *behind* the potential subjective surfaces but were shallow (indicating target pop-out) when they appeared in front. A target item in which the notched circle appeared behind (so that it can be amodally completed behind the modally completed figure) can be seen by fusing the left and central images in Figure 7-5B, with uncrossed fusion (the resulting appearance for nonfusers is cartooned in Fig. 7-5C, left). A target item with the notched circle appearing in front instead can be viewed by fusing the central and right images of Figure 7-5B in the same manner (appearance cartooned in Fig.7-5C, right). Various control conditions confirmed that a difficult search was specific to apparent occlusion of the notched targets by modally completed squares rather than simply to searching in the back plane. Moreover, these control conditions also ruled out trivial accounts of the effect of the modally completed squares in terms of low spatial-frequency blurring or the mere alignment of inducing edges with the notched circle target.

Analogously to the results of He and Nakayama (1992) and Rensink and Enns (1998), these findings imply that amodal completion (of the notched target) can occur in parallel vision and may do so even when counter to the observer's intention. Davis and Driver's (1998) data further suggest that both of these assertions apply also to the formation of subjective squares via *modal* completion. Such subjective squares can act as occluders in parallel vision, and do so even when this is highly detrimental to search performance.

Taken together, all these search results imply that both amodal and modal completion may arise within parallel vision without requiring serial attentional scrutiny of the inducing stimuli. Moreover, they can do so automatically, even when counter to the observer's intentions and the prescribed task. These search results therefore demonstrate some objective consequences of modal and amodal completion for performance, but thus far, these consequences have not differed for the two forms of completion. Indeed, these visual search results might instead be added to the long list of similarities between the two forms of completion (modal and amodal), as previously articulated by Kellman and Shipley

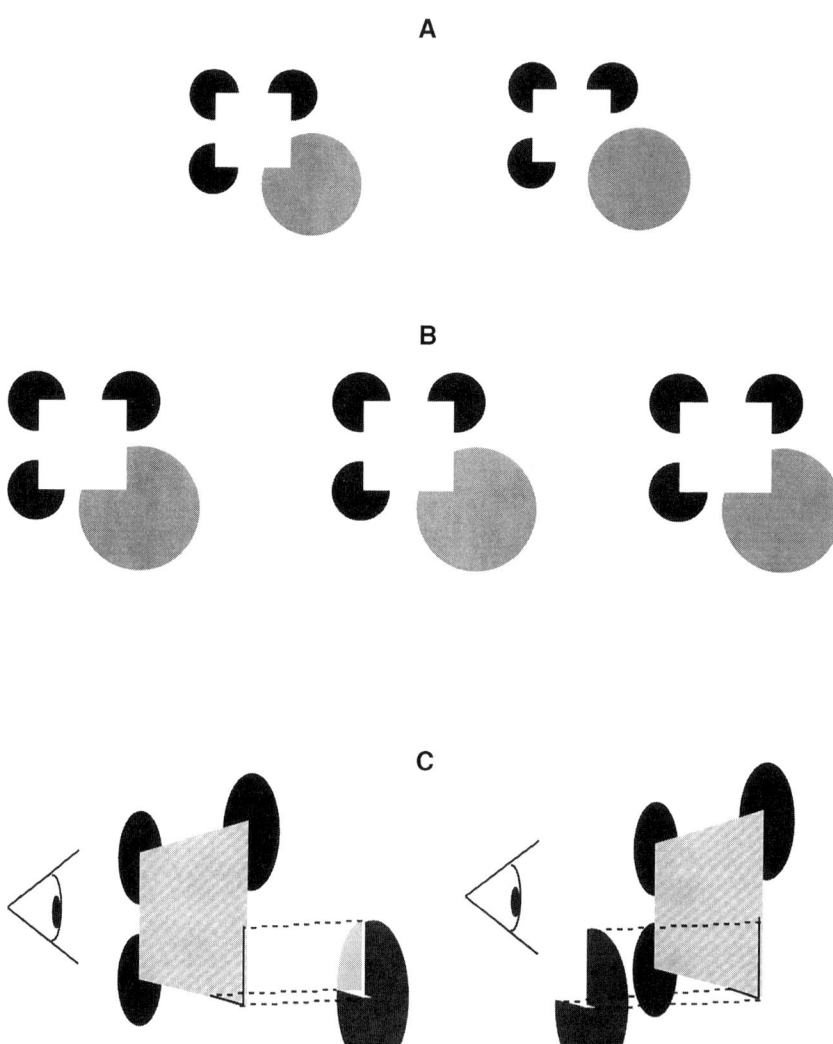

**Figure 7-5.** (A) Target (left) and nontarget stimuli employed by Davis and Driver (1998). (B) Illustration of manipulation of depth relations by Davis and Driver (1998a). When the left and central patterns of the stimuli are fused with uncrossed fusion, the gray notched circle appears farther away than the black pacmen elements and the modally completed square. Under these conditions, the gray notched circle appears, with unrestricted viewing, to be amodally completed as a complete circle that is partially occluded by the illusory modally completed square (appearance cartooned in C, left). However, when instead the central and right images are fused, the gray notched circle appears nearer than the modally completed white square, so the gray notched circle can no longer become amodally completed to form a complete, partly occluded circle (appearance cartooned in C, right).

(1992). However, we now turn to a recent search study that found some initial evidence that modal and amodal completion can in fact sometimes have differential effects within parallel vision, affecting search performance in different ways. In this experiment, we took advantage of a well-established subjective difference between modal and amodal completion related to the perception of transparency.

Kanizsa (1979) and Van Tuijl and De Weert (1979) demonstrated that for simple patterns comprising three luminance levels, *modal* completion of transparent subjective figures is constrained by the luminance profile of the inducing stimuli in a way that *amodal* completion is not (see also Nakayama and Shimojo, 1992). We will refer to this constraint as the *Metelli Rule*, since it stems from Metelli's (1974) description of the luminance conditions constraining transparency perception. In order for the elements of an inducing stimulus to form part of a transparent, modally completed surface, the luminance of these inducing elements must fall between the luminance of the surround and the luminance of the inner region over which the subjective figure is formed. For example, the stimulus in Figure 7-6A satisfies these constraints. The luminance of the four small gray sectors on the otherwise black circles falls between that of the white inner region and the black surround of the circles. These gray sectors can therefore be seen to form part of a transparent, modally completed surface. However, the stimulus in Figure 7-6B fails to satisfy Metelli Rule's prescription for the luminance relations. The luminance of the small, dark sectors on the otherwise gray circles does *not* fall between the luminance level of the gray surrounding regions and the white inner region, being less than both. Thus, the dark sectors cannot form parts of a modally completed transparent surface.

This dependence of modal completion upon the luminance profile of the stimulus makes functional sense when one considers the optics of transparent surfaces (see Metelli, 1974; Nakayama and Shimojo, 1992) and also that modal completion processes may serve to encode partly camouflaged surfaces (e.g., Ramachandran, 1987; Davis and Driver, 1994); see Driver et al. (2001) for further discussion. However, the critical point for our purposes is that the Metelli transparency constraint does *not* apply to amodal completion, as that concerns apparently occluded surfaces rather than apparently transparent surfaces in the front plane (e.g., Kanizsa, 1979; Nakayama and Shimojo, 1992). For example, the two notched-ring elements at the far left of Figures 7-6D and 7-6E are both amodally completed to form complete rings that appear partially occluded by the abutting rectangles, even though the luminance configuration in 7-6E is not compatible with the Metelli Rule.

In a new series of studies, we recently tested (Davis et al., in prep; see also Driver et al., 2001) whether the Metelli constraint on modal but not amodal completion arises differentially within the parallel vision tapped by appropriate search tasks. Subjects searched for notched rings (i.e., like those in Figs. 7-6D and 7-6E) among physically complete unnotched rings in four different search conditions. The luminance profile of the displays was either consistent (Fig. 7-6D) or inconsistent (Fig. 7-6E) with the Metelli Rule, and orthogonally to this, stereo

142  Fast-Acting Filling-In in Normal Vision

disparity was arranged so that all the rings lay either farther away than the rectangles or nearer than them. When the rings appeared farther away, the notched rings could be *amodally* completed to form complete rings (with unrestricted viewing) irrespective of whether the luminance profile was inconsistent or consistent with the Metelli Rule. Impressions of typical target items with this depth arrangement can be perceived by free fusing (with uncrossed fusion, as for previous figures) the left and central images of Figures 7-6D or 7-6E. In both Figure 7-6D (luminance profile consistent with the Metelli Rule) and Figure 7-6E

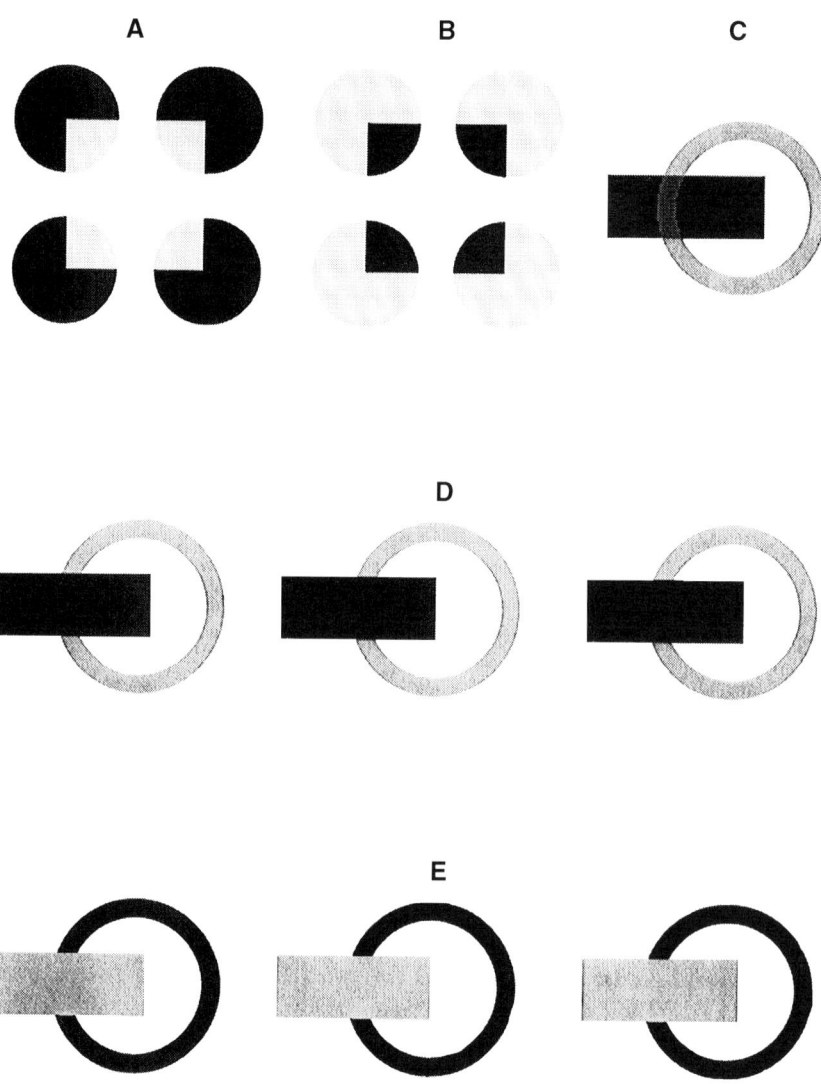

# Effects of Modal versus Amodal Completion Upon Visual Attention 143

(luminance profile inconsistent with the Metelli Rule), the notched ring element appears amodally completed to form a complete, partially occluded ring. However, in two further conditions, where the rings now appeared nearer, notched rings could only be *modally* completed to form a modally complete ring (appearance cartooned in Fig. 7-6C) when the luminance configuration was consistent with the Metelli Rule (free-fuse the central and right images of Fig. 7-6D). When the luminance profile was inconsistent with the Metelli Rule, no modal completion could occur and the ring thus appeared as a notched circle (as can be perceived by free-fusing the central and right images of Fig. 7-6E).

The results showed efficient parallel search (i.e., pop-out of the notched target) only when the rings lay in the front plane with a luminance profile that was *inconsistent* with the Metelli Rule (Fig. 7-6E, fusing the central and right images; no completion of the notched ring takes place). In the other three conditions, inefficient search with steep search slopes was found. The implication is that in these latter three conditions, completion of the notched target arose in parallel vision (thus making it hard to distinguish from the physically complete, unnotched nontarget rings), even though this was highly detrimental to performance

**Figure 7-6.** Demonstrations of the Metelli Rule applying to cases of modal but not amodal completion. (A) Kanizsa pattern in which the four gray inner sectors are modally completed to form a transparent gray rectangle. Note that modal completion can occur in this pattern because the luminance of the gray sectors falls between that of the black pacmen and the white background. (B) Same pattern as in (A) except that the luminances of the inner segments and pacmen are now reversed. Now the luminance of the inner sectors does not fall between the luminance of the three-quarter circles and of the background, breaking the Metelli Rule. Consequently, the inner segments are *not* modally completed to form a single transparent square. (C) Cartooned phenomenal appearance of a typical target item employed by Davis et al. (in prep.), in which the notched circle appeared nearer than the rectangle and the luminance profile is consistent with the Metelli Rule. Under such conditions, the notched ring element is modally completed as a complete ring with unrestricted viewing, with the region where the ring and rectangle overlapped becoming filled-in with illusory gray color. (D) Typical target stimuli in which the luminance profile is consistent with the Metelli Rule. When the central and left images are fused with uncrossed fusion, the notched-ring element in the fused image appears farther away than the rectangle and is amodally completed to form a complete ring. When, instead, the central and right images are fused, the notched ring appears nearer than the rectangle and is modally completed. In the modal completion case, the region where the perceived ring and rectangle overlap is filled-in with illusory gray (cartooned in 6C). (E) Typical target stimuli in which the luminance profile is inconsistent with the Metelli Rule. When the central and left images are fused with uncrossed fusion, the notched-ring element in the fused image appears farther away than the rectangle and is still amodally completed to form a complete ring (as amodal completion is insensitive to the Metelli Rule with unrestricted viewing). However, when, the central and right images are fused, the notched ring appears nearer than the rectangle but cannot be modally completed, as the luminance profile is inconsistent with the Metelli Rule (and modal completion is constrained by the Metelli Rule).

and thus counter to the observer's intentions. Amodal completion (of notched circles apparently lying behind the abutting rectangles) was unaffected by the Metelli constraints. By contrast, modal completion (i.e., of notched circles lying in front of the abutting rectangles) was highly dependent on the Metelli Rule even in parallel vision, taking place only when the luminance profile was consistent with the constraints on perception of a subjective transparent surface. When the Metelli Rule was violated, no modal completion took place, so the target popped out as the only incomplete ring in the display.

These results indicate that the Metelli Rule for the perception of transparency, which relates to the real-world optics of transparent surfaces (see Driver et al., 2001), can operate within parallel vision as tapped by appropriate visual-search tasks. Moreover, the data suggest that modal versus amodal completion may operate according to different constraints within such parallel vision, in a manner consistent with the differential impact of the Metelli Rule on phenomenology that is apparent when each item is inspected in an unspeeded manner with free vision (see Fig. 7-6).

In sum, the visual-search findings reviewed above suggest that both modal and amodal completion may arise within parallel vision, even when counter to the observer's intention. Moreover, recent results provide preliminary evidence that the two forms of completion may be subject to different constraints (in relation to the Metelli Rule) even at this level of vision. On conventional interpretations of visual search data, these results would be taken to indicate that modal and amodal completion can both arise preattentively (i.e., in parallel for many objects at once, without requiring serial attentional scrutiny, even when counter to intentions) and also that they may be differentiated preattentively. In our final review section, we consider whether the two forms of completion may have different impacts upon the distribution of attention.

## *Differential Impact of Modal versus Amodal Completion on the Spreading of Attention*

Many studies have indicated that segmentation of visual input into distinct perceptual *objects* or surfaces can constrain how our attention is spatially allocated within a given scene (e.g., Duncan, 1984; Egly et al., 1994; see Lavie and Driver, 1996, for review). In particular, when attention is cued to one part of a perceptual object or visible surface, attention may typically *spread* to incorporate all of it (e.g., Egly et al., 1994; He and Nakayama, 1995; Behrmann et al., 1998; Braun and Snowden, 2000). Attention may likewise spread to spatially separate items with a similar color or brightness (e.g., Baylis and Driver, 1993).

This tendency for attention to spread between regions belonging to the same visible object or surface, and to grouped items with similar surface properties, led us to predict differential patterns of attention-spreading across modally versus amodally completed surfaces. For the example of amodal completion shown in Figure 7-7A, three spatially separated gray fragments are perceived to form a single elliptical gray surface that is occluded near the center by two white bars.

Effects of Modal versus Amodal Completion Upon Visual Attention    145

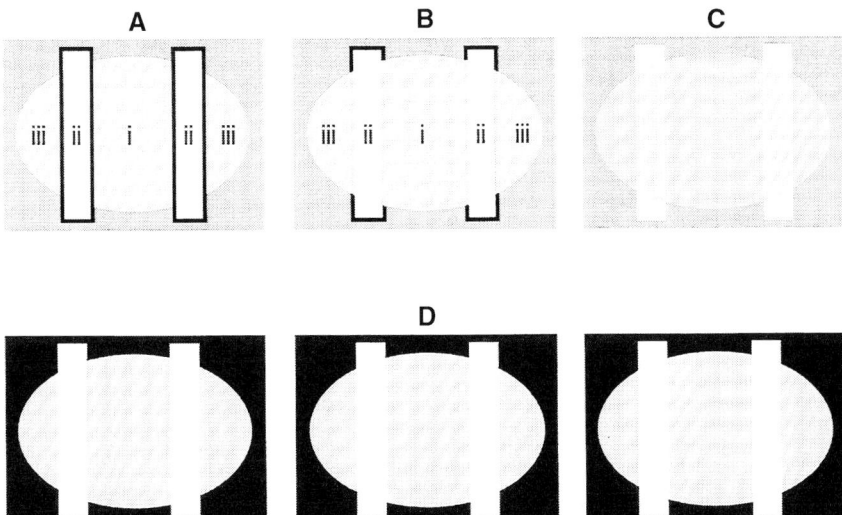

**Figure 7-7.** (A) The gray sectors in the image are amodally completed to form a partially occluded ellipse. No filling-in occurs where the perceived ellipse overlaps with the white bars. (B) Similar stimulus to (A) in which the sectors now undergo modal completion to form a transparent ellipse overlapping in front of the white bars. Here, filling-in *does* occur where the perceived ellipse overlaps with the white bars. (C) Cartoon of the phenomenal appearance of the modally completed ellipse, and the associated filling-in perceived where the ellipse overlapped with the two white bars in Davis and Driver's (1997) experiments. (D) When the left and central images are fused with uncrossed fusion, the gray elements appear farther away than the white bars and are amodally completed to form a partially occluded ellipse: There is no filling-in where the ellipse and bars overlap. However, when instead the central and right images are fused, the gray sectors now appear nearer than the white bars and are modally completed as a transparent ellipse. Now the regions where the ellipse overlaps with the bars are filled-in with illusory color (as cartooned in C).

If attention were cued to the central gray sector (labeled *i* in the figure), then based on the attention-spreading experiments described above, one might expect attention to spread readily to the left and right gray regions (each labeled *iii*), since these regions appear to form part of a single surface and have the same physical color and brightness as the central gray sector. Indeed, recent evidence from attention-cueing studies with amodally completed stimuli has documented an effect of exactly this type (e.g., Moore et al., 1998; Braun and Snowden, 2000; see also Mattingley et al., 1997, for a neuropsychological analog). A similar spreading of attention would be expected for an analogous case of modal completion, such as that shown in Figure 7-7B. If attention was cued to the central gray sector (again labeled *i* in the figure), then it would be expected to spread to the left and right gray sectors also (labeled *iii*), which again appear to belong to the same perceptual surface and have the same physical color. Neuropsychological evidence consistent with this was found by Mattingley et al. (1997).

Attention-spreading between the *physically present fragments* inducing a completed shape may therefore be similar for modally and amodally completed surfaces. But the critical question for our present concerns is whether the two cases might differ for attention-spreading from the physically present segment to the *completed region* of each shape (i.e., to the regions labeled *ii* in Figs. 7-7A and 7-7B). Davis and Driver (1997, 1998b) examined this question in several experiments. They used displays like those in Figure 7-7 (note: the numerals were not presented), but with a manipulation of stereoscopic depth. An example of the stimulus eliciting amodal completion can be viewed by cross-fusing the left and central patterns of Figure 7-7D; and an example of the modal-completion stimulus can be seen by cross-fusing its right and central patterns. Note that these modal and amodal stimuli are identical in 2D structure, differing only in terms of the perceived depth of the vertical white bars. When the white bars appear closer to the observer than the gray regions abutting them, the gray regions become amodally completed as a gray ellipse partly occluded by the bars. Note that there is no filling-in of illusory color/brightness where the perceived ellipse falls behind the bar. However, when the bars instead appear farther away than the gray segments, observers see a modally completed transparent ellipse that apparently overlaps in front of the white bars. Critically, in contrast to the amodal-completion stimulus, filled-in illusory gray coloring is now perceived at the central region where the ellipse and bars overlap (appearance cartooned in Fig. 7-7C). Thus, filling-in of illusory color/brightness takes place for the completed region only in the *modally* completed case, not in the otherwise comparable amodal case, as we have emphasised throughout this chapter.

What Davis and Driver (1997, 1998b) found, using the methods summarized below, was that when attention is cued or directed to the central, physically present gray fragment of an *amodally completed* surface (e.g., region *i* in Fig. 7-7A), it does not spread to the completed regions of that surface (labeled *ii* in the figure), which yield no filling-in of illusory color/brightness. By contrast, such spreading is found for the completed region (again, region *ii*) in the *modally completed* case, in which filling-in does occur. An analogous difference was also found for the reverse direction of attention-spreading (i.e., from the completed region to the inducing fragments, which again occurred for modal but not amodal completion). Thus, the presence or absence of filling-in (i.e., in modal but not amodal completion) was associated with a corresponding presence versus absence of attention-spreading between inducing regions and completed regions.

Davis and Driver (1997) demonstrated this using measures of distractor interference. In one study, we placed a target character on the central gray sector and distractor characters on the white bars on either side of it. Subjects were instructed to attend just to the central gray region, as that was where the target character would appear, while trying not to let their attention spread to the completed regions of the ellipse (i.e., where the ellipse and bars overlapped), as that was where the distractor characters would appear. Using the effects of target–distractor congruence upon reaction time (RT) as an index of attention-spreading to the ellipse's completed region (with larger congruent effects implying more attention spreading, i.e., less effective exclusion of the distractors from performance), we found that distractors produced more interference in the modal-completion condition than in the amodal-completion condition. This suggested that when observers tried to attend just to the central gray sector of the modally completed ellipse (see Fig. 7-7C), their attention also spread to neighboring, completed areas of the ellipse where filling-in was present (e.g., the regions labeled *ii* in Fig. 7-7B). This spreading of attention to completed regions did not occur to the same extent for amodal completion, where no filling-in took place.

To ensure that the differential attention-spreading found in modal versus amodal completion conditions was indeed associated with the presence of filling-in for modal completion only, rather than just with the difference in depth relations between the two cases, we also conducted additional control experiments. These new studies replicated exactly the conditions in our original experiment (including an identical manipulation of depth relations between the bars and gray segments), except that there was now a narrow gap between the gray segments and white bars in each display. This gap prevented any modal or amodal completion of an ellipse, irrespective of depth. We now found no difference between the two depth arrangements, suggesting that depth alone could not account for the greater spreading of attention for modal stimuli in our original experiment.

In another set of studies (Davis and Driver, 1998b) we made a similar point, but now using a different attentional measure. We cued attention to the bars, or to the physically present gray segments of the ellipse, by transiently altering their shape. We then measured the effect of this cueing on RT to subsequent target characters, which could be presented either on physically present or completed regions. In the modal-completion condition, the results suggested that cueing the physically gray segments of the ellipse attracted attention to its completed (illusory gray) regions also, whereas in the amodal-completion case this did not occur. Control stimuli, with gaps to prevent completion, again showed that this effect was not due to differences in depth per se between modal and amodal cases, but rather was associated with the presence of filling-in for the modal case only.

These experiments on attention-spreading thus show that filling-in of illusory color/brightness in the case of modal completion, but not amodal completion, is associated with differential effects on the distribution of attention in objective performance tasks. Modal and amodal completion may be similar in many other respects (e.g., the shape-completion processes they induce may indeed be identical, as Kellman and Shipley [1992] and others have suggested). Nevertheless, they can differ in their functional consequences, in a manner that seems to be associated with the important phenomenal difference between them, in terms of the presence versus absence of illusory filling-in for the completed regions.

## Discussion

We have suggested that a close comparison of modal versus amodal completion may be particularly revealing regarding the possible functions of filling in, since the two forms of completion are highly similar in many respects (e.g., in terms of the inducing stimuli and in the shape completion they induce, just as Kellman and Shipley [1992] emphasized), yet they differ dramatically in terms of whether illusory surface properties are perceived phenomenally in the completed region. Here we have focused on possible functional differences between modal and amodal completion in relation to visual attention. A review of visual-search experiments suggests that both modal and amodal completion may arise preattentively, that is, at parallel stages of vision, and even when counter to the observer's intentions. However, the two forms of completion may then differ in their effect upon attention, with attention tending to spread between inducing fragments and completed regions only for the case of modal completion, for which filling-in arises in the completed region.

Filling-in may serve to mark the completed region as potentially visible, and thus of potential relevance to the observer whenever the inducing fragments (that appear to belong to the same visible surface) attract attention. A real-world example of this might arise when highly visible parts of an animal attract attention, while better-camouflaged (but still resolvable) regions of the same animal appear less salient but should also be attended to. By contrast, when the visible fragments of an amodally completed object attract attention, the completed regions are occluded and thus can only project information about the occluder. This occluder may be an irrelevant object that is quite unrelated to the occludee (e.g., a tree in front of the animal), and so should not necessarily be attended to jointly with the latter. Whether or not these proposals turn out to be correct in detail, our existing results already show that there are some objective functional consequences to the difference between modal and amodal completion. The presence of filling-in, for the modal case only, does not seem to be merely a superficial difference in illusory phenomenal appearance, but rather a difference with very real functional effects.

*Acknowledgments*

This work was supported by the Royal Society and the BBSRC (UK). JD holds a Royal Society-Wolfson Research Merit award. GD holds a Royal Society Research Fellowship.

## References

Baylis G and Driver J (1993) Visual attention and objects: Evidence for hierarchical coding of location. *J Exp Psychol (Hum Percept)* 19:451–470.

Behrmann M, Zemel R, and Mozer M (1998) Object-based attention and occlusion: Evidence from normal participants and a computational model. *J Exp Psychol (Hum Percept)* 24:1011–1036.

Braun P and Snowden R (2000) Attention to overlapping objects: Detection and discrimination of luminance changes. *J Exp Psychol (Hum Percept)* 26:342–358.

Brewster D (1832) *Letters in Natural Magic.* London: John Murray.

Davis G and Driver J (1994) Parallel detection of Kanizsa subjective figures in the human visual system. *Nature* 371:791–793.

Davis G and Driver J (1997) Spreading of visual attention across modally versus amodally completed surfaces. *Psychol Sci* 8:275–281.

Davis G and Driver J (1998a) Kanizsa subjective figures can act as occluding surfaces in preattentive human vision. *J Exp Psychol (Hum Percept)* 24:169–184.

Davis G and Driver J (1998b) A functional rôle for filling-in in the control of visual attention. *Perception* 26:1397–1411.

Dennett DC (1991) *Consciousness Explained.* Boston: Little, Brown, and Company.

Driver J, Davis G, Russell C, Turatto M, and Freeman E (2001) Segmentation attention and phenomenal visual objects. *Cognition* 80:61–95.

Duncan J (1984) Selective attention and the organisation of visual information. *J Exp Psychol (Gen)* 113:501–517.

Durgin FH, Tripathy SP, and Levi DM (1995) On the filling in of the blind spot: Some rules of thumb. *Perception* 24:827–840.

Egly R, Driver J, and Rafal R (1994) Shifting visual attention between objects and locations: Normality and pathology. *J Exp Psychol (Gen)* 123:161–177

Grabowecky M and Toeisman A (1989) Attention and fixation in subjective contour perception. *Investigative Opthalmology and Visual Science* 30:457.

Gurnsey R, Poirier FJAM, and Gascon E (1996) There is no evidence than Kanizsa-type subjective contours can be detected in parallel. *Perception* 25:861–874.

He ZJ and Nakayama K (1992) Surfaces versus features in visual search. *Nature* 359:231–233.

He ZJ and Nakayama K (1995) Visual attention to surfaces in 3–dimensional space. *Proc Natl Acad Sci USA* 92:11155–11159.

Kanizsa G (1979) *Organization in Vision.* New York: Praeger Publishers.

Kellman PJ and Shipley TF (1992) Perceiving objects across gaps in space and time. *Curr Dir Psychol Sci* 1:193–199.

Lavie N and Driver J (1996) On the spatial extent of attention in object-based visual selection. *Percept Psychophys* 58:1238–1251.

Mattingley JB, Davis G, and Driver J (1997) Preattentive filling-in of visual surfaces in parietal extinction. *Science* 275:671–673.

Metelli F (1974) The perception of transparency. *Sci Am* 230:90–98.

Michotte A, Thines G, and Crabbe G (1964) Les compliments amodaux des structures perceptives. *Studia Psycol*

Moore C, Yantis S, and Vaughan B (1998) Object-based visual selection: Evidence from perceptual completion. *Psychol Sci* 9:104–110.

Nakayama K and Shimojo S (1992) Experiencing and perceiving visual surfaces. *Science* 257:1357–1363.

Pessoa L, Thompson E, and Noë A (1998) Finding out about filling-in: A guide to perceptual completion for visual science and the philosophy of perception. *Behav Brain Sci* 21:723–802.

Petry S and Meyer GE (Eds) (1987) *The Perception of Illusory Contours.* New York: Springer-Verlag.

Ramachandran VS (1987) Visual perception of surfaces: A biological theory. In: S Petry and GE Meyer, eds, *The Perception of Illusory Contours.* New York: Springer-Verlag, pp 91–104.

Ramachandran VS and Gregory RL (1991) Perceptual filling-in of artificial scotomas in human vision. *Nature* 350:699–702.

Rensink RA and Enns JT (1998) Early completion of occluded objects. *Vision Res* 38:2489–2505.

Treisman A and Gelade G (1980) A feature-integration theory of attention. *Cogn Psychol* 12:97–136.

Van Tuijl HF and De Weert CM (1979) Sensory conditions for the occurrence of the neon spreading illusion. *Perception* 8:211–215.

Watanabe T (1995) Orientation and color processing for partially occluded objects. *Vision Res* 35:647–655.

# 8

## Completion Phenomena in Vision:
## A Computational Approach

### HEIKO NEUMANN

How does the brain manage to form invariant representations of objects in the environment that are relevant for the current behavioral task? Spatiotemporal arrangements of patterns that signal coherent surface arrangements must somehow be reliably detected and grouped into elementary items. Such mechanisms must work robustly in variable environmental situations of stimulus acquisition. For example, surface properties must be acquired under variable illumination conditions, view positions, and scenic object arrangements. Recent findings support the belief that the underlying processing succeeds by first delineating boundaries and measuring local contrast properties at neighboring regions. At a later stage, figure and ground are segregated and elementary visual items are integrated to generate a neural representation of object properties (e.g., Gegenfurtner, 1999; Baylis and Driver, 2001).

Experimental studies suggest that visual processing proceeds by initially detecting outlines of shape and form and by subsequently assigning invariant surface attributes to homogeneous regions. The results of oriented contrast detection are subsequently grouped over spatially long distances to generate outlines of visual shape that are consistent with the input measures (Grossberg and Mingolla, 1985). Once the boundaries are extracted, the regions that are partitioned by the boundaries need to be assigned surface features, such as lightness, brightness, color, or transparency. The emerging picture from experimental investigations suggests that, in order to achieve an invariant representation of homogeneous regions, localized measurements need to be integrated over spatial distances of varying size. Several perceptual completion phenomena (see Pessoa et al., 1998, for a recent overview) suggest that, on a functional level, regions inherit local border contrast information by means of *spreading mechanisms*, or *filling-in* (e.g., Paradiso and Nakayama, 1991).

In this chapter, we outline a computational framework of recurrent processing emphasizing the need and computational role for mechanisms of spatial integration. We argue that, in boundary processing, feedback is utilized in order to find the most likely and consistent interpretation of degraded input measurements by assessing and combining contrast items. This computational framework is also proposed to apply for the estimation of coherent motion by integrating local ambiguous flow estimates. Mechanisms of lateral spreading are suggested to fill-in properties from boundaries into the interior of regions. Such a computational principle was originally intended to generate a dense representation of perceptual surface properties. Combined junction/boundary grouping helps to determine occlusion boundaries and closed shapes. The propagation of contrasts induced at junctions and high curvature locations is suggested to realize a mechanism of assigning border ownership. Finally, we propose that an extended filling-in mechanism can account for the perceptual integration of partially occluded regions by processes of amodal completion.

## Mechanisms of Completion for Surface Perception

### Coding Principles and Neural Mechanisms for Boundary and Surface Processing

Many researchers have investigated the question of how the visual system might utilize an efficient representation of visual layout by eliminating redundancies from the visual signal. For example, regions of a continuous color signal object continuity and, thus, contain no extra information in addition to that available at region boundaries (Barlow, 1961; Field, 1994). Furthermore, straight edges connecting distant corners are redundant in the sense that the contrast relations are unambiguously determined near the corner locations (Zetzsche and Barth, 1990). It has been conjectured that such features (which resemble changes in the luminance stimulus in two or more independent directions) alone are sufficient for a complete representation of the input luminance. In all, an information-theoretic point of view for analyzing cortical processing of luminance stimuli suggests that a sparse representation can be employed in which only key points such as corners, junctions, and line terminations are represented. Such features, in turn, are considered sufficient, in principle, to perform subsequent computational tasks, since these features contain all information to fully recover the original luminance stimulus.

The question remains whether mechanisms for surface perception and object recognition only rely on such a sparse feature representation by using these features directly. Consider, for example, the pattern depicted in Figure 8-1 (left). This stimulus shows a Kanizsa pattern in which a central bright square is perceived that lies in front of four dark circular disks, each of which has one sector occluded by the square. A coding strategy, such as the one discussed, investigates the extraction of particular key points that are sufficient to reconstruct the original luminance pattern. However, the perception of the Kanizsa pattern is much richer than a mere reconstruction of the input luminance distribution. The cen-

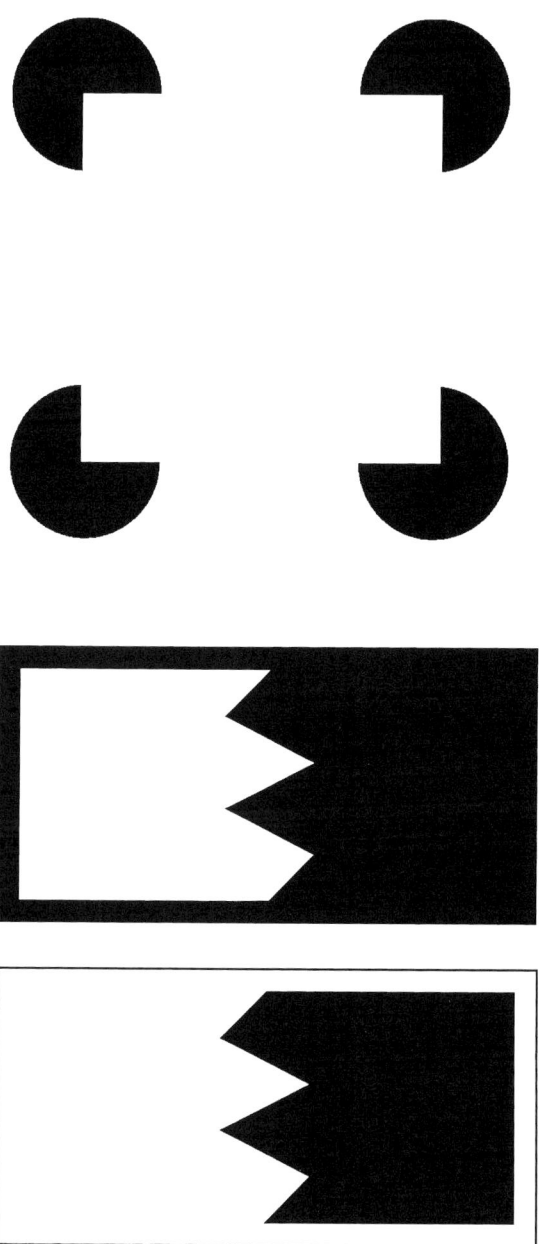

**Figure 8-1.** Examples of spatial integration of stimulus components for perceptual surface formation. Left: Illusory contours as a result of boundary formation in the Kanizsa square. Right: Border ownership of the central vertical contour is changed, depending on spatially remote manipulations of the shape outline. Note that the shape and contrast polarity of the central contour are left unchanged after the transformation (adapted from Baylis and Driver, 2001).

tral white patch appears to hover in front of the background with a slightly increased brightness than the surround. Illusory contours are completed between the aligned inducers. These inducers, in turn, appear as partially occluded disks whose surface quality is amodally completed behind the central square. Figure 8-1 (right) illustrates another example in which global mechanisms are required to assign surface-related properties to figural patterns. The assignment of border ownership and, thus, figure–ground direction in surface perception for the vertical boundary in the image center depends on contour/region properties of the whole figure. Here, the region that is bounded by the closed contour inside the image frame appears as the figure (against the ground) irrespective of the contrast polarity (Baylis and Driver, 2001). Again, local curvature maxima along the contour taken in isolation may be useful to reconstruct the luminance stimulus. In order to find the figure–ground direction, however, one must decide which region alongside the central contour "owns" the boundary and thus defines the surface border. In all, the underlying neural processes generate a richer representation than is predicted by a simple coding approach.

These examples illustrate that it is important to analyze computational mechanisms of early feature extraction in the context of object and surface perception. In order for object representations to be invariant under varying viewing and scene conditions, initial local measurements have to be completed to provide richer representations of contours and surfaces. From the standpoint of efficient coding, these computations add redundancy to the representation, but we suggest that they are necessary to achieve the robustness of rich perceptual units that are the building blocks for invariant object representations. This does not necessarily imply that the underlying neural completion mechanisms are designed to generate an internal representation that is spatially isomorphic with the external stimulus. Instead, we suggest that completion mechanisms for boundary finding and surface filling-in are a means to incorporate the local and global constraints of generating a perceptual judgment, as in the example of figure–ground assignment. These mechanisms may be implemented using the following key principles: (1) convergent feedforward integration over several areas; (2) lateral integration utilizing long-range, horizontal connections; or (3) a recurrent mechanism of converging feedforward and feedback integration.

## Boundary Finding and Completion

Several neural models of contour detection and grouping have been developed based on feedforward processing alone (Heitger et al., 1998) or on recurrent interactions based on feedforward as well as feedback processing (Grossberg and Mingolla, 1985; Gove et al., 1995; Grossberg et al., 1997). These models suggest that initial estimates of oriented contrast or higher-order features, such as corners and line ends, are grouped at a stage of long-range integration utilizing bipartite, or bipole, weighting functions (also called *association fields*; Field et al., 1993) to gather input from segregated subfields. The strength of support for the presence of a target feature can be expressed using a compatibility, or relatability, measure that is encoded in the association field. For example, Zucker and coworkers (Parent and Zucker, 1989) have proposed sampling a compatibility measure that is derived from differential geometry of smooth circular arcs. In general, grouping mechanisms invoke principles of selective integration of more localized measurements along feature dimensions, such as orientation (see Neumann and Mingolla, 2001). Such processing creates boundary representations that complete over gaps to group fragmented items and generates illusory contours at partial surface occlusions.

The computational role of cortical feedback as a hierarchical predictor has been investigated by Rao and Ballard (1999) (cf. Mumford, 1991, for an outline of the general idea). These authors suggest that feedback pathways of recurrent loops carry top-down predictions of contour coherence and continuity. In general, large-scale receptive fields at a higher cortical area frequently receive input from coactivated small-scale receptive fields (in a lower area) of the same orientation and at corresponding locations. During a learning period, likely input patterns can be associated to determine template pattern activities, which in turn will be carried along the feedback pathway for input pattern matching. This principle has been hypothesized to explain cortical end-stopped responses: Top-down predictions of a continuous contour (represented by the activity of cells with large-scale receptive fields in the higher area) are compared with bottom-up contour activation (represented by cells with small-scale receptive fields in the lower area) to generate a residual activity pattern. The residuum is small when the prediction is close to the input signal, whereas in the case of line endings the prediction of a continuous contour fails and large residual responses remain. These, in turn, are suggested to correspond with the responses of oriented end-stopped cells.

## A Unified Computational Framework for Filling-In

We propose a computational theory of recurrent processing that provides a unified account for boundary detection, completion, and segregation from noisy backgrounds. This approach combines computational mechanisms for grouping elementary items with the idea of predictive coding via feedback processing. To introduce concepts, consider a stage of oriented contrast measurement utilizing oriented kernels. This can be considered as a stage of feature detection in which activity is propagated bottom up to be subsequently integrated from a larger surround (Fig. 8-2, left). We suggest that the integration occurs at a higher-level cortical area and carries model information of likely visual patterns and their attributes. Considering shape outlines, the a priori visual *knowledge* is represented in *templates* of boundary segments of various possible curvatures. The above-mentioned bipole kernels are examples of such a mechanism whereby the expected most likely patterns are encoded in their weighting patterns. These patterns encode the sampled compatibility measure derived from the geometry of smooth shape segments and could, therefore, be considered a model of the typ-

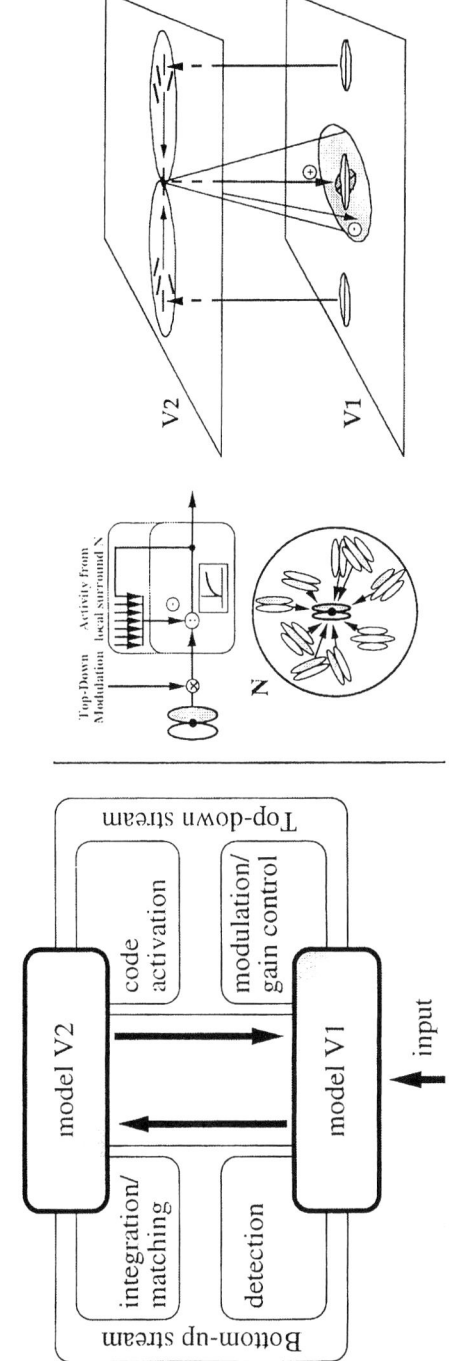

**Figure 8-2.** Computational principles for recurrent boundary finding. Left: Sketch of functional building blocks of the feedforward and feedback streams of processing. Contrasts are detected and subsequently integrated utilizing a larger spatial context. The result of this integration is used to modulate activities that are consistent with the larger context of integration via a gain control mechanism. Right: This abstract computational framework is instantiated in a model of recurrent cortical boundary processing of areas V1 and V2. The icons indicate different stages of processing. Initial responses from oriented contrast detection are normalized through shunting competition against pooled activity in a spatial neighborhood. Individual responses from area V1 are integrated by V2 contour cells. These contour activations modulate V1 activities with the same position and orientation via a mechanism of gain control and inhibit nonmatching activations. The recurrent interaction biases those activities that are consistent with the spatial context that is generated by the contour arrangement. (*Source:* Reprinted by permission from Neumann and Sepp, 1999)

ical appearance of boundary segments. In order to evaluate the significance of a particular input pattern, these templates are simultaneously matched by correlating the current input arrangement with the bipole weightings (cf. Ullman, 1995). The result of this correlation represents a signature of the degree of similarity between model and data. The resulting activation is propagated along the feedback pathway to enhance those activities at the low-level visual area that are consistent with the shape segments encoded in the contour templates (cf. Grossberg, 1980; Mumford, 1991). We suggest that this enhancement is achieved by a neural gain control mechanism that modulates non-zero activities through converging feedback activation from a broader context that has been determined by the shape outline of the current stimulus pattern (Fig. 8-2, left). The recurrence achieves a *weak loop*, in the terminology of Crick and Koch (1998), since feedback does not generate a driving input to the earlier processing stages but, rather, modulates already existing activation. The enhanced patterns of activity are subsequently fed through a stage of on-center/off-surround competition between cells in the lower area. Here, cell activities around a target location and with similar orientation preferences are inhibited by the activities of cells that were pooled over a larger neighborhood of the target location in the space-orientation domain. We employ a *shunting* mechanism in which the inhibition is divisive to achieve activity normalization (cf. Grossberg, 1980; Heeger, 1992). Through competition, those activities that receive strong modulatory feedback are favored over those that receive little or none. As a consequence, cell responses that are enhanced via top-down feedback are further contrast enhanced such that they can suppress other cell activities in their neighborhood that do not form salient shape arrangements.

This model has been particularly applied to cortical boundary processing in visual areas V1 and V2 (Fig. 8-2, right). Localized features are detected by orientation-selective V1 complex cells. These initial estimates are normalized through competitive shunting center–surround interaction, as sketched above. The resulting normalized activity patterns are integrated by V2 cells with oriented receptive fields built upon weightings in a space-orientation neighborhood. In order to be consistent with the data on V2 contour cell responses to illusory contour stimuli (von der Heydt et al., 1984), the model utilizes a mechanism of contour integration based on bipole cells with segregated collinear subfields. In order to activate a target cell at the stage of V2, inputs must drive the subfields at both ends. Consequently, on a functional level, a V2 contour cell completes the activity between inducers that are spatially separated but that, according to the expected outline information represented in the weighting patterns of the contour cells (Neumann and Sepp, 1999), can be related and therefore completed perceptually. The code patterns that are generated by activity at the matching stage are fed back from V2 to V1. In this way, activity of a V2 contour cell excites cells with smaller V1 receptive fields at the same position and corresponding orientation, while activities of nonmatching position and orientation are inhibited (Fig. 8-2, right). Figure 8-3 shows processing results of the proposed model (Neumann and Sepp, 1999).

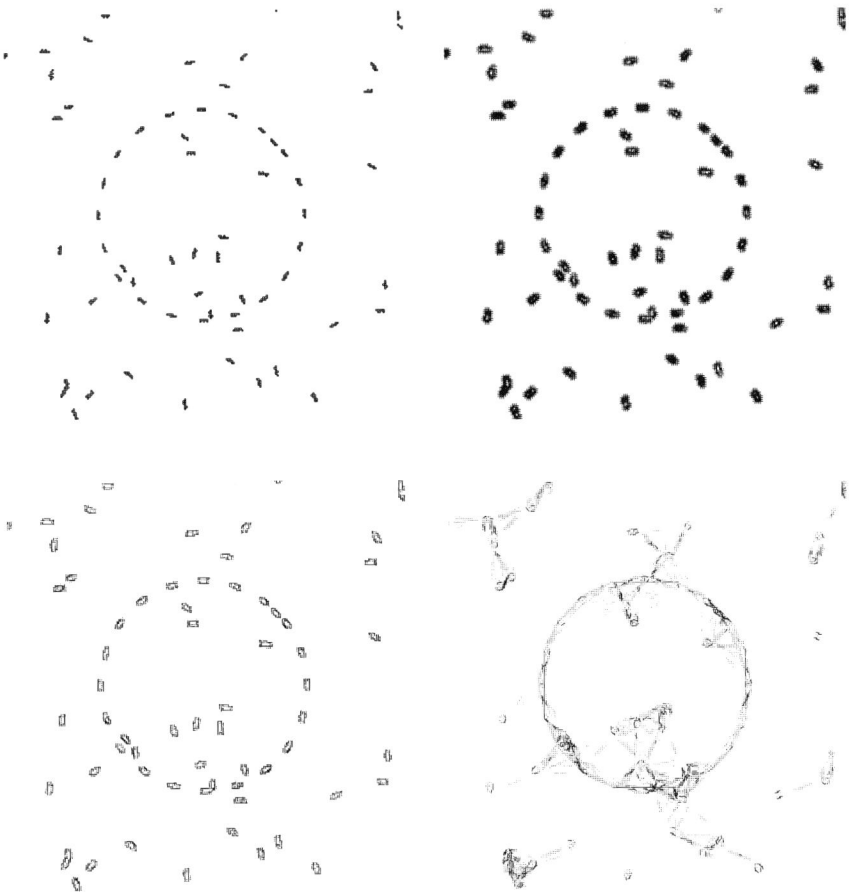

**Figure 8-3.** Simulation results. Integration of contour measures for a fragmented circular contour arrangement. The input image shows initial coarse estimates of oriented contrast, equilibrated model V1 responses lead to sharpened detail, and equilibrated model V2 responses with integrated contour responses show the interpolation of fragmented contour segments (from top left to bottom right).

Neumann and Sepp (2000) show that the generation of illusory contours for phase-shifted grid patterns is an emergent phenomenon of the recurrent interaction. In this case, initial contrast responses at line ends are uncertain and only weakly drive V2 contour cells. During the course of long-range integration of (weak) aligned contrast responses, feedback kicks in and enhances those responses oriented orthogonal to the line ends. As a consequence, the boundary that segregates two regions of parallel bars gets stronger. The integration of localized measurements for the generation of a dense boundary representation results as a net effect of recurrent interaction.

We will now discuss how the feedback processing proposed above achieves a predictive coding mechanism. It was argued above that feedback stabilizes and enhances weak measurements based on their coherent arrangement, even in cases of low contrast and noisy situations. In other words, input patterns in the full range of input contrast are evaluated in a flexible manner based on their matching with a range of expected boundary shapes. The resulting activities, which represent the degree of similarity between the input and the curved contour outlines (stored in the weightings of V2 contour cell receptive fields to define the expected a priori shape model), drive a competitive on-center/off-surround feedback mechanism to modulate V1 complex cells. This gain-control scheme is complemented by an additional mechanism of feedforward center–surround shunting competition. As a net effect, the competitive interaction between responses of oriented contrast cells achieves a nonlinear compressive mapping of input activations (Fig. 8-2, right). An analysis of model V1 steady-state responses demonstrates that the sensitivity of network responses (and the mapping of activities) during competition is adaptively controlled by the strength of excitatory and inhibitory feedback from V2 to V1. The sensitivity curve of V1 cells is tuned, depending on the balance between excitatory and inhibitory feedback activation. It is pushed toward the saturation level even for low-amplitude input activations when the feedback is strong, whereas it is flattened out when inhibitory feedback gets stronger. The model therefore realizes a predictive coding principle. Depending on the activity that has been generated on the higher cortical stage (V2 in our case), the resulting gain field increases or decreases the sensitivity of the neural input stage. Thus, a prediction is generated of where to increase or to decrease the sensitivity of the processing, or, in other words, of where to devote more selectivity and processing capacity.

## *Filling-In for the Completion of Surface Properties*

### *Evidence for Early Active Processes of Region Completion*
Recent results from empirical investigations support the view that the assignment of attributes to the interior of regions is based on an active process that laterally spreads local measures from boundaries. Such a mechanism of filling-in was originally suggested by Cohen and Grossberg (1984) and was subsequently adopted and extended by Grossberg and Todorovic (1988) to explain a rich set of brightness data. The idea that lateral spreading processes are involved in generating a filled-in region representation was suggested by clinical studies and stabilized image experiments (Krauskopf, 1963; Gerrits and Vendrik, 1970). More recent psychophysical studies have investigated the details of such an active process in which localized quantities (initially measured at boundary locations) are propagated to region interiors. Because such a process takes time, investigators reasoned that neural signal propagation could be disrupted by proper masking or temporal modulation of the input stimulus to unravel the propagation of activity (Paradiso and Nakayama, 1991; Davey et al., 1998; see Pessoa and Neumann, 1998, for a detailed discussion). Further evidence has been gained from physiological investigations by Paradiso and coworkers (MacEvoy et al., 1998) show-

ing that surface brightness information is represented inside homogeneous regions by neurons (as early as in V1) that are distant from any boundaries (see Chapter 4).

*Diffusion as a Computational Metaphor for Active Filling-In*

We propose a framework that relates filling-in of perceptual quantities (brightness in particular) to the problem of diffusion and to the mathematical framework of approximation and interpolation. Functionally, such a process interpolates between local measurements to signal coherent and dense surface properties. Consider a chain of laterally interconnected cells. Each cell can receive a driving input that injects local measurements of luminance contrast near boundaries. These activities, in turn, can be propagated via lateral connections to neighboring cells. Passive decay forces the activity to a resting state. Efficacy of the lateral spreading of activity is modulated by an auxiliary mechanism that is fed by the boundary process discussed in the previous section. As a result, the activity that is induced by the driving inputs can spread laterally as long there is no boundary activity to block the spread. Such a process can be described by a spatially variant diffusion mechanism with an additional (reaction) term that is defined by a driving input and a passive decay mechanism (both define the source and the sink component, respectively).

Figure 8-4 (left) shows an example stimulus of a light region on a darker background. Initial processing of such a stimulus utilizing center–surround interactions produces local contrast activations in the vicinity of the contrast edges (Fig. 8-4, middle). The lateral spreading, or diffusion, process smoothly interpolates localized measurements at the boundaries (Fig. 8-4, right) to "paint" the region's interior. Neumann et al. (2001) investigated the filling-in process in terms of a regularization principle for generating a dense representation of surface regions with features. It is shown that, computationally, the underlying variational

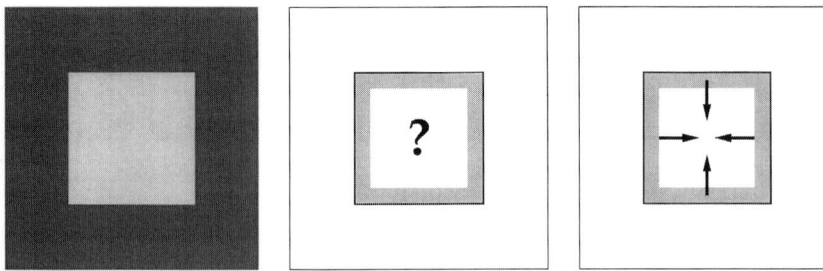

**Figure 8-4.** Computational mechanism of filling-in for region completion processes. A light region on a dark background (left) is initially processed by a center–surround mechanism. Significant responses are arranged along the spatial discontinuities; at the same time, homogeneous regions are suppressed (middle). Filling-in processes are suggested to propagate localized responses (ON contrast in this case) into the region's interior and generate a dense representation of perceptual surface brightness (right).

mechanism finds a balance between the closeness of the result to the initial contrast data (measured at the boundaries) and the smoothness of the region's representation by integrating distant measures across a region. Figure 8-5 shows the results of the filling-in model when a square wave pattern generated by Craik-O'Brien-Cornsweet (COC) cusps of alternating contrast polarities is used as an input stimulus. Initial center–surround interactions generate localized contrast responses near the cusps. They serve as inputs for the diffusive filling-in network. ON- and OFF-contrast activities are propagated into the interiors of the rectangular bounded regions to yield the final brightness appearance.

## Discounting the Illuminant and Constraints on Neural Filling-In Mechanisms

What are the computational principles of a processing strategy that first discards information of homogeneous regions by taking only local contrast measures along boundaries and subsequently integrates these local measures to generate a representation of homogeneous surface features? Consider a surface of constant reflectance, such as a table that is illuminated by a source emitting an inhomogeneous light distribution. The resulting spatially varying luminance distribution depends on the position of the light source over the surface and (at least partially) on the viewer's position. As a consequence, a direct analysis of intensities in homogeneous regions is prone to error due to the variability of the imaging conditions, namely, illumination and noise. In order to achieve a perceptually invariant representation of the surface, the illuminant should be *discounted* (see Chapter 2) by measuring luminance ratios along the region boundaries that correspond to the surface borders and by suppressing the gradually varying luminances within the regions (cf. Land, 1983).

The stages of initial center–surround processing at the retina and lateral geniculate nucleus (LGN) implement the key mechanisms for discounting the illuminant. These cells respond only very weakly (or not at all) to luminance gradients of constant slope, whereas they respond vigorously at sharply localized luminance

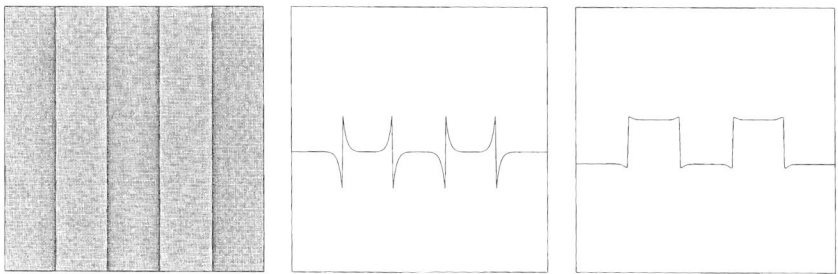

**Figure 8-5.** Simulation results: regional filling-in for a Craik-O'Brien-Cornsweet (COC) square wave stimulus: Input stimulus (left), profile of input (middle), and profile of simulation result (right). (*Source:* Reprinted with permission from Neumann et al., 2001)

changes, or edges. In terms of signal theory, center–surround processing resembles a bandpass filter that suppresses low- as well as high-frequency components of the luminance stimulus. As a result, any information about the reference level of local contrast measures (namely, the average luminance signal) is discarded at the output of this processing stage. In order to illustrate the related perceptual consequences, consider two luminance stimuli (Fig. 8-6, left). The first is composed of a sequence of four cusps of the same contrast polarity with constant regions of the average luminance level in between, and the second stimulus is a luminance staircase with discontinuities at the same spatial positions as the cusps in the first pattern. The results of initial center–surround processing (bandpass filtering) of these stimuli look almost indistinguishable since the luminance plateaus of the staircase as well as the constant regions of the cusp pattern will be discarded, while the edge responses for the cusps and the luminance steps result in a pattern of juxtaposed ON- and OFF-contrast responses. Since the perceptual appearance of the cusp pattern and the staircase is different, the visual system must somehow gain access to a reference level, or luminance anchor, in order to generate different brightness representations despite the same intermediate contrast measures at boundaries. A related problem of brightness anchoring is illustrated with two other luminance stimuli (Fig. 8-6, right). Both stimuli contain a central patch with the same luminance. Whereas the patch at the top is solely embedded in a surround of constant luminance, the bottom stimulus has a richer context. In the latter case, the neighboring surround of the center patch is itself enclosed by two plateaus with different luminance levels such that they make different step heights at the outer edges. In this case, the local contrasts measured at the central patch are ambiguous, and global information is required to estimate a brightness baseline and to assign the proper brightness levels.

The Retinex algorithm for lightness integration (Land, 1983) accounts for these observations by integrating contrasts along several pathways of different lengths or, alternatively, by numerically inverting the differentiated luminance stimulus. Under certain conditions, a unique solution exists and can be determined by numerical techniques (Hurlbert, 1986). The mechanisms are, however, often unsta-

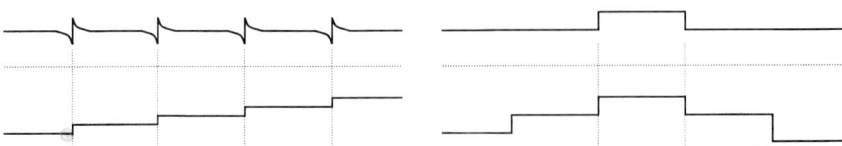

**Figure 8-6.** Example patterns illustrating the necessity for brightness *anchors* in addition to local contrast measures that are integrated by filling-in. Left: Sequence of four luminance cusps of equal contrast polarity (top) and a luminance staircase with edges at the same positions as the cusps (bottom). Right: A bright region in the center is flanked by plateaus of equal luminance (top); the same bright region and its flanking regions are now surrounded by a different context defined by luminance regions of different levels (bottom). See text for discussion.

ble and can lead to results that are inconsistent with the percept. In order to enable filling-in models to assign proper brightness levels, several computational approaches utilize an auxiliary (compressed) luminance signal to get the spatial modulation of amplitude levels with the local contrast signals being superimposed (Grossberg and Todorovic, 1988; Pessoa et al., 1995; Neumann, 1996). Arrington (1996) proposed a modified diffusion mechanism that utilizes semipermeable boundaries: ON filling-in activities are allowed to pass successive incremental contrast edges, whereas OFF activities pass decremental transitions. This directional leakage of filled-in activity at boundaries provides a baseline for *anchoring* the edges in the brightness representation. This model predicts the same brightness appearance for the stimuli depicted in Figure 8-6 (left), which is not confirmed perceptually. In order to propagate local contrast information over larger distances to bridge regions of high spatial frequency content, Sepp and Neumann (1999) proposed a multiscale filling-in scheme. Weighting functions of large spatial size provide contrast information over different spatial scales, or contexts, which help to get a baseline of the brightness through filling-in at larger grids. Spatial detail is added from smaller scales utilizing smaller weighting functions (for contrast measures) and smaller grids for filling-in of contrast signals.

## Completion Mechanisms for Integrating Perceptual Items

### The Aperture Problem and the Coherent Computation of Image Flow

Along elongated contour segments, temporal changes of a moving pattern can only be estimated in a direction normal to the local contrast orientation (the so-called aperture problem). Flow direction can be unambiguously estimated at image locations where multiple contrast orientations occur within the aperture—for example, at line ends (terminators) or corners and junctions. Global rigid motion of an object can be estimated under the assumption that the fragments of individual measurements belong to a connected object. Then the normal flows estimated at different locations define several constraint lines in the two-dimensional (2D)-image velocity space. Their intersection defines the coherent flow direction (e.g., Adelson and Movshon, 1982). The question remains of how the visual system solves the aperture problem to generate a representation of coherent motion. Pack et al. (2000) have investigated the time course of neural responses in area MT of the behaving macaque. They found that MT cells, when probed by elongated bars of a given orientation, show an early response in the direction orthogonal to the contrast orientation. Later, the responses are adaptively changed such that the preference now coincides with the true motion direction that is integrated from the ends of the bar. Areas V2 and V4 (in the ventral pathway) contribute to the disambiguation of motion signals as static occlusion features significantly change the integration of localized motion measurements (Lorenceau and Shiffrar, 1992; see Lidén and Pack, 1999, and Grossberg et al., 2000, for modeling approaches).

In order to generate a coherent representation of region motion, activities that correspond to the most likely motion direction must be propagated to help disambiguate the estimation from earlier stages. We suggest that for the computation of the moving boundary, a higher cortical stage such as MST (in the dorsal pathway) contributes to this integration mechanism via feedback. In area MT, pools of direction-sensitive cells exist with broad tuning properties that respond to movement directions in a range below ±90 degrees around the preferred direction. Individual estimates compete before they feed forward to the next higher stage of integration. Cells at a higher cortical stage, such as those in area MSTd, integrate activities from a large surround of remote spatial locations. Such cells, which are sensitive to different movement directions, in turn compete against each other in order to sharpen their tuning and to normalize their activity. Modulatory feedback to MT cells with a corresponding direction preference will enhance their activities that were weak due to the aperture problem of initial measurement. This proposal follows the same basic principle as the one discussed above for static boundary integration. Conceptually, the integration of motion signals from a large pool of direction-selective cells helps to get more "votes" from locations where unambiguous motions signals were estimated. Excitatory feedback is suggested to provide a top-down gain-control mechanism, which will enhance those activities of cells at corresponding locations and direction preferences that are compatible with the integrated signal from the higher stage of processing.

Again, on a computational level, this scheme of recurrent interaction can be interpreted as a mechanism of predictive coding. Consider, for example, an opaque rectangular region that moves in front of a homogeneous background. Unambiguous motion estimates will be extracted at locations around the corners, whereas along the straight boundaries, the resulting estimates will remain ambiguous due to the aperture problem. Long-range integration of motions signals ensures that unambiguous estimates will be pooled together with those that are ambiguous in such a way that the resulting activation signals the degree of similarity with expected (model) flow patterns. Top-down activation will, in turn, bias the competition between direction-selective cells such that the unambiguous motion direction propagates inward along the contrast boundaries of the rectangular region. An implementation of such mechanisms demonstrates the disambiguation of motion signals in a recently discovered motion illusion (Bayerl and Neumann, 2002).

*Border Ownership and Spatial Occlusion*
The Gestaltists observed that surfaces possess boundary ownership in which the boundary of a figural part is detached from the background and belongs to the foreground surface (Koffka, 1935). In other words, the boundary between a figure and the ground belongs to (is owned by) the figure. The segregation of a figure from the background is an important perceptual step. Once it has been decided what constitutes a figure and what belongs to the background, surface properties can be assigned by selectively integrating the local contrast measures that reliably signal, for example, luminance contrasts between spatially neighboring surfaces. Since initial center–surround mechanisms measure luminance differences only locally at edges irrespective of their figural belongingness, their

subsequent integration for assigning surface properties from contrasts may lead to perceptually erroneous results. Consider, for example, a gray surface that moves over a textured background whose average reflectance gradually varies like a sinusoid. The contrasts computed along the occlusion boundary change over time, depending on the properties of the background. Consequently, if contrast signals are integrated irrespective of the figure–ground assignment of the boundaries, the brightness of the occluding surface will oscillate over time. In order to achieve an invariant surface representation, those contrast measures that signal accidental configurations need to be discarded.

A possible neural substrate for the suppression of contrast signals along occlusion boundaries is an inhibitory feedback signal generated within the ventral pathway for object processing (Desimone and Ungerleider, 1989) implemented in the interactions between areas V1, V2, V3, and V4. We suggest that this inhibition is generated by an OFF-surround mechanism similar to the modulatory feedback described above for the boundary formation system. In boundary processing, however, excitatory and inhibitory interactions contribute to the processing of contours and surface borders. The computational principle suggested here for the suppression of interfering contrast signals (that lead to inconsistent information for contrast integration) necessitates an interaction between several channels and mechanisms, namely, boundary processing, junction *tagging*, and contrast integration by filling-in.

For example, T-junction configurations signal the presence of spatial occlusion and segregation in depth. We suggest a computational mechanism for shape processing in which contrast signals (and measures of local motion) along the top of a T-configuration are suppressed. Such a mechanism does not act purely locally but requires long-range integration of pairwise occlusion signals; otherwise, it cannot be decided on which side along the T-bar the contrast signals should be extinguished before they contribute potentially erroneous features for the integration process. Figure 8-7 (left) illustrates this idea. Local T-junction configurations signal the presence of occlusions. The conjunctive response of V1 and V2 contour cells signals the presence of T-junctions in a distributed fashion without the need for specialized detector neurons. (Forward projections of oriented V1 and V2 contrast cells converge in area V3, which contains contrast-sensitive cells with multipeaked orientation-/direction-tuning [Felleman and Van Essen, 1987].) We suggest that individual junctions trigger signals that can be grouped pairwise via oriented completion along paths determined by V2 cells. Occlusion signals need, however, an assignment of occlusion direction to distinguish the side where the stem touches the top of the T. A candidate mechanism sensitive to orientation discontinuities generates activities at the ending of the stem. In the case of Figure 8-7 (left), the groupings are generated at both sides along the occluding surface region between pairs of T-junction locations. Once the contrast signals that may lead to erroneous feature integration are extinguished by the inhibitory action of the groupings along the occlusion boundary, region filling-in mechanisms can integrate the remaining input and generate a brightness representation that is invariant against sudden background changes.

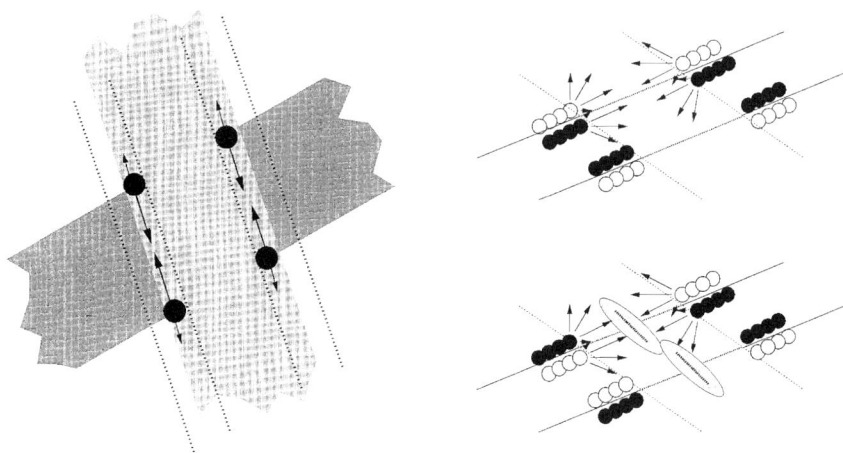

**Figure 8-7.** Left: Spatial arrangement of luminance regions for a dark surface patch that is partially occluded by a brighter surface. T-junctions indicate occlusions at the region boundaries where pairs of equally oriented junctions indicate the occluding segment. We suggest that trigger signals are generated at the end of the T-stems (circles) to propagate at the side of those boundaries that form the roofs of the T (dashed lines). Right: Filling-in mechanism for amodal completion (the dotted lines denote the boundaries of the occluding surface patch). Compatible contrast ON- and OFF-contrast responses are completed behind the occluder and form a fuzzy boundary (dense dotted line, top); incompatible contrast responses generated by opposite contrast polarities (at either side of the occluder) spread behind the occluder and form segments of a fuzzy shape boundary (dense dotted line, bottom). Contrary to the case of relatable regions, opposite contrast activities meet at the center and generate an additional contrast that is oriented orthogonal to the completed shape (elliptic gray shapes). These activities are suggested to segregate the facing regions and prevent them from grouping behind occluders (see text).

The suggested mechanisms of junction grouping and suppression of contrast signals are similar to the model of lightness integration proposed by Ross and Pessoa (2000). These authors suggest that an image is partially segmented into different context domains in which the segmentation is triggered by the presence of T-junctions. The scheme proposed above generalizes the Ross/Pessoa model in that it does not rely on an explicit T-junction detection stage but rather on surface-related occlusions including illusory contours, and that it further suggests an interaction between different contour representations that are also useful for selectively inhibiting local motion estimates.

A complete specification of the mechanisms involved in occlusion detection and junction grouping needs to take into account several constraints. The long-range integration of T-junction locations along boundaries should be insensitive to other types of junctions, as boundaries with orientation discontinuities should be processed as well. The tagging of boundary segments as occlusion fragments uses the conjunction of a boundary representation (from V2) and a grouping process that is triggered by simultaneous V1 and V2 activities. The grouping of junctions is guided by oriented boundaries such that grouping can occur along visible boundaries that are extracted at earlier stages. There is a computational need for selectivity with respect to the T-junction orientation. An occlusion is signaled by T's whose stems point away from the occluding surface. Thus, an ownership process and a suppression mechanism should integrate between these locations, irrespective of any other discontinuities and junctions that are part of the occluding surface. Since the integration always occurs along boundary segments, these representations may be used to guide the integration at the stage of junction selectivity. Although this is speculative, we suggest that this basic computational principle of junction/boundary grouping may also explain the rapid assignment of border ownership for figures of variable shape and size. For a bounded surface region, the conjunctive junction groupings and boundary activations from V1 and V2 may be integrated in IT cortex. We suggest that coarse-grained V4 responses generated at locations of high contour curvature and at acute junctions are spatially propagated by a completion mechanism. Contour cells, preferentially in area TE, control filling-in to prevent it from spreading across shape outlines. Furthermore, these cells are suggested to be selective to gradient directions of input activities. For example, consider Figure 8-1 (right). The gradient direction of integrated high-curvature responses along the central vertical contour switches with the changes of figure–ground direction in the upper and lower figures. The assignment of border ownership can thus be generated by a contour mechanism utilizing spatial long-range integration based on filling-in. Feedback may again modulate boundary activations as early as in V1 and V2 to generate figure–ground assignments to contour representations.

The mechanisms for signaling segments of occlusion boundaries and for assigning boundary ownership do not act in an all-or-none fashion. It has been demonstrated that occlusion phenomena and related perceptual completions are contrast dependent (see the discussion in Grossberg, 1997). We therefore suggest that the inhibitory mechanisms for suppressing contrast and motion signals (prior to integration) are controlled by the graded responses of the boundary representation. Also, the suggested mechanism of border ownership assignment is predicted to be dependent on the strength of boundary and junction signals.

*Amodal Completion*
In the same way that T-junctions help to suppress disparate measures of unreliable contrast and motion signals, the endings of partially occluded surface regions trigger processes of amodal completion. Kellman et al. (1998) suggest that such mechanisms follow the same principles as grouping in modal spatial completion processes. We suggest that for partially occluded patterns, the stems of the T-junctions feed into bipole kernels signaling far disparity, which generates a representation of amodally completed boundaries. There have been, however, arguments against the existence of a shared mechanism of modal and amodal completion based on boundary computation alone. For example, Shapley and Gordon's (1987) results suggest that the spatial range of boundary completion is

limited and, therefore, that a mechanism for completion behind occluders of various sizes and shapes might suffer from this limitation (see also Chapter 7). We propose a combination of long-range boundary integration and an extended version of the contrast filling-in mechanism to achieve the computational flexibility for amodal completion behind occluders of variable sizes.

Recent investigations by Shipley and colleagues (Yin et al., 1997) show that in amodal completion the surface properties on either side of the occluded surface must be consistent; otherwise, the perceptual strength of grouping regions behind an occluder is reduced. Figure 8-7 (right, top) sketches a configuration in which the sign relationships of contrast responses are consistent along the visible boundary segments for a partially occluded homogeneous surface. In the case of two accidentally aligned surfaces, the contrast responses are inconsistent (Fig. 8-7 (right, bottom) and, therefore, opposite contrast polarities occur on either side of the occluder. In the computational scheme described above, the lateral spreading of contrast activities is guided by the boundary activations that define the compartments for regions that will be filled-in. Conversely, features can freely diffuse when boundaries are missing. Therefore, a filling-in based mechanism for amodal completion will potentially suffer from the missing guidance of any boundaries. In order to overcome this limitation, we suggest that the boundary-driven modulation be augmented by an extra mechanism in which ON and OFF filling-in systems mutually inhibit each other. This idea is similar to the proposal of Gerrits and Vendrik (1970), who suggested that ON and OFF contrast diffusion mechanisms are mutually inhibitory in order to generate a representation of form with the property of rapidly completing a cortical scotoma. Here, we suggest a center–surround mechanism in which ON-center filling-in activity is inhibited by OFF filling-in activity in the spatial surround. The same principle suggests an antagonistic mechanism for OFF-center activation that is inhibited by ON-surround filling-in activity.

A contrast mechanism is suggested that samples juxtaposed ON- and OFF-center filling-in cells in order to selectively measure incompatible contrasts from remote measurement sites that are unobscured by the occluding surface patch. This principle is illustrated in Figure 8-7 (right): Juxtaposed ON and OFF filling-in activities at both sides of the occluder guide the spreading to generate a fuzzy shape boundary behind the occluder (the effective drift of the diffusion is shown by the arrows of different lengths). If same-polarity contrast measures approach from both sides, their activities will be merged—possibly generating a smooth gradient in the distribution of responses (Fig. 8-7 right, top). In case of region fragments with nonrelatable surface properties, denoted by opposite contrast polarities, the diffusive filling-in process starts in the same fashion as in the case of consistent polarities. However, activities of opposite polarities meet at locations about halfway distant from the inducing boundaries at the occluder. Where the spreading ON- and OFF-activations meet, extra contrasts are generated that are oriented orthogonal to the fuzzy shape outline along the completion boundary. We suggest that this extra contrast signal represents a signature that separates the homogeneous regions of the partially occluded background into two separate parts. In other words, the lack of such contrasts enables the grouping of disconnected but relatable surface patches on both sides of the occluder.

We suggest that this newly proposed mechanism provides an adaptive means for the grouping of surface patches in the case of partial occlusion. This principle demonstrates the usefulness of filling-in to augment the processing of localized mechanisms in the case of occlusion phenomena. In order to flexibly handle occlusions of variable sizes and shapes, a grouping and decision mechanism must integrate activities from spatially disparate locations. Lateral spreading is a means to transport localized measures providing the necessary input for localized mechanisms with a limited range of integration. This prediction may be tested in a psychophysical experiment. Consider an arrangement of shapes that are partially occluded by a homogeneous surface patch whose width is one of the key parameters of the experimental setting. The proposed mechanism predicts that the time needed to decide whether or not two surface patches can be related depends on the width of the occluder. Similar to the reasoning of Paradiso and Nakayama's (1991) paradigm, relatedness should be reliably judged for brief exposures when the width of the occluder is small. When the width of the occluder gets bigger, a longer exposure is needed to make a reliable decision.

## Summary

We have outlined a computational framework for boundary and region processing for preattentive segmentation and figure–ground processing. We argue that boundary processing (for static form perception) and the computation of rigid shape motion are examples of a neural principle of predictive coding. The underlying principle is based on the matching of local measures against a model of likely, and therefore expected, shape or flow patterns. The similarity between input (from the lower area) and expected patterns (which are stored in the weighting functions of integrating cells in the higher area) is measured by a correlation function. The matching is performed in a stimulus-adaptive fashion utilizing the context defined by a more coarse-grained integration of local measurements. The activity generated by this matching process defines a signature of the degree of similarity, which is subsequently used to assess the significance of initial localized measures based on the broader visual context. A gain control mechanism modulates cell activities in the lower area. In conjunction with subsequent competitive interactions, this processing principle enhances those measures consistent with visual context, while others are suppressed. Complementary computations for the integration of surface properties are instantiated by lateral completion mechanisms. Initial measures of localized contrast at luminance edges are propagated into the regions' interiors in order to generate a dense representation of surface regions. Computationally, the generation of such a representation follows a variational principle of smooth interpolation of activities between the contrast measures at the boundaries irrespective of the size of the region.

While the basic processes discussed in this chapter represent models of low-level mechanisms of vision, we have extended the computational framework to mid-level vision where surface properties are generated from reliable feature measurements and where partially occluded surface patches are integrated. We suggest that the initial processing mechanisms can be partially extended in their functionality such that they can help to assess initial contrast measures and to disambiguate local motion signals. We argue that T-junction configurations can be detected by a distributed mechanism that selectively tags boundary segments of occluding surface regions by means of a conjunctive junction/boundary grouping mechanism. Along occluding surface boundaries, contrast signals (that may lead to erroneous input for computing surface brightness from contrasts) will be extinguished, as motion signals will be suppressed before they are integrated along extrinsic terminators (at occluding surface segments).

Occlusion patterns also determine border ownership and figure–ground direction and trigger amodal completion. We suggest that an extended version of the filling-in mechanism allows the integration of related surface regions over a variety of distances. The augmented contrast mechanism helps to generate a representation that indicates the grouping or dissociation of regions in amodal completion processes. Filling-in mechanisms may provide a flexible means to deal with considerably variable sizes and shapes of occluding surfaces. Together with the integration of contrast measures over regions of (previously suppressed) luminance gradients, filling-in generates mid-level representations of perceptual surface information that are invariant against changes in size, shape, and illumination conditions. Furthermore, we propose that activity generated by junction/boundary grouping processes can also fill-in bounded shapes in order to determine border ownership. In all, these suggestions clarify why the visual system generates representations that are redundant from the standpoint of sparse coding. The proposed mid-level processes provide a testable explanation of the need for an ensemble of several computational mechanisms of spatial integration (or filling-in) and the principle of localized processing. This clearly shifts the focus from the discussion of whether or not there is a homunculus to watch internal representations (of dense surface properties) toward a functional interpretation of completion processes in the brain.

*Acknowledgments*

Parts of the research presented in this chapter benefited from discussions with Steve Grossberg and Jim Williamson during the author's sabbatical (fall 1999 to spring 2000) at the Center for Adaptive Systems at Boston University. The discussions with Mark Rubin and Andrzej Przybyszewski on the investigation and analysis of cortical feedback processes are gratefully acknowledged. I thank Thorsten Hansen and Matthias Keil for fruitful discussions on this research. Luiz Pessoa's and Peter De Weerd's critical comments on earlier versions of the manuscript helped improve the line of argumentation. This work was supported in part by a grant from the Volkswagen-Stiftung (VW I/75967).

# References

Adelson EH and Movshon J (1982) Phenomenal coherence of moving visual patterns. *Nature* 300:523–525.
Arrington KF (1996) Directional filling-in. *Neural Comput* 8:300–318.
Barlow HB (1961) Possible principles underlying the transformations of sensory mes-

sages. In: Rosenbluth WA (ed), *Sensory Communication.* Cambridge, MA: MIT Press, pp 217–234.

Bayerl P and Neumann H (2002) Recurrent processing in the dorsal pathway underlies the robust integration and segregation of motion pattern. *Proceedings of the second annual meeting of the Vision Sciences Society*, Sarasota, Florida, May 10–15, pp. 226–227.

Baylis GC and Driver J (2001) Shape-coding in IT cells generalizes over contrast and mirror reversal, but not figure–ground reversal. *Nat Neurosci* 4:937–942.

Cohen M and Grossberg S (1984) Neural dynamics of brightness perception: Features, boundaries, diffusion, and resonance. *Percept Psychophys* 36:428–456.

Crick F and Koch C (1998) Constraints on cortical and thalamic projections: The no-strong-loop hypothesis. *Nature* 391:245–250.

Davey MP, Maddess T, and Srinivasan MV (1998) The spatiotemporal properties of the Craik-O'Brien-Cornsweet effect are consistent with "filling-in." *Vision Res* 38:2037–2046.

Desimone R and Ungerleider LG (1989) Neural mechanisms of visual perception in monkeys. In: Boller F and Grafman J (eds), *Handbook of Neuropsychology*, Vol 2. Amsterdam: Elsevier Science Publishers, pp 267–299.

Felleman DJ and Van Essen, DC (1987). Receptive field properties of neurons in area V3 of macaque monkey extrastriate cortex. *J Neurophysiol* 57:889–920.

Field DJ (1994) What is the goal of sensory coding? *Neural Comput* 6:559–601.

Field DJ, Hayes A, and Hess RF (1993) Contour integration by the human visual system: Evidence for a local "association field." *Vision Res* 33:173–193.

Gegenfurtner KR (1999) Reflections on color constancy. *Nature* 402:855–856.

Gerrits H and Vendrik A (1970) Simultaneous contrast, filling-in process and information processing in man's visual system. *Exp Brain Res* 11:411–430.

Gove A, Grossberg S, and Mingolla E (1995) Brightness perception, illusory contours, and corticogeniculate feedback. *Vis Neurosci* 12:1027–1052.

Grossberg S (1980) How does the brain build a cognitive code? *Psychol Rev* 87:1–51.

Grossberg S (1997) Cortical dynamics of three-dimensional figure–ground perception of two-dimensional pictures. *Psychol Rev* 104:618–658.

Grossberg S and Mingolla E (1985) Neural dynamics of form perception: Boundary completion, illusory figures, and neon color spreading. *Psychol Rev* 92:173–211.

Grossberg S, Mingolla E, and Ross WD (1997) Visual brain and visual perception: How does the cortex do perceptual grouping? *Trends Neurosci* 20:106–111.

Grossberg S, Mingolla E, and Viswanathan L (2000) *Neural Dynamics of Motion Integration and Segmentation Within and Across Apertures.* Technical Report CAS/CNS-2000–004. Boston: Boston University, Center for Adaptive Systems, Department of Cognitive and Neural Systems.

Grossberg S and Todorovic D (1988) Neural dynamics of 1–D and 2–D brightness perception: A unified model of classical and recent phenomena. *Percept Psychophys* 43:723–742.

Heeger DJ (1992). Normalization of cell responses in cat striate cortex. *Vis Neurosci* 9:184–197.

Heitger F, von der Heydt R, Peterhans E, Rosenthaler L, and Kübler O (1998) Simulation of neural contour mechanisms: Representing anomalous contours. *Image Vision Comput* 16:407–421.

Hurlbert A (1986) Formal connections between lightness algorithms. *J Opt Soc Am A* 3:1684–1693.

Kellman PJ, Yin C, and Shipley TF (1998) A common mechanism for illusory and occluded object completion. *J Exp Psychol Percept Perform* 24:859–869.
Koffka K (1935) *Principles of Gestalt Psychology.* London: Routledge and Kegan Paul Ltd.
Krauskopf J (1963) Effect of retinal image stabilization on the appearance of heterochromatic targets. *J Opt Soc Am A* 53:741–744.
Land E (1983) Recent advances in retinex theory and some implications for cortical computations: Color vision and the natural image. *Proc Natl Acad Sci USA* 80:5163–5169.
Lidén L and Pack C (1999) The role of terminators and occlusion cues in motion integration and segmentation: A neural network model. *Vision Res* 39:3301–3320.
Lorenceau J and Shiffrar M (1992) The influence of terminators on motion integration across space. *Vision Res* 32:263–273.
MacEvoy SP, Kim W, and Paradiso MA (1998) Integration of surface information in primary visual cortex. *Nat Neurosci* 1:616–620.
Mumford D (1991) On the computational architecture of the neocortex II: The role of cortico-cortical loop. *Biol Cybernet* 65:241–251.
Neumann H (1996) Mechanisms of neural architecture for visual contrast and brightness perception. *Neural Networks* 9:921–936.
Neumann H and Mingolla E (2001) Computational neural models of spatial integration mechanisms for perceptual grouping. In: Shipley TF and Kellman PJ (eds), *From Fragments to Objects: Segmentation and Grouping in Vision.* Amsterdam: Elsevier Science Publishers, pp 353–400.
Neumann H, Pessoa L, and Hansen T (2001) Visual filling-in for computing perceptual surface properties. *Biol Cybernet* 85:355–369.
Neumann H and Sepp W (1999) Recurrent V1–V2 interaction in early visual boundary processing. *Biol Cybernet* 81:425–444.
Neumann H and Sepp W (2000) Perceptual strength and time course of illusory contour generation explained by a neural model of recurrent cortico-cortical interaction. *Perception* 29(Suppl):64.
Pack C, Abrams PL, and Born RT (2000) Neural and behavioral correlates of ambiguous local motion measurements in cortical visual area MT. *Perception* 29(Suppl):81.
Paradiso M and Nakayama K (1991) Brightness perception and filling-in. *Vision Res* 31:1221–1236.
Parent P and Zucker S (1989) Trace inference, curvature consistency, and curve detection. *IEEE Trans PAMI* 11:823–839.
Pessoa L, Mingolla E, and Neumann H (1995) A contrast- and luminance-driven multiscale network model of brightness perception. *Vision Res* 35:2201–2223.
Pessoa L and Neumann H (1998) Why does the brain fill-in? *Trends Cogn Sci* 2:422–424.
Pessoa L, Thompson E, and Noe A (1998). Finding out about filling-in: A guide to perceptual completion for visual science and the philosophy of perception. *Behav Brain Sci* 21:723–802.
Rao RPN and Ballard DH (1999) Predictive coding in the visual cortex: A functional interpretation of some extra-classical receptive-field effects. *Nat Neurosci* 2:79–87.
Ross WD and Pessoa L (2000) Lightness from contrast: A selective integration model. *Percept Psychophys* 62:1160–1181.
Sepp W and Neumann H (1999) A multi-resolution filling-in model for brightness perception. IEE Conf. Publ. No. 470. *Proceedings of the 9th International Conference on Artificial Neural Networks (ICANN-99)*, Edinburgh, UK, Sept. 7–10, pp 461–466.
Shapley R and Gordon J (1987) The existence of interpolated illusory contours depends

on contrast and spatial separation. In: Petry S and Meyer GE (eds), *The Perception of Illusory Contours.* New York: Springer, pp 109–115.

Ullman S (1995) Sequence seeking and counter streams: A computational model for bidirectional information flow in the visual cortex. *Cereb Cortex* 1:1–11.

von der Heydt R, Peterhans E, and Baumgartner G (1984) Illusory contours and cortical neuron responses. *Science* 224:1260–1262.

Yin C, Kellman PJ, and Shipley TF (1997) Surface completion complements boundary interpolation in the visual integration of partly occluded objects. *Perception* 26:1459–1479.

Zetzsche C and Barth E (1990) Fundamental limits of linear filters in the visual processing of two-dimensional signals. *Vision Res* 30:1111–1117.

# II

# FROM PERMANENT SCOTOMAS TO CORTICAL REORGANIZATION

# 9

## Completion Through a Permanent Scotoma:
### Fast Interpolation Across the Blind Spot and the Processing of Occlusion

MARIO FIORANI, JR., LETICIA DE OLIVEIRA,
ELIANE VOLCHAN, LUIZ PESSOA,
RICARDO GATTASS, AND
CARLOS EDUARDO ROCHA-MIRANDA

In the human retina, there is a large region naturally devoid of photoreceptors called the *blind spot*. It corresponds to the optic nerve head and has an elliptical shape approximately 7.5 degrees in height and 5.0 degrees in width and is located about 15 degrees from the fovea (see Figs. 9-2A, a1, and 9-2A, a2). This discontinuity in the receptive surface, however, under normal circumstances, is not accompanied by abnormal perception, even under monocular conditions (Fig. 9-1). Two types of this unusual "normal" perception at the blind spot can be distinguished: First, straight lines are *completed*; second, homogeneous backgrounds are *filled-in*. Both phenomena are generally called *perceptual filling-in* or *perceptual completion*. Interestingly, behavioral studies have shown that perceptual filling-in at the blind spot also occurs in monkeys (e.g., Komatsu and Murakami, 1994; see also Chapter 6).

Somewhere between our retinas and our perception, the retinotopic discontinuity due to the blind spot is converted into visuotopic continuity. Where in the brain does the conversion take place? Some investigators have suggested that this process may be *cognitive* (Gregory, 1972; Rock and Anson, 1979). As discussed below, however, recent data implicate low-level visual processing in the generation of perceptual filling-in. In any case, the discussion about the neural substrates of filling-in is highly controversial (see Pessoa et al., 1998).

The existence of perceptual completion is well documented by a wealth of psychophysical studies, perhaps only rivaled by the many different interpretations of the underlying mechanisms. In this chapter we shall argue that some forms of completion are likely implemented early in the visual system. We re-

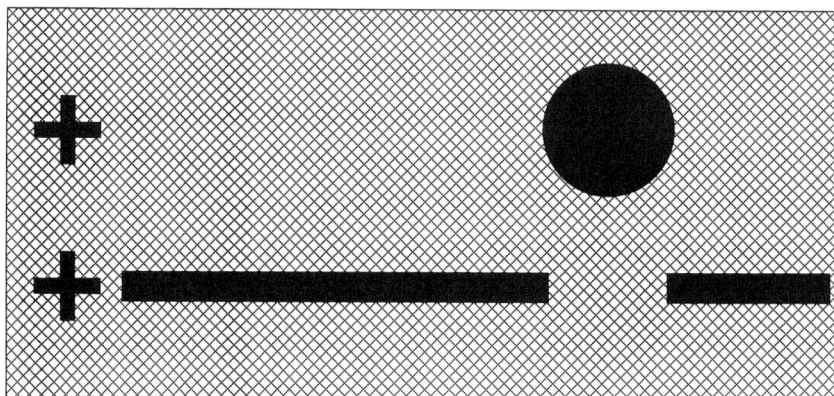

**Figure 9-1.** Filling-in at the blind spot. The right-eye blind spot can be revealed by closing the left eye and fixating the upper cross with the right eye. Starting with the book at about 25 cm from the eye, move it back and forth slowly; the circle on the right will disappear when imaged on the blind spot. If the right eye now fixates the lower cross, the gap in the horizontal bar is imaged on the blind spot and the bar is perceived as continuous. Note that in the upper demonstration the missing circle is perceptually filled-in with the texture (pattern) around it, and in the lower one the black line is completed across the blind spot.

**Figure 9-2.** Interpolated receptive fields (RFs) in neurons at the blind spot representation in primate V1. (A) To map RFs at the right blind spot representation, long moving bars are swept in different orientations in the region around the blind spot projection in the right visual field (a1) while a recording microelectrode is placed at the blind spot representation in the left V1 (a5). (a1) Representation of the right visual field showing the projection of the right-eye blind spot over the horizontal meridian (HM). VM = vertical meridian; ★ = fixation spot. (a2) Schematic representation of a dorsal view of the eyes showing the blind spot and the fovea (★). (a3) Schematic view of the contalateral lateral geniculate nucleus (dLGN) showing the afferent projection from the right optic nerve and the efferent projection to the left primary visual cortex (V1). (a4) Tangential view of layer 4c of the left (contralateral) primate V1 showing schematically the ocular dominance stripes and the blind spot (box) revealed by cytochrome oxidase histochemistry (see text). Dark stripes correspond to the contralateral eye (the one with the blind spot). (a5) Enlargement of the blind spot region in V1 illustrating a microelectrode placed at the blind spot representation. Note the absence of right (contralateral) eye inputs in the blind spot representation (revealed by an absence of dark stripes). (B and C) Long bars in different orientations are swept over the blind spot projection and neuronal responses, depicted by the dashed lines (response region), are systematically evoked along the stimulus trajectory. (D) An interpolated RF can be revealed at the intersection of the two responsive regions. Note that the cell used distinct regions around the blind spot to interpolate the RF, depending on the stimulus orientation (h = horizontal; v = vertical). (F) No response is elicited when a bar smaller than the blind spot is swept over the interpolated RF.

view experimental data showing completion-like properties across the blind spot representation in the striate cortex of monkeys. This property seems to be based on interpolation of spatially collinear stimuli. Experimental evidence will also be presented for interpolation not restricted to natural scotomata like the blind spot. Additionally, we will present findings of spatial interpolation from striate cortex cells of the opossum, a more primitive mammal.

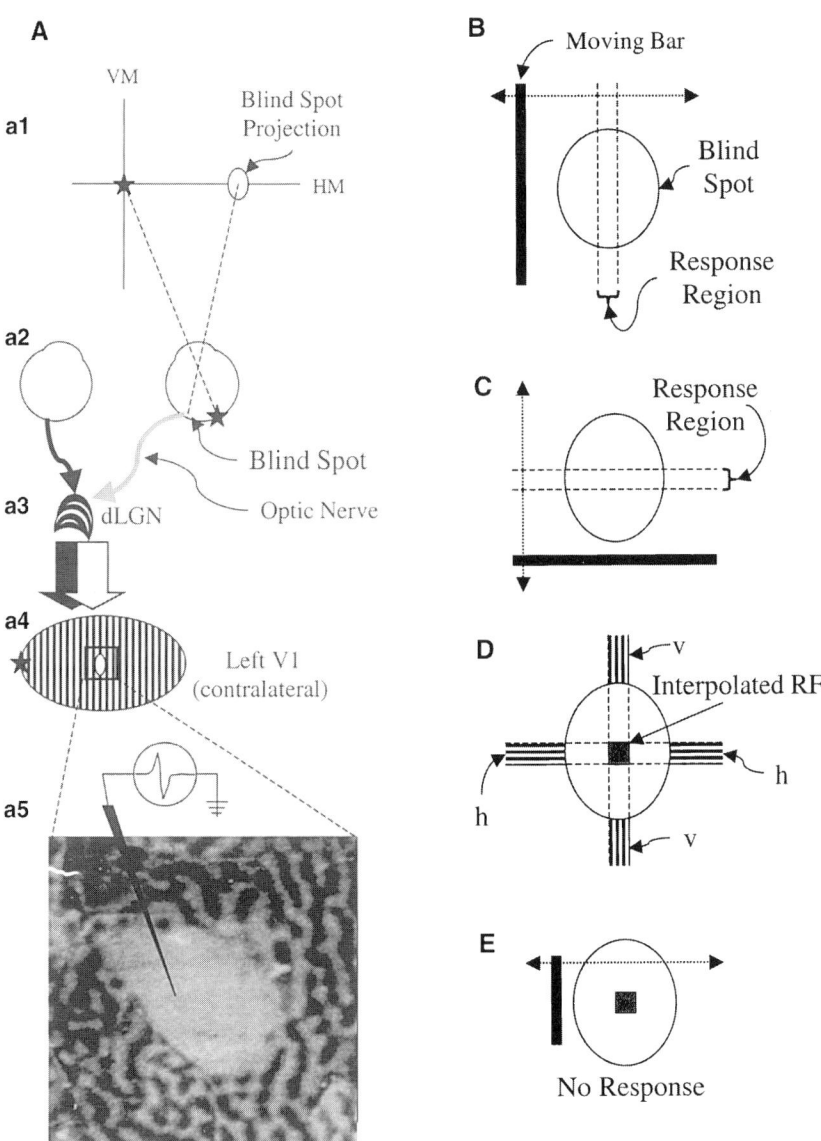

## Review of Experimental Findings

Anatomical data show that the sensorial gap in the retina due to the blind spot is reflected in the afferent layer (4c) of the primary visual cortex (V1) in humans and nonhuman primates (Rosa et al., 1988; Horton et al., 1990). Cytochrome oxidase studies after monocular deprivation show a pattern of alternating ocular dominance (OD) patches along layer 4c (Fig. 9-2A, a5). Each alternate patch receives direct projections predominantly from one retina via the dorsal lateral geniculate nucleus (Fig. 9-2A, a3). Functionally, cells located inside a given eye-projecting patch belong to a given OD column. Cells within an OD column tend to give better responses to that eye but usually also respond to the other eye (Rosa et al., 1992). In tangent cytochrome oxidase preparations, the blind spot representation is easily identifiable as a large area without direct retinogeniculate input from the contralateral eye (Fig. 9-2A, a5). (Rosa et al., 1988, 1992). The demonstration of a retinal sensorial gap reflected in the afferent layer in V1 makes this area the lowermost level candidate for the neural filling-in of the blind spot.

Fiorani and collaborators (1992; 2001) found cells within the cortical representation of the blind spot that unexpectedly responded to elongated stimuli presented to the contralateral eye. In fact, during the presentation of long, oriented bars (exceeding the size of the blind spot), these cells showed responses when the bars crossed the blind spot representation (Fig. 9-2B–D). When tested with small stimuli restricted to the blind spot, as expected, the cells showed no response (Fig. 9-2E). Moreover, they showed reduced or no response to stimulation with *half-bars*, that is, bars extending to only one side of the blind spot. Critically, the sum of the responses to the half-bars was significantly smaller than the response to the full bar. These results indicate that the cells were effectively integrating, that is, *interpolating*, the bar segments in a nonlinear manner (see Fig. 3 in Fiorani et al., 1992). Furthermore, the interpolated receptive fields (RFs) were topographically organized, showing that the interpolation was associated with a precise visuotopic position (see Fig. 1 in Fiorani et al., 1992; see also Fiorani et al., 2001). In sum, the cortical representation of visual contours crossing the blind spot generates a spatially continuous representation that preserves topographical organization. These findings argue in favor of a contribution of early visual circuits in the integration of contours imaged at the blind spot.

The suggested contribution of V1 cells to the perception of interpolated contours is strengthened by the finding of Fiorani et al. (1992) that integration of contours is not restricted to a natural scotoma like the blind spot. Some neurons in the primary visual cortex gave clear responses to stimulation of areas outside the mapped RF when it was masked (i.e., an artificial scotoma was produced). Given that cell responses were elicited by the simultaneous stimulation of the extra-RF regions along the same collinear axis, the authors proposed that these cells could be involved in contour integration in general.

Although contour integration is often discussed in the context of form perception, it may also play an important role in the planning and execution of visually guided movement. Goodale and Milner (1996), taking an evolutionary perspective, have proposed that "vision may not have evolved to provide perception of the world in any obvious sense, but rather to provide distal sensory control of the movements that the animal makes in order to survive and reproduce in that world." The detection of a contour in a visual scene with which the animal is interacting is relevant for its visuomotor acts. For effective visually guided behavior, it must be possible for action to be steered by objects that are occluded (e.g., von der Heydt, 1995). In this vein, one should expect most species to detect occluded contours. These ideas prompted Oliveira et al. (1998) to investigate cell properties in the primary visual cortex of the opossum, a primitive mammal with a less specialized visual system. They showed that, for a group of cells in V1, masking the RF and sweeping a long bar over it elicited robust responses. Similar to the work of Fiorani et al. (1992) in monkeys, these cells also showed reduced responses to stimulation with half-bars. Likewise, the sum of the half-bar responses was significantly smaller than the response to the full bar, indicating that the animals were interpolating the bar segments in a nonlinear fashion. This study revealed that primary visual cortex cells of the opossum can interpolate large gaps consistent with conditions of physical occlusion.

About 30% of the cells in V1 exhibited integration properties in both the monkey and the opossum (Fiorani et al., 1992; Oliveira et al., 1998). The presence of similar mechanisms for stimulus integration in such distantly related species raises the interesting possibility that interpolation is a basic building block of contour integration in mammals rather than a high-level cognitive mechanism, which might be expected in more advanced animals.

The results of Fiorani et al. (1992) and of Oliveira et al. (1998) are consistent with the RF structure shown in Figure 9-3. The region outside the RF along the preferred orientation does not have an effect when unilaterally stimulated (Fig. 9-3C). However, the simultaneous stimulation of *both* sides in a collinear fashion can drive the cell to an excitatory response even without stimulation of the classical RF per se (Fig. 9-3D). When *both* stimuli are present, they sum up in a *nonlinear* fashion. Under this condition, enlarging the gap over the RF by increasing the distance between stimuli leads to a response decrease, indicating a greater influence of the regions immediately surrounding the RF (Fig. 9-3E); that is, a distance-dependent mechanism is assumed. This structure is compatible with the model proposed by Grossberg and Mingolla (1985) for *bipole* cells that would be involved in the perception of illusory contours (see Chapters 2 and 8).

Our results follow a long tradition of studies that probe nonclassical RF properties, originating with the investigation of Nelson and Frost (1985). More recent investigations have demonstrated that RFs in V1 have highly context-dependent, dynamic properties (Redies et al., 1987; Grosof et al., 1993; Rossi et al., 1996; Zipser et al., 1996; MacEvoy et al., 1998; Das and Gilbert, 1999; see also Chapter 4). Electrophysiological studies in cats and monkeys have found cells responsive to illusory contours (abutting gratings) in the primary visual cortex (Redies et al., 1987; Grossof et al., 1993), although von der Heydt and Peterhans (1989; Peterhans and von der Heydt, 1989) and Baumann et al. (1997) found cells with such properties only in the secondary visual cortex.

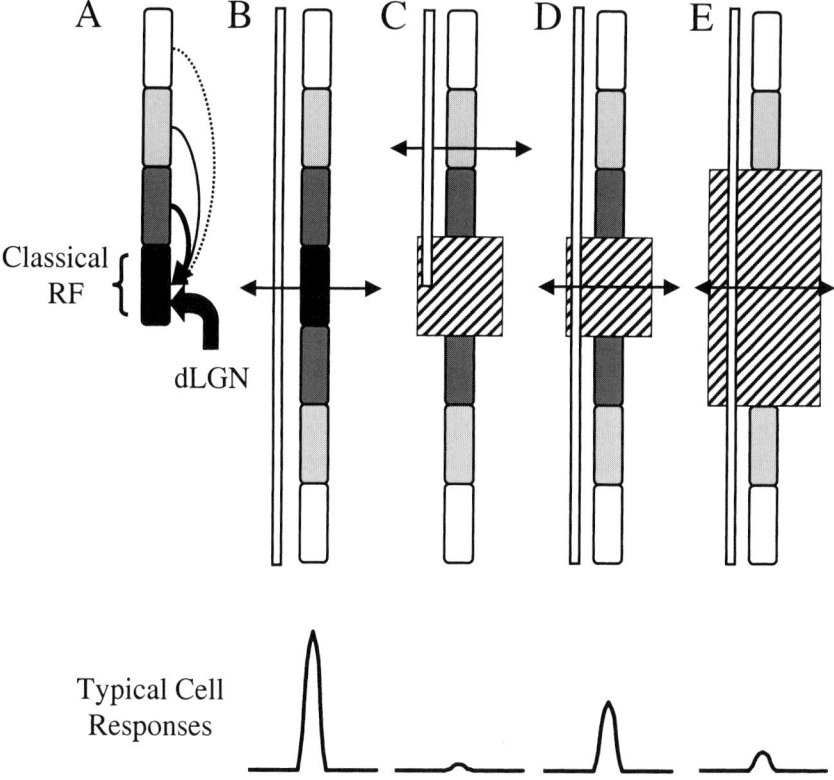

**Figure 9-3.** Structure of interpolation receptive field (RF). (A) Schematic figure showing influences over the classical RF (black rectangle). The bigger influence comes from the retina via the lateral geniculate nucleus of the thalamus (dLGN); there is also weak influences coming from cortical regions (V1 or other areas) aligned with the classical RF. Note that the cortical influences decrease with increasing distance to the classical RF (gray scale and arrows). (B–E) Some stimuli configurations (top) and typical cell responses (bottom). Sweeping a long bar centered on the classical RF elicits a robust response (B). Masking the classical RF (hatched region) and stimulating just one side of the modulatory surround RF elicits almost no response (C). When both modulatory sides of a masked RF are simultaneously stimulated, a nonlinear summation evokes a significant response (D). Increasing the mask largely reduces the cell responses (E).

The existence of cells that respond to illusory contours in V1 is still a matter of debate (see also Chapter 3).

Recent studies in behaving monkeys have shown that the collinear arrangement of contour segments is a key factor in the modulation of V1 cells. Kapadia et al. (1995) showed that some complex cells in V1 of the rhesus monkey were facilitated when a second bar was placed outside the classical RF while a similarly oriented bar stimulated the RF. In parallel with psychophysical results, the facilitation decreased when the bar outside the RF was noncollinear or had a different orientation. Also, in the awake monkey, Polat et al. (1998) showed that similar facilitation occurs when a near-threshold stimulus inside the RF is flanked by collinear elements with higher contrast in the surrounding region of visual space (see also Sengpiel et al., 1997).

Another context-dependent property of V1 neurons is dynamic RF expansion, described by Gilbert and collaborators in area V1 of anesthetized cats and monkeys (Gilbert and Wiesel, 1990, 1992; Gilbert, 1992; Pettet and Gilbert, 1992; Das and Gilbert, 1995, 1999; Volchan and Gilbert, 1995). RF expansion occurs when the RF and immediate surrounding regions are masked and the background is stimulated for some time. This masking can lead to a five-fold average increase in the RF area. Subsequent stimulation of the expanded RF shrinks it back to its original size. Gilbert and collaborators have suggested that this type of RF expansion may provide the neural basis for several perceptual filling-in effects.

At present, there is no consensus regarding the mechanisms responsible for dynamic RF properties in V1. There is evidence that horizontal, lateral connections are involved (see Gilbert, 1992). Hirsch and Gilbert (1991) found that both excitatory and inhibitory influences of the surround might be produced by horizontal connections. They suggest that "the state dependence of horizontal connections could be responsible for nonlinear interactions between the lateral and interlaminar inputs," indicating that these connections may mediate some of the context dependency of RFs. In an interesting study in support of this possibility is the demonstration of Bosking et al. (1997) that in the tree shrew, cells in the superficial layers are connected to other neurons not only having the same orientation preference but also placed in the visual field representation along the axis of the preferred orientation. In fact, this result fits quite well with the scheme shown in Figure 9-3. It should also be noted that feedback interactions may play an important role in the dynamic properties of V1 RFs, particularly those related to more cognitive influences, such as attention (Gilbert et al., 2000).

## Conclusions

The neural substrates of, and the regions responsible for, perceptual filling-in are still a matter of debate. Gregory (1972) and Rock and Anson (1979) proposed that perceptual filling-in is a high-level cognitive process. Along similar lines, Kawabata (1984) has argued that completion occurs only after similarity grouping has been achieved, that is, at a higher level than contour analysis. More recent evidence has implicated more basic perceptual processes at the core of a range of filling-in effects. For example, Murakami (1995) showed that the motion aftereffect is also found at the blind spot, suggesting that filling-in of this region is processed at an early stage in the visual system. Other results also have indicated that completion of occluded objects occurs early in the visual system (Rensink and Enns, 1998; Greene and Brown, 2000). Finally, it is interesting to note that newborn infants (less than 1 month old) can perceive partly occluded gratings (Kawabata et al., 1999), which suggests that the perception of occlusion may not need much learning or may even be innate.

The evidence reviewed in this chapter for contour interpolation in the primary visual cortex of primates and opossums has some important implications. First, it shows that interpolated information across the blind spot is available at the initial stages of visual cortical processing. This suggests that perceptual completion of contours across the blind spot may start at an early processing level. Second, the observation of interpolation outside the blind spot, that is, interpolation across masks, suggests that the associated mechanisms may be involved in contour integration in general. Third, the presence of interpolation in the striate cortex of a primitive mammal, such as the opossum, suggests that this property evolved early in phylogeny as part of a general mechanism for contour analysis. Fourth, the interpolation property we studied fits well with a key feature of primary visual cortex, namely, the generation of a detailed visuotopic representation. Despite the fact that signals originating from a large region of the retinal surface must be integrated to allow for interpolation, a continuous and precise representation of the visual field is built up. Thus, early in visual cortical processing, the discontinuous retinal image is converted into a continuous visuotopic representation.

## References

Baumann R, van der Zwan R, and Peterhans E (1997) Figure–ground segregation at contours: A neural mechanism in the visual cortex of the alert monkey. *Eur J Neurosci* 9:1290–1303.

Bosking WH, Zhang Y, Schofield B, and Fitzpatrick D (1997) Orientation selectivity and the arrangement of horizontal connections in tree shrew striate cortex. *J Neurosci* 17:2112–2127.

Das A and Gilbert CD (1995) Receptive field expansion in adult visual cortex is linked to dynamic changes in strength of cortical connections. *J Neurophysiol* 74:779–792.

Das A and Gilbert CD (1999) Topography of contextual modulations mediated by short-range interactions in primary visual cortex. *Nature* 339:655–661.

Fiorani M, Rosa MGP, Gattass R, and Rocha-Miranda CE (1992) Dynamic surrounds of receptive fields in primate striate cortex: A physiological basis for perceptual completion. *Proc Natl Acad Sci USA* 89:8547–8551.

Fiorani M, Azzi JCB, and Gattass R (2001) Primate V1 has a visuotopic rather than a retinotopic organization: The topographic organization of the blind spot (BS) in V1. *Soc Neurosci Abstr* 27: Prog. No 619.46.

Gilbert CD (1992) Horizontal integration and cortical dynamics. *Neuron* 9:1–13.

Gilbert CD and Wiesel TN (1990) The influence of contextual stimuli on the orientation selectivity of cells in primary visual cortex of the cat. *Vision Res* 30;1689–1701.

Gilbert CD and Wiesel TN (1992) Receptive field dynamics in adult primary visual cortex. *Nature* 356:150–152.

Gilbert CD, Ito M, Kapadia M, and Westheimer G (2000) Interactions between attention, context and learning in primary visualcortex. *Vision Res* 40:1217–1226.

Greene HH and Brown JM (2000) Amodal completion and localization. *Vision Res* 40:383–390.
Goodale MA and Milner AD (1996) The visual brain in action, Oxford Psychology Series no 27. Oxford University Press.
Gregory RL (1972) Cognitive contours. *Nature* 238:51–52.
Grosof D, Shapley R, and Hawken M (1993) Macaque V1 neurons can signal "illusory" contours. *Nature* 365:550–552.
Grossberg S and Mingolla E (1985) Neural dynamics of form perception: Boundary completion, illusory figures, and neon color spreading. *Psychol Rev* 92:173–211.
Hirsch JA and Gilbert CD (1991) Synaptic physiology of horizontal connections in the cat's visual cortex. *J Neurosci* 11:1800–1809.
Horton JC, Dagi LR, McGrane EP, and Monasterio F (1990) Arrangement of ocular dominance columns in human visual cortex. *Arch Ophthalmol* 108:1025–1031.
Kapadia MK, Ito M, Gilbert CD, and Westheimer G (1995) Improvement in visual sensitivity by changes in local context: Parallel studies in human observers and in V1 of alert monkeys. *Neuron* 15:843–856.
Kawabata N (1984) Perception at the blind spot and similarity grouping. *Percept Psychophys* 36:151–158.
Kawabata H, Gyoba J, Inoue H, and Ohtsubo, H (1999) Visual completion of partly occluded grating in infants under 1 month of age. *Vision Res* 39:3586–3591.
Komatsu H and Murakami I (1994) Behavioral evidence of filling-in at the blind spot of the monkey. *Vis Neurosci* 11:1103–1113.
MacEvoy SP, Kim W, and Paradiso MA (1998) Integration of surface information in primary visual cortex. *Nat Neurosci* 1:616–620.
Murakami I (1995) Motion aftereffect after monocular adaptation to filled-in motion at the blind spot. *Vision Res* 35:1041–1045.
Nelson JI and Frost BJ (1985) Intracortical facilitation among co-oriented, co-axially aligned simple cells in cat striate cortex. *Exp Brain Res* 61:54–61.
Oliveira L, Volchan E, Pessoa L, Pantoja JH, Joffily M, Souza-Netto D, Marques RF, and Rocha-Miranda CE. Contour integration in the primary visual cortex of the opossum. *Neuro Report*, in press.
Oliveira L, Volchan E, Souza AO, Pantoja JH, Penetra LJS, Marques RF, Pereira A, Gawryszenski LG, Bernardes RF, and Rocha-Miranda CE (1998) Amodal completion in the opossum primary visual cortex. *Soc Neurosci Abstr* 24:646.
Pessoa L, Thompson E, and Nöe A (1998) Finding out about filling-in: A guide to perceptual completion for visual science and the philosophy of perception. *Behav Brain Sci* 21:723–802.
Peterhans E and von der Heydt R (1989) Mechanisms of contour perception in monkey visual cortex. II. Contours bridging gaps. *J Neurosci* 9:1749–1763.
Pettet MW and Gilbert CD (1992) Dynamic changes in receptive-field size in cat primary visual cortex. *Proc Natl Acad Sci USA* 89:8366–8370.
Polat U, Mizobe K, Pettet MW, Kasamatsu T, and Norcia AM (1998) Collinear stimuli regulate visual responses depending on cell's contrast threshold. *Nature* 391:580–584.
Redies C, Crook JM, and Creutzfeld OD (1987) Neuronal responses to borders with and without luminance gradients in cat visual cortex and dorsal lateral geniculate nucleus. *Exp Brain Res* 61:469–481.
Rensink RA and Enns JT (1998) Early completion of the occluded objects. *Vision Res* 38:2489–2505.

Rock I and Anson R (1979) Illusory contours as a solution to a problem. *Perception* 8:665–681.

Rosa MGP, Gattass R, and Fiorani M Jr (1988) Complete pattern of ocular dominance stripes in V1 of a New World monkey *Cebus apella*. *Exp Brain Res* 72:645–648.

Rosa MGP, Gattass R, Fiorani M Jr, and Soares JGM (1992) Laminar, columnar and topographic aspects of ocular dominance in the primary visual cortex of the *Cebus* monkeys. *Exp Brain Res* 88:249–264.

Rossi AF, Rittenhouse CD, and Paradiso MA (1996) The representation of brightness in primary visual cortex. *Science* 273:1104–1107.

Sengpiel F, Sen A, and Blakemore C (1997) Characteristics of surround inhibition in cat area 17. *Exp Brain Res* 116:216–228.

Volchan E and Gilbert CD (1995) Interocular transfer of receptive field expansion in cat visual cortex. *Vision Res* 35:1–6.

von der Heydt R (1995) Form analysis in visual cortex. In: Gazzaniga MS (ed), *The Cognitive Neurosciences*. Cambridge, MA: MIT Press, pp 365–382.

von der Heydt R and Peterhans E (1989) Mechanisms of contour perception in monkey visual cortex. I. Lines of pattern discontinuity. *J Neurosci* 9:1731–1748.

Zipser K, Lamme V, and Schiller P (1996) Contextual modulation in primary visual cortex. *J Neurosci* 16:7375–7389.

# 10

## The Reactivation and Reorganization of Retinotopic Maps in Visual Cortex of Adult Mammals After Retinal and Cortical Lesions

JON H. KAAS, CHRISTINE E. COLLINS, AND YUZO M. CHINO

The mammalian visual system is characterized by a hierarchy of processing stations that tend to preserve and reflect the spatial order of outputs from the retina of each eye. The optic nerve fibers maintain much of the spatial organization as they leave the eye, and refine that order as they terminate in their major brainstem targets, the dorsal lateral geniculate nucleus (LGN) and the superior colliculus. A retinotopic pattern is preserved in the LGN projections to primary visual cortex and in at least several other areas devoted to the early stages of cortical processing of visual information. The question we address here is, what happens to these orderly representations of the retinal outputs when some part of the retina is missing? A commonsense answer to that question is "not much." Obviously, neurons in central structures such as the LGN and primary visual cortex (V1) cannot respond to missing parts of the retina, so neurons totally deprived of visual activation after binocular lesioning, would be expected to respond not at all, and neurons missing inputs from only one eye would be expected to respond from visuotopically equivalent or matched positions of the intact eye. This commonsense outcome is so expected that when we and our coworkers submitted a paper on cortical reorganization after retinal lesioning some years ago (Kaas et al 1990), a reviewer protested that our finding that neurons in the deprived region of the cortex acquired new receptive fields and became responsive to intact portions of the retina could not be valid, because only the developing visual system could have that much plasticity. It seemed to matter little that reorganization of similar topographic representations of the contralateral body surface in primary somatosensory cortex had already been known to reorganize after a loss of afferents as a result of nerve damage (Merzenich et al., 1983a, 1983b, 1984). Many investigators appeared to think that visual and somatosensory systems were different, in that only the somatosensory system was plastic in adults, or perhaps they questioned the results from the somatosensory system.

Fortunately, the paper was published, and soon similar results appeared from two other laboratories (Kaas et al., 1990; Heinen and Skavenski, 1991; Gilbert and Wiesel, 1992). The reality of such plasticity in the brains of adult cats and monkeys no longer seems in doubt, and researchers have gone on to subsidiary questions. Investigators now want to know if retinotopic maps in all structures are plastic, the extents and types of plasticity in these structures, the conditions and rates of reorganization, the response properties of reactivated neurons and their functional roles, and the mechanisms of recovery. Investigators also want to know if reorganization in retinotopic representations occurs if part of their map is damaged or if part of the activity in retinotopic input from another area is removed. The possibility of such reorganization in visual cortex is suggested by evidence of local reorganization around small lesions in somatosensory cortex (Jenkins and Merzenich, 1987; Doetch et al., 1990) and from reorganization of the second somatosensory area, S2, after partial lesioning of the first area, S1 (Pons et al., 1988). In this review, we address research related to some of these issues.

## Reorganization of Visual Cortex Following Damage to Inputs

Visual cortex has been deprived of retinal activation in cats and monkeys in several ways. The conceptually simple approach has been to create small but visuotopically matching lesions in the retina of each eye so that a small portion of visual cortex is totally deprived of its normal sources of retinal activation (see Gilbert and Wiesel, 1992; Chino et al., 1995; Darian-Smith and Gilbert, 1995). Since it can be difficult to match the two lesions precisely, a related approach has been to remove all visual input from one eye while placing a small lesion in the retina of the other eye (Kaas et al., 1990; Chino et al., 1992; Schmid et al., 1996). Thus, visual cortex becomes essentially monocular, and the retinal lesion produces a hole in the monocular relay of retinal positions. A third approach has been to lesion the retina of only one eye (Chino et al., 1992; Schmid et al., 1996; Chino, 1997; Calford et al., 1999, 2000). These monocular lesions do not totally deprive any region of visual cortex of visual activation, but the responses to the lesioned and intact eyes could be compared in binocular neurons.

The experiments listed above raised and addressed several basic questions: (1) Would cortex in the retinotopic representations in primary visual cortex (striate cortex) and elsewhere that is deprived of normal activation by binocular lesions recover responsiveness to intact surrounding portions of the retina? (2) If recovery occurs, is it rapid or slow? In each case, what are the implied mechanisms of recovery? What hard evidence can be obtained about the mechanisms of recovery? (3) Do reorganizational changes in the retina or LGN contribute to cortical recovery? (4) What are the response properties of reactivated neurons? Are they extremely abnormal or do they have some of the response features of neurons in normal visual cortex? (5) After monocular lesioning, do neurons in deprived cortex respond to only the retina of the intact eye or to both eyes but possibly preferentially to the intact eye? If neurons respond to both eyes, do individual neurons respond to both eyes with mismatched receptive fields for each eye or only to one eye? (6) Finally, what are the perceptual consequences of retinal lesions and any subsequent cortical reorganization? Obviously, retinal lesions would produce monocular or binocular blind spots, but such blind spots often escape awareness and the blind area is filled-in by the visual surround. Can such filling-in be explained by changes in the cortex after lesions?

## The Recovery of Responsiveness

One might expect bilateral matching lesions of the retina of each eye to produce zones of visual cortex where neurons are totally and permanently unresponsive to visual stimuli. Neurons in the deprived cortex would no longer have access to the parts of the retina that created their normal receptive fields. To become responsive to visual stimulation, they would need to acquire new sources of activation, either as a result of previously existing but not above-threshold connections becoming effective or as a result of the growth of new connections. The surprising result from the early experiments was that deprived neurons became responsive to visual stimulation, and they acquired new receptive fields dispersed around the margins of the retinal lesion. The reactivated neurons often responded vigorously to visual stimuli, appeared to have at least roughly normal response properties, and had receptive fields of roughly normal sizes. Thus, Kaas et al. (1990) reported that after 2–6 months of recovery in cats, deprived "neurons were activated by visual stimuli and had receptive fields of normal sizes." However, some neurons had two receptive fields, one on either side of the lesion. Similarly, Gilbert and Wiesel (1992), recording from adult cats and monkeys after creating matched retinal lesions in the two eyes, found deprived neurons to be highly responsive to visual stimuli, with displaced receptive fields of normal sizes located around the margin of the lesions. They also noted bipartite receptive fields spanning the lesion and mismatched receptive fields for the two eyes (also see Chino et al., 1995). Heinen and Skavenski (1991) deactivated a larger sector of visual cortex in adult monkeys by producing bilateral foveal lesions and found that after 75 days of recovery, many neurons in the totally deprived zone of striate cortex were vigorously responsive to stimuli. The neurons had receptive fields that were much larger (up to 5 degrees in diameter) than the very small receptive fields expected for foveal striate cortex neurons but only somewhat larger than one might expect from parafoveal activation. Many of the reactivated neurons had receptive fields with diffuse borders, and they were less responsive than normal neurons. Possibly with the larger cortical deactivation produced by foveal lesions in monkeys, recovery was less complete.

Altogether, the results indicate a remarkable capacity for neurons in visual cortex of the mature brain to acquire new receptive fields and new activating inputs from nearby retinal locations when totally deprived of their normal sources of retinal input. The new receptive fields are often roughly normal in size. However, the nature of the reactivation may depend on the size of the retinal lesions and the portion of visual cortex deactivated. The monocular sector of V1 representing the extreme of peripheral vision appears to reactivate only to a very limited extent after retinal lesioning (Clarke et al., 1992; Rosa et al., 1995).

## The Sequence of Reactivation

The immediate consequence of producing matched bilateral lesions of the retina is to deactivate neurons in the core of the deprived zone. When, for example, Heinen and Skavenski (1991) recorded immediately after lesioning the fovea of each eye in monkeys, a region of foveal striate cortex was found in which "all neurons were unresponsive to any . . . visual stimuli presented anywhere within five degrees of arc of the center of the visual field." The "totally unresponsive zone" was bordered by a fringe of cortex where some cells could be driven, apparently because they retained some of their activating inputs. Gilbert and Wiesel (1992) noted that immediately after bilaterally matched paracentral retinal lesions were produced in adult cats, neurons in the core of the deactivated striate cortex were completely unresponsive to visual stimuli. However, neurons near the margin of the deprived zone of cortex did respond to visual stimuli. These neurons had greatly expanded receptive fields that were shifted in position from just inside to just outside the retinal lesion.

Thus, a fringe of deprived cortical neurons started to become reactivated and acquired new receptive fields immediately after total loss of suprathreshold activating inputs due to retinal lesioning of both eyes. The location of these neurons on the fringe of the deactivated zone suggests that they receive more subthreshold activating inputs that can be raised to above the threshold. The rapid changes in the effective receptive fields for these neurons suggest that the retinal lesions reduced the inhibition in the deprived cortex so that weak activating inputs from the intact retina become suprathreshold.

Over days to months, more neurons become responsive to intact portions of the retina until deprived regions of cortex several millimeters in diameter become reactivated throughout. Larger regions of deactivation may not completely fill-in or they may require longer periods of recovery than have been studied. The small portion of primary visual cortex that represents the monocular crescent of the contralateral eye may be special in that it seems to have only limited potential for reactivation.

## The Effects of Restricted Monocular Lesions

In early studies of the effects of monocular lesions on the responses of neurons in visual cortex, there was little evidence of cortical plasticity (Kaas et al., 1990;

Chino et al., 1992; Gilbert and Wiesel, 1992; Komatsu and Murakami, 1994; Chino, 1997). Kaas et al. (1990) concluded that monocular lesions revealed only the effect of removing one of two sources of activation to binocular cortical neurons rather than any basic reorganization. Thus, deprived neurons responded with retinotopically appropriate receptive fields for the intact eye and not with mismatched receptive fields displaced to the surround of the lesion in the lesioned eye, even after months of recovery (Chino et al., 1992). A latent reorganization in cortex was revealed by enucleating the intact eye in animals that had chronic lesions in the other eye (Chino et al., 1992). In these cats, the now totally deprived neurons in primary visual cortex immediately acquired displaced receptive fields in the retina around the retinal lesion. Thus, a connectional framework for such displaced receptive fields either always existed or developed during the recovery period. This framework was cryptic and was suppressed by inputs from the normal eye.

The results of subsequent studies suggest that some reorganization of visual cortex does develop over time after focused monocular lesions. Schmid et al. (1996) lesioned one eye in adult cats and found, 8–33 days later, as had previous investigators, that neurons in the deprived zone of cortex were largely unresponsive to the lesioned eye while being quite responsive to the intact eye. However, they also found some neurons with weak, rapidly habituating responses to the lesioned eye, with responses coming from retinal locations around the lesion. These neurons were most frequently located along the fringe of the deprived zone, suggesting that these neurons may not have been totally deprived. These neurons exhibited very weak responses that could be masked by the (Schmid et al., 1996; also see Chino et al., 1992) inhibitory influence of activity evoked from the intact eye. Recently, Calford et al. (1999) have provided evidence that the normally inhibited and subthreshold activation of neurons in visual cortex by stimuli beyond their normal receptive fields can rise above threshold within hours. After focal lesioning of one eye in adult cats, neurons in the deprived zone of primary visual cortex were normally responsive to stimulation of the intact eye but were unresponsive or weakly responsive to stimulation of the lesioned eye. However, responses to the lesioned eye strengthened over hours after lesioning. Most notably, neurons along an electrode tract in deprived cortex that were totally unresponsive to the lesioned eye 3 hours after lesioning became responsive after 7 hours of deprivation. The reactivated neurons had large, displaced receptive fields. The results suggest that weak connections can be potentiated over a period of hours, but it is not clear why such connections were expressed in these experiments and not in others.

The fact that the responses of monocularly deprived neurons to the lesioned eye are typically weak, absent, or fragile does not diminish their importance. In a quantitative study, Chino (1997) described the characteristics of the binocular signal interactions that resulted from the stimulation of the receptive field for the nonlesioned eye and the simultaneous stimulation of a discrete intact region surrounding the lesion. The binocular signal interactions were either excitatory or suppressive, and the strength of binocular interactions decreased as the visual stimulation moved away from the edge of the scotoma in the lesioned eye. The experiment illustrated in Figure 10-1 demonstrates the existence of such weak signals from the lesioned eye in deprived visual cortex. In an adult cat that received a unilateral lesion 3 months prior to the recording experiment, no receptive fields could be mapped, as expected, for the neurons normally receiving input from the lesioned area of the retina, while normal receptive fields of these units were found for the nonlesioned eye (Fig. 10-1A, top and middle). However, under our dichoptic stimulation conditions, there were considerable *excitatory* binocular signal interactions between the receptive fields of the nonlesioned eye (arrow in the top panel) and a discrete intact region surrounding the scotoma (arrow with stimulation area in the middle panel) (Fig. 10-1B). More important, upon removal of *all* activity from the nonlesioned eye by injecting lidocaine into the vitreous during the same penetration, receptive fields could be mapped by stimulating the lesioned eye at the recording sites where no driven activity was recorded before silencing the nonlesioned eye (receptive fields with thick lines in Fig. 10-1A, bottom). Also, newly activated units were very responsive and showed normal orientation/direction tunings and spatial frequency tunings (Fig. 10-1C).

Even more extensive reorganization appears to emerge when monocular lesions are placed in younger animals and longer recovery times are allowed. In a preliminary study, Mori et al. (2000) demonstrated that if a monocular lesion was produced at 8 weeks of age in kittens, the map reorganization was complete and no silent area of the brain was found following an extraordinarily long recovery period (>3 years) (Fig. 10-2). The receptive fields of newly activated cells have normal orientation and spatial frequency tuning properties that are very similar to those found for the receptive fields of the nonlesioned eye. Moreover, there were substantial signal interactions between the two eyes under dichoptic stimulation conditions that were either excitatory or inhibitory in nature.

---

**Figure 10-1.** (A) Cortical map for nonlesioned (top) and lesioned (middle) eyes during a single penetration through the medial bank of the posterolateral gyrus of an adult cat. Shaded circles indicate a scotoma created by the lesion. At the end of the penetration, the activity from the nonlesioned eye was completely suppressed by an intravitreous injection of lidocaine while the electrode stayed in the brain. When no activity was recorded from the nonlesioned eye, the electrode was retracted, and at every 200 $\mu$m, receptive fields were mapped (bottom). Note that receptive fields could be mapped at the sites that were unresponsive prior to silencing the nonlesioned eye (fields with thick lines) (Mori et al., 2000). (B) Binocular interactions between the receptive field of a unit to stimulation of the nonlesioned eye (arrow in A) and the eight discrete normal regions surrounding the scotoma (A, middle). Data points inside the circle indicate binocular suppression and those outside indicate the excitatory interactions. Note that a significant excitatory interaction was found for the upper left edge of the scotoma (Chino, 1997). (C) Orientation/direction tuning functions and spatial frequency tuning functions for the unit studied in (A, top) before silencing the activity (top) and a reactivated unit after silencing the nonlesioned eye (bottom) (Chino, 1997).

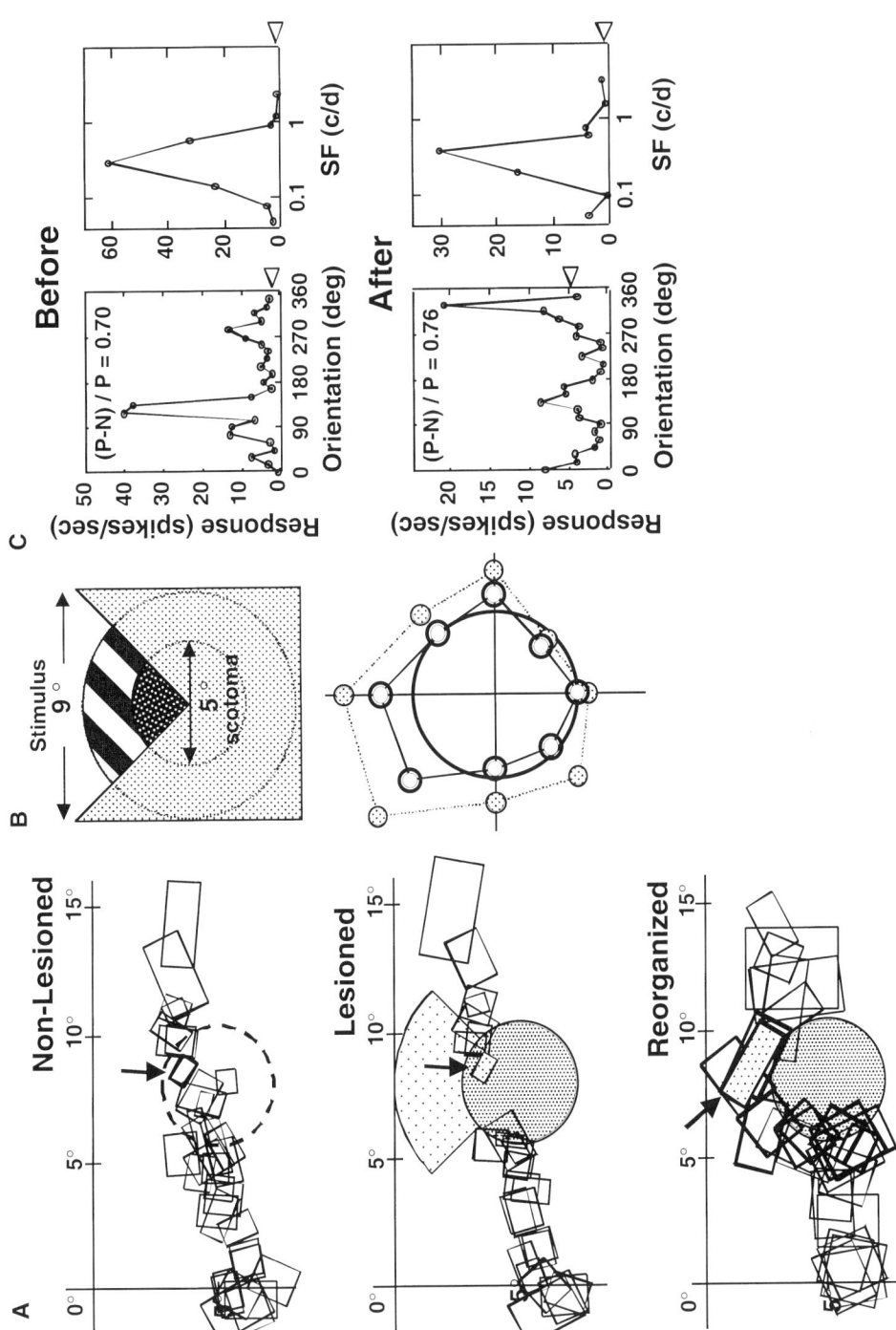

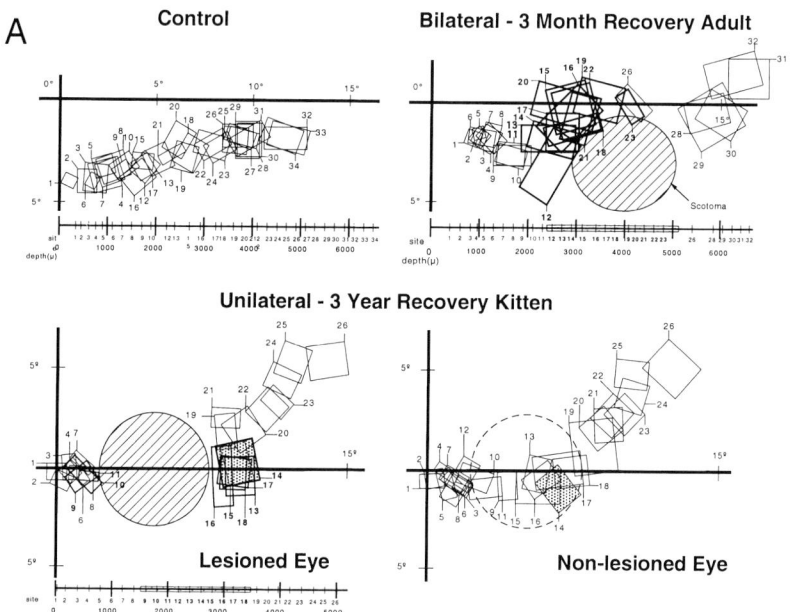
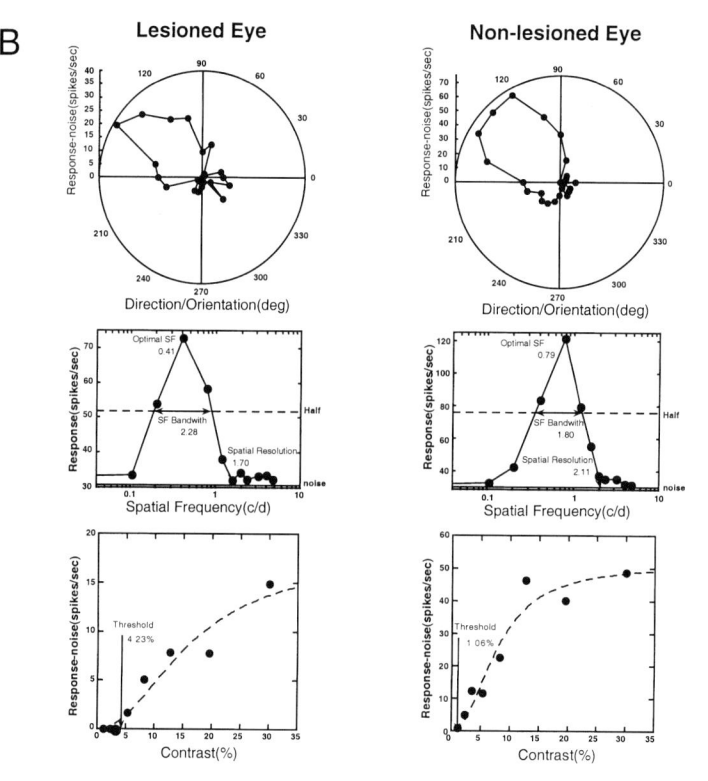

These findings provide evidence for a system of weak lateral activation in visual cortex that emerges after retinal lesioning but is normally suppressed. In the absence of suppressive influence from the normal eye, neurons in the monocularly deprived zone of cortex can express these weak connections. Moreover the strengthening of such connections by prolonged use could account for the more profound reactivations of binocularly deprived neurons due to plasticity that exists in the adult brain (Kaas et al., 1990; Chino et al., 1992; Darian-Smith and Gilbert, 1994; Chino, 1997; Matsuura et al., 1999).

## Effects of Restricted Retinal Lesions on Neurons in the LGN

In principle, all of the reorganization expressed in primary visual cortex after foveal retinal lesions could occur in the LGN or even the eye itself. Horton and Hocking (1998), for example, contend that the delayed cortical recovery after retinal lesioning is related to retinal healing. However, both the retina and the LGN as possible sites of significant reorganization seem to be ruled out by studies of the effects of retinal lesions on the activation of LGN neurons (also see Fig. 10-3). Long before the cortical effects of retinal lesions were known, Eysel and coworkers (1980, 1981) found that small monocular retinal lesions of the retina of cats left a permanent core of unresponsive neurons in the deprived layers of the LGN. These unresponsive cores were bordered by a narrow transition zone of neurons that over weeks of recovery acquired new receptive fields just outside the lesion in the retina. Thus, there was some reorganization of the retinotopy of the deprived geniculate layers and some reactivation of neurons. Yet, this reactivation was too limited in extent to account for the cortical reorganization.

This point was again demonstrated by Darian-Smith and Gilbert (1995) when they made binocularly matched foveal lesions in the retinas of cats and

**Figure 10-2.** (A) Receptive field maps of units encountered during the electrode penetration through area 17 in a normal control cat (top left) and in an adult cat that received bilateral retinal lesions and was mapped after 3 months of recovery (top right) (Chino et al., 1995). This map was obtained in the same cat described in Figure 10-1. Receptive fields with thick lines indicate the reactivated neurons. Similar cortical maps for the lesioned eye (left bottom) and the nonlesioned eye (right bottom) for a cat that received a unilateral lesion and over 3 years of recovery (Mori et al., 2000). Hatched circles indicate the cortical scotoma created by retinal lesions, and the open circle with dotted lines shows the area of the visual field for the nonlesioned eye that retinotopically matches that in the scotoma for the lesioned eye. The response properties of the neuron having the filled receptive fields are illustrated in (B). (B) Similarity in the response properties of the marked unit in (A) during stimulation of the reactivated receptive field of the lesioned eye (left) and the normal receptive field of the nonlesioned eye (right). Direction/orientation tuning (top), spatial frequency tuning (middle) and contrast-response functions (bottom) (Mori et al., 2000).

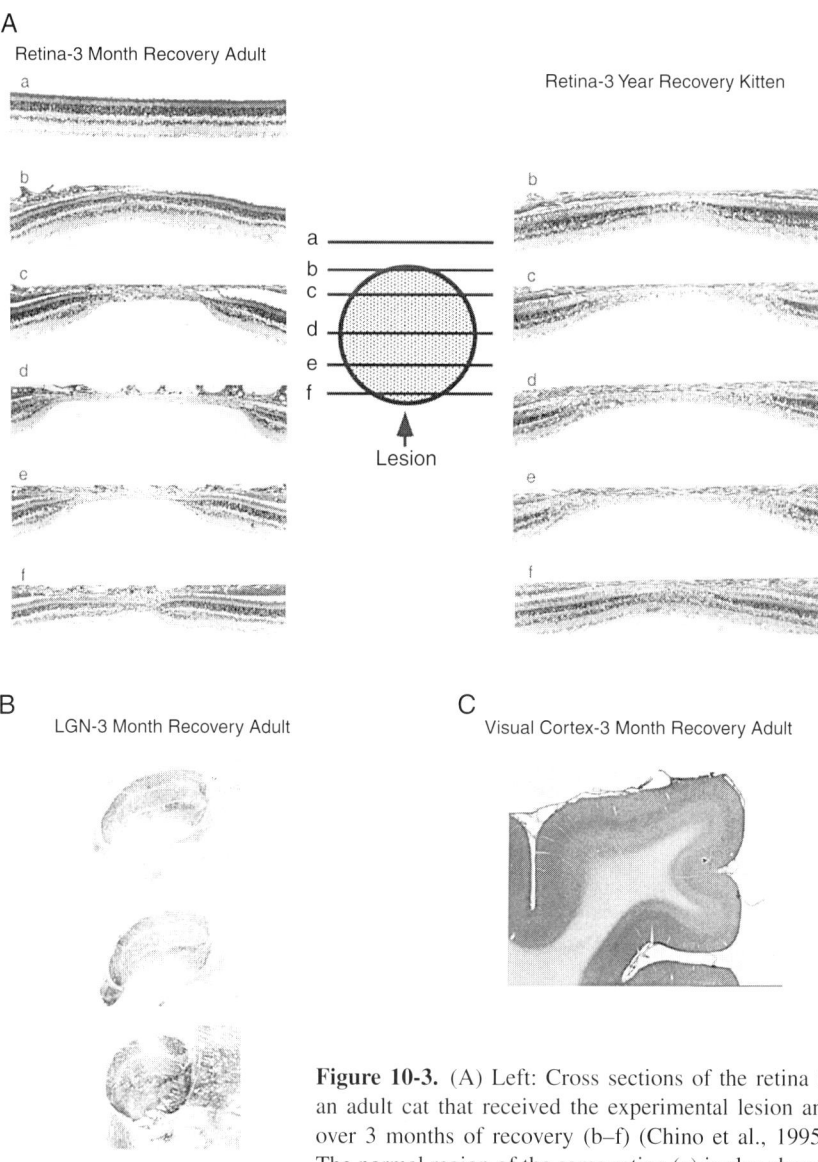

**Figure 10-3.** (A) Left: Cross sections of the retina in an adult cat that received the experimental lesion and over 3 months of recovery (b–f) (Chino et al., 1995). The normal region of the same retina (a) is also shown. Middle: The diagram shows the approximate locations from which each section was taken. Right: Similar cross sections of the retina in a cat that received a comparable lesion and over 3 years of recovery (b–f) (Mori et al., 2000). (B) Coronal LGN sections stained with cytochrome oxidase (CO) in the same cat as in (A) that received a bilateral experimental lesion in the contralateral eye and a larger lesion in the ipsilateral eye. Note the clear reduction in CO activity in layers A and A1 of the LGN that corresponded to the size and location of the lesion (most obviously in the bottom section) (Y. Chino, unpublished data). (C) Coronal section of areas 17 and 18 stained with CO in the same cat as in (A) and (B). The arrow head indicates a lesion made by the electrode track. Note the absence of regions showing a clear reduction in CO activity (Y. Chino, unpublished data).

monkeys and recorded from the LGN and cortex in the same animals after months of recovery. Their conclusion was that at a time when cortical reorganization is complete, a silent area of the LGN persists (Fig. 10-3B), indicating that the changes in cortical topography are due to alterations that are intrinsic to cortex. Thus, some of the slowly emerging changes observed in cortex may be relayed from the LGN, but clearly most are not. Only a narrow fringe zone of cortical recovery along the margins of the deprived cortex can be attributed to a geniculate relay. These observations on the limits of plasticity in the LGN also clearly indicate that the reorganization of cortex is not a relay of changes in the retina as a result of "healing" or retinal reorganization (e.g., Figs. 10-3A, 10-3B), since the LGN reorganization should then be as extensive as that observed in cortex. The limited LGN reactivation that emerges slowly (Eysel et al., 1981) seems to depend on increased synaptic effectiveness of intact retinal afferents on the distal dendrites of deprived neurons that extend into the innervated portions of the LGN rather than local sprouting of preserved retinal afferents into the denervated zones (Stelzner and Keating, 1977; Baisden et al., 1980; Eysel, 1982).

## The Response Properties of Reactivated Cortical Neurons

The properties of reactivated cortical neurons after focused retinal lesions depend on the recovery time. The few initial responses of neurons, apparently as a result of the potentiation of sparse preserved inputs due to reduced inhibition, are weak, inconsistent, and rapidly habituating (Schmid et al., 1996). These responses are clearly abnormal. However, after weeks to months of recovery, neurons recorded in the deprived zone of cortex have been described as having roughly normal responses to visual stimuli (Kaas et al., 1990; Chino et al., 1992; Gilbert and Wiesel, 1992). These subjective impressions of the recovery of normal responsiveness with abnormal receptive field locations have been supported to a large extent by the results of a quantitative study of single-neuron response properties in deprived cortex of adult cats 2.5 to 3 months after the placement of retinotopically matched lesions in each retina (Chino et al., 1995). In the deactivated zone, over 98% of recorded neurons responded to visual stimuli and had new, displaced receptive fields. The reactivated neurons displayed normal orientation tuning, direction selectivity, and spatial frequency tuning when tested with high-contrast stimuli. However, the neurons as a group were abnormal in that stimulus contrast thresholds were elevated and the maximal responses to optimal stimuli were reduced. Thus, the neurons were capable of generating normal signals, except for spatial location, but they were generally less responsive to optimal visual stimuli than normal neurons. Interestingly, a longer recovery period following retinal lesions (e.g., >3 years) was reported to improve the overall responsiveness of the reactivated units (Matsuura et al., 1999). Further studies are needed to evaluate the time course of recovery and the influences of retinal lesion size. In addition, data from monkeys as well as cats would be valuable.

## Mechanisms of Recovery

The immediate responses of deprived neurons after retinal lesioning reveal the presence of previously existing but subthreshold inputs to cortical neurons. The presence of such connections can be revealed in intact animals by several procedures that reduce cortical inhibition. One procedure is to induce an artificial scotoma by masking a portion of the visual field during visual stimulation. When tested during these conditions, neurons in the deprived region of cortex visually demonstrate enlarged receptive fields after a few minutes of masking (Fiorani et al., 1992; Pettet and Gilbert, 1992). The deprivation effect is even seen when binocular neurons are deprived in one eye and tested in the other eye, providing clear evidence that the relevant changes in responsiveness are due to cortical mechanisms (Volchan and Gilbert, 1995).

The responses of cortical neurons to stimuli within the receptive field are altered by stimuli beyond the classical receptive field (Allman et al., 1985; Das and Gilbert, 1995b, 1999), indicating a powerful role for horizontal connections in normal cortex. Subthreshold facilitation and suppression effects of stimuli presented outside the receptive field have also been revealed by optical imaging techniques (Toth et al., 1996). The connections that mediate such effects could have a role in cortical reactivation as they would be potentiated after retinal lesions reduce the activation of inhibitory neurons within the deprived cortex. As another mechanism for recovery, synaptic strengths and neuron response properties can be rapidly altered by associative conditioning procedures (McLean and Palmer, 1998). Thus, even short periods of visual experience would potentiate weak connections. Finally, other possibilities for weak but immediate responses in deprived cortex need to be considered. A few neurons with ectopic receptive fields may exist in normal cortex, and there are weak but measurable effects of the lateral spread of excitation in the retina (McIlwain, 1966; Barlow et al., 1977).

Longer-term effects that restore nearly normal response properties to deprived neurons may depend in part on conditioning effects that selectively strengthen some of the synapses (Eysel et al., 1998; Matsuura et al., 1999). In addition, the decreased activity, sometimes reflected in reduced cytochrome oxidase activity (Horton and Hocking, 1998), appears to downregulate the expression of the inhibitory neurotransmitter gamma-aminobutyric acid (GABA) and receptors for GABA (Rosier et al., 1995; Arckens et al., 1998), thereby increasing the chances for subthreshold excitatory synapses to be expressed in neuronal responses. Furthermore, the effectiveness of horizontal cortical connections may be increased by the actual growth of new connections, as reported for reorganized primary visual cortex of cats after retinal lesions (Darian-Smith and Gilbert, 1994) and in primary somatosensory cortex of monkeys after peripheral nerve damage (Florence et al., 1998). The growth of new connections may be mediated by activity-sensitive changes in gene expression. The deprived zones of visual cortex thereby express more neurotrophins and growth-associated proteins as early as 2 days after lesioning (Obata et al., 1999).

## Functional Consequences of Retinal Lesions

The reactivation of cortical neurons could alter perception in two different ways. First, deprived neurons acquire new receptive fields that overlap those of nearby neurons in normally activated cortex. This creates a substantial increase in the number of neurons with receptive fields corresponding to the immediate surround of the retinal lesion. Devoting more neurons to a task could produce better performance. Thus, improved perception could exist for the region of the retina surrounding the lesion. While more study is needed, there is some evidence in monkeys for such improved performance, as supersensitivity develops for retinal locations surrounding the lesion (Weiskrantz and Cowey, 1967).

The second expected perceptual consequence of cortical reorganization following bilateral lesioning is that visual stimuli would be mislocated, since the reactivated neurons would signal the wrong visual field location for visual stimuli. In cases of forelimb amputation in humans, touch on the stump of the amputated limb activates neurons in primary somatosensory cortex that normally respond to the upper arm and neurons in reactivated cortex that normally respond to the hand (Davis et al., 1998; Kaas et al., 1999). In humans with retinal lesions, stimuli in the surround of the lesion may also be seen within the portion of the visual field covered by the lesion, so that the blind spot is filled-in and not seen by the patient (Gerrits and Timmerman, 1969; Sergent, 1988). We would expect better filling-in in the core of a binocular than a monocular scotoma, although for small lesions filling-in is extensive even with a monocular scotoma if lesions are due to congenital defects or occur very early in life, since binocular interactions do appear to occur in the region of a monocular congenital scotoma in humans (Tripathy and Levi, 1999). For monocular lesions, there also may be other mechanisms for filling-in (see De Weerd et al., 1995; Murakami et al., 1997).

## The Reactivation of Extrastriate Visual Cortex After Focal Lesioning of Primary Visual Cortex

What happens to extrastriate visual cortex after lesioning of primary visual cortex is not yet fully apparent. Since striate cortex provides direct or indirect activating input to areas of extrastriate cortex, such lesioning could abolish all visually evoked activity. Alternatively, to the extent that other thalamic inputs from the LGN or visual pulvinar are normally effective, evoked visual responses could remain in extrastriate cortex immediately after lesions. As another possibility, such thalamic inputs could be initially subthreshold but could be raised to above-threshold levels over recovery times. Finally, if such thalamic sources of activation are missing or insufficient, inputs from remaining portions of the striate cortex could enlarge their extrastriate zones of activation, either immediately, due to a reduction of lateral inhibition, or more slowly, due to a number of recovery mechanisms possibly including the growth of new horizontal connections. To date, the most relevant studies have been in monkeys, in which few lateral geniculate projections target extrastriate areas (see Bullier et al., 1994; Stepniewska et al., 1999) and in which lesioning and cooling of striate cortex deactivate large regions of extrastriate cortex (e.g., Schiller and Malpeli, 1977; Girard et al., 1991).

As one of the major targets of V1 projections, the middle temporal (MT) visual area, has been repeatedly studied after partial or complete lesioning or deactivation of V1. The results seem somewhat inconsistent and confusing, possibly because of the different protocols of the investigators and possibly because of the different species of monkeys that were studied. The effects of striate cortex lesioning on the responsiveness of extrastriate neurons may vary from one cortical area to another or even with species for the same area. Most relevant for the present issue of the potential for plasticity in extrastriate cortex is that there is evidence for the expansion of the activating territories in MT of the remaining parts of area 17 after incomplete lesioning. Several investigators have reported that neurons in MT remain responsive to visual stimuli after lesioning or inactivation of striate cortex in macaque monkeys, either after weeks of recovery (Rodman et al., 1989) or within hours (Girard et al., 1992). This responsiveness has been attributed to an alternative pathway from the superior colliculus to the pulvinar and then to cortex (Rodman et al., 1990). These results contrast with the findings of Maunsell et al. (1990), who reported that MT neuron responsiveness depended on the LGN, presumably via a relay through striate cortex. In New World owl monkeys, Kaas and Krubitzer (1992) found zones of completely unresponsive neurons in MT immediately after partial striate cortex lesioning. However, some neurons along the fringe of the deprived zone in MT responded to remaining inputs from area 17 with slightly displaced receptive fields. Thus, there was some evidence for rapid plasticity in a marginal zone of cortex.

Other studies examined the responsiveness of deprived MT neurons in New World monkeys after weeks or more of recovery. Collins et al. (1999) tested the responsiveness of MT neurons in adult owl monkeys 2 months or more after striate cortex lesioning. This study revealed a normally responsive MT 2 months after production of a small striate cortex lesion in the lower visual quadrant, suggesting complete filling-in of the scotoma. However, a persistent lack of responsiveness of MT neurons was found in the core of the deprived zone in MT after a more extensive striate cortex ablation (Fig. 10-4). With a large ablation, neurons along the margin of the deprived portion of MT were responsive to visual stimuli and were often direction and speed selective, but in many cases were rapidly habituating (Fig. 10-4B). All visual activity in responsive MT neurons could be related to intact portions of V1.

A study by Rosa et al. (2000) reported displaced receptive fields in more than half of MT neurons weeks after a partial striate cortex ablation in marmosets. The receptive fields were shifted to represent the visual field immediately surrounding the scotoma. Thus, there is further evidence that preserved parts of area 17 expand their territories in MT over recovery times. The report also stated that 20% of MT neurons with receptive fields within the scotoma were normally responsive. This recovery appears to be substantially less than that previously re-

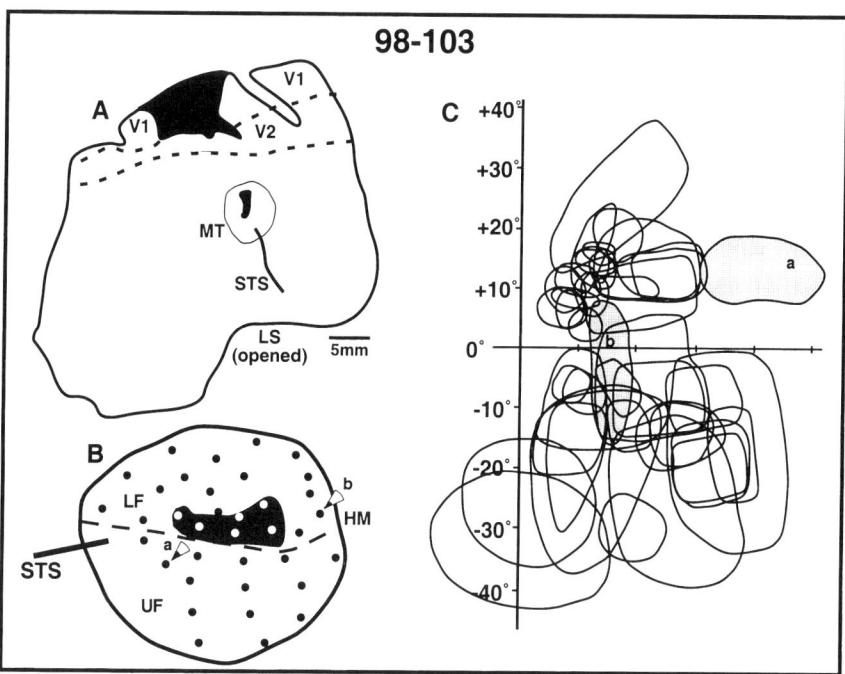

**Figure 10-4.** (A) A surface-view drawing of flattened neocortex of one hemisphere of an owl monkey (case 98-103) with a V1 lesion. The drawing was made from a cytochrome oxidase–stained section cut parallel to the surface of flattened cortex. The area shaded in black is the location of the V1 lesion. The affected portion of MT is also black. The superior temporal sulcus (STS) is indicated, and the lateral sulcus (LS) is opened. (B) An enlarged drawing of MT from case 98-103 shows recording electrode penetration sites marked by black dots. The black area surrounding 6 penetration sites indicates that neurons at those sites were unresponsive to visual stimuli. Arrowheads indicate two electrode penetration sites, near the unresponsive zone of cortex, where rapidly habituating responses to visual stimuli were noted. (C) Receptive fields of MT neurons 77 days after V1 lesioning. Two light gray shaded receptive fields, a, and b, correspond to electrode penetrations marked with arrowheads in (B) where rapidly habituating responses were noted.

ported by Rodman et al. (1989) after area 17 lesioning in macaque monkeys. Again, the authors suggest that this remaining responsiveness in MT is attributable to an alternative input that is effective when striate cortex is removed. Given the methodological and species differences across these few studies of extrastriate cortex reorganization after striate cortex ablation, it is not yet possible to draw definitive conclusions about the pattern, extent, and mechanisms of reorganization following cortical lesioning. Issues remaining to be addressed concern (1) the size and retinotopic position of striate cortex ablations across studies; (2) whether or not an alternative pathway to extrastriate cortex becomes activated in the absence of striate cortex; (3) whether there is increased sensitivity to portions of the visual field surrounding the cortical ablation due to shifting receptive fields; and (4) species differences. However, suggestive evidence for retinotopic reorganization of parts of MT was present in each study. Some of the neurons deprived of their normal sources of activation by partial lesioning of area 17 appeared to acquire new receptive fields based on preserved inputs from area 17.

## The Roles of Striate and Extrastriate Cortex in the Filling-In of a Scotoma

In the field of visual neuroscience, it has lately become important to know how much and in what way V1 neurons, as opposed to neurons in the extrastriate visual areas, are involved in visual perceptual experience. For example, our ability to perceive a three-dimensional percept of the world based on a pair of two-dimensional images (stereopsis) has been shown to require more than the normal presence of V1 neurons sensitive to interocular image disparity; higher-order neurons in the extrastriate areas must integrate local disparity information from V1 (Cumming and Parker, 2000). Similarly, an increasing number of studies suggest that perceptual rivalry is a *multistable phenomenon* of perceptual dominance that requires higher-level perceptual processes beyond the binocular signal combinations found at early cortical sites (Leopold and Logothetis, 1996; Logothetis et al., 1996; Lee and Blake, 1999). Competing theories also exist to explain how a monocular blind spot is perceptually filled-in. One possibility is that the functional connections of the primary visual cortex, either the feedforward or intrinsic long-range horizontal connections, are altered, and thus the blind spot is actively *sewn up* at the low levels (e.g., V1/V2) of cortical processing (Tripathy and Levi, 1999). The findings that have been summarized thus far in adult and developing cats and monkeys certainly support this hypothesis. Another possibility is that perceptual filling-in depends on high-level cognitive or *associative* processes while spatial values around the blind spot are maintained (i.e., do not depend on low-level topographic map reorganization or sewing-up processes) (Dennett, 1991; Ramachandran, 1992; Komatsu and Murakami, 1994). Perhaps both types of mechanisms are involved, but reorganizations within V1, and V2 and MT, the immediate targets of V1, seem capable of mediating much of the filling-in.

## References

Allman J, Miezin F, and McGuinness E (1985) Stimulus specific responses from beyond the classical receptive field: Neurophysiological mechanisms for local-global comparisons in visual neurons. *Annu Rev Neurosci* 8:407–430.
Arckens L, Eysel UT, Vanderhaeghen J-J, Orban GA, and Vandesande F (1998) Effect of sensory deafferentation on the GABAergic circuitry of the adult cat visual system. *Neuroscience* 83:381–391.

Baisden RH, Polley EH, Goodman DC, and Wolf ED (1980) Absence of sprouting by retinogeniculate axons after chronic focal lesions in the adult cat retina. *Neurosci Lett* 17:33–38.

Barlow HB, Dessington AM, Harris LR, and Lennie P (1977) The effects of remote retinal stimulation on the responses of cat retinal ganglion cells. *J Physiol* 269:177–194.

Bullier J, Girard P, and Salin P-A (1994) The role of area 17 in the transfer of information to extrastriate visual cortex. In: Peters A and Rockland KS (eds), *Cerebral Cortex: Primary Visual Cortex in Primates*, Vol 10. New York: Plenum Press. pp 301–330

Calford MB, Schmid LM, and Rosa MGP (1999) Monocular focal retinal lesions induce short-term topographic plasticity in adult cat visual cortex. *Proc R Soc Lond B Biol Sci* 266:499–507.

Calford MB, Wang C, Taglianetti V, Waleszczyk WJ, Burke W, and Dreher B (2000) Plasticity in adult cat visual cortex (area 17) following circumscribed monocular lesions of all retinal layers. *J Physiol* 524:587–602.

Chino YM (1995) Adult plasticity in the visual system. *Can J Physiol Pharmacol* 73:1323–1338.

Chino YM (1997) Receptive field plasticity in the adult visual cortex; dynamic signal rerouting or experience-dependent plasticity. *Semin Neurosci* 9:24–46.

Chino YM, Kaas JH, Smith EL 3d, Langston AL, and Cheng H (1992) Rapid reorganization of cortical maps in adult cats following restricted deafferentation in retina. *Vision Res* 32:789–796.

Chino YM, Smith EL 3d, Kaas JH, Sasaki Y, and Cheng H (1995) Receptive-field properties of deafferented visual cortical neurons after topographic map reorganization in adult cats. *J Neurosci* 15:2417–2433.

Clarke RJ, Datskovsky BW, Grigonis AM, and Hazel Murphy E (1992) The effects of monocular enucleation on visual topography in area 17 in the rabbit. *Exp Brain Res* 91:303–310.

Collins CE, Lyon DC, and Kaas JH (1999) Responses of neurons in MT after longstanding lesions of V1 in adult owl monkeys. *Soc Neurosci Abstr* 25:673.

Cumming BG and Parker AJ (2000) Local disparity not perceived depth is signaled by binocular neurons in cortical area V1 of the macaque. *J Neurosci* 40:3324–3333.

Darian-Smith C and Gilbert CD (1994) Axonal sprouting accompanies functional reorganization in adult cat striate cortex. *Nature* 368:737–740.

Darian-Smith C and Gilbert CD (1995) Topographic reorganization in the striate cortex of the adult cat and monkey is cortically mediated. *J Neurosci* 15:1631–1647.

Das A and Gilbert CD (1995a) Long-range horizontal connections and their role in cortical reorganization revealed by optical recording of cat primary visual cortex. *Nature* 375:780–784.

Das A and Gilbert CD (1995b) Receptive field expansion in adult visual cortex is linked to dynamic changes in strength of cortical connections. *J Neurophysiol* 74:779–792.

Das A and Gilbert CD (1999) Topography of contextual modifications mediated by short-range interactions in primary visual cortex. *Nature* 399:655–661.

Davis KD, Kiss ZH, Luo L, Tasker RR, Lozano AM, and Dostrovsky JO (1998) Phantom sensations generated by thalamic microstimulation. *Nature* 391:385–387.

Dennett DC (1991) *Consciousness Explained.* Boston: Little, Brown, and Company.

De Weerd P, Gattass R, Desimone R, and Ungerleider LG (1995) Responses of cells in monkey visual cortex during perceptual filling-in of an artificial scotoma. *Nature* 377:731–734.

Doetsch GS, Johnston KW, and Hannan CJ Jr (1990) Physiological changes in the somatosensory forepaw cerebral cortex of adult raccoons following lesions of a single cortical digit representation. *Exp Neurol* 108:162–175.

Eysel UT (1982) Functional reconnections without new axonal growth in a partially denervated visual relay nucleus. *Nature* 299:442–444.

Eysel UT, Eyding D, and Schweigart G (1998) Receptive optical stimulation elicits fast receptive field changes in mature visual cortex. *Neuroreport* 9:949–954.

Eysel UT, Gonzalez-Aguillar F, and Mayer U (1980) A functional sign of reorganization in the visual system of adult cats: Lateral geniculate neurons with displaced receptive fields after lesions of the nasal retina. *Brain Res* 191:285–300.

Eysel UT, Gonzalez-Aguilar F, and Mayer U (1981) Time-dependent decrease in the extent of visual deafferentation in the lateral geniculate nucleus of adult cats with small retinal lesions. *Exp Brain Res* 41:256–263.

Eysel UT and Neubacher U (1984) Recovery of function is not associated with proliferation of retinogeniculate synapses after chronic deafferentation in the dorsal lateral geniculate nucleus of the adult cat. *Neurosci Lett* 49:181–186.

Eysel UT and Schweigart G. (1999) Increased receptive field size in the surround of chronic lesions in the adult cat visual cortex. *Cereb Cortex* 2:101–109.

Fiorani M Jr, Rosa MGP, Gattass R, and Rocha-Miranda CE (1992) Dynamic surrounds of receptive fields in primate striate cortex: A physiological basis for perceptual completion? *Proc Natl Acad Sci USA* 89:8547–8551.

Florence SL, Taub HB, and Kaas JH (1998) Large-scale sprouting of cortical connections after peripheral injury in adult macaque monkeys. *Science* 282:1117–1121.

Gerrits HJ and Timmerman GJ (1969) The filling-in process in patients with retinal scotomata. *Vision Res* 9:439–442.

Gilbert CD (1983) Microcircuitry of the visual cortex. *Annu Rev Neurosci* 6:217–247.

Gilbert CD and Wiesel TN (1979) Morphology and intracortical projections of functionally charaterised neurones in the cat visual cortex. *Nature* 280:120–125.

Gilbert CD and Wiesel TN (1992) Receptive field dynamics in adult primary visual cortex. *Nature* 356:150–152.

Girard P, Salin PA, and Bullier J (1991) Visual activity in areas V3a and V3 during reversible inactivation of area V1 in the macaque monkey. *J Neurophysiol* 66:1493–1503.

Girard P, Salin PA, and Bullier J (1992) Response selectivity of neurons in area MT of the macaque monkey during reversible inactivation of area V1. *J Neurophysiol* 67:1437–1446.

Heinen SJ and Skavenski AA (1991) Recovery of visual responses in foveal V1 neurons following bilateral foveal lesions in adult monkey. *Exp Brain Res* 83:670–674.

Horton J and Hocking D (1998) Monocular core zones and binocular border strips in primate striate cortex revealed by the contrasting effects of enucleation, eyelid suture, and retinal laser lesions on cytochrome oxidase activity. *J Neurosci* 18:5433–5455.

Jenkins WM and Merzenich MM (1987) Reorganization of neocortical representations after brain injury: A neurophysiological model of the bases of recovery from stroke. *Prog Brain Res* 71:249–266.

Kaas JH, Florence SL, and Jain N (1999) Subcortical contributions to massive cortical reorganizations. *Neuron* 22:657–660.

Kaas JH and Krubitzer LA (1992) Area 17 lesions deactivate area MT in owl monkeys. *Vis Neurosci* 9:399–407.

Kaas JH, Krubitzer LA, Chino YM, Langston AL, Polley EH, and Blair N (1990). Reorganization of retinotopic cortical maps in adult mammals after lesions of the retina. *Science* 248:229–231.

Komatsu H and Murakami I (1994) Behavioral evidence of filling-in at the blind spot of the monkey. *Vis Neurosci* 11:1103–1113.

Lee SH and Blake R (1999) Rival ideas about binocular rivalry. *Vision Res* 39:1447–1454.

Leopold DA and Logothetis N (1996) Activity changes in early visual cortex reflects monkey's percepts during binocular rivalry. *Nature* 379:549–553.

LeVay S, Wiesel TN, and Hubel DH (1980) The development of ocular dominance columns in normal and visually deprived monkeys. *J Comp Neurol* 191:1–51.

Logothetis N, Leopold DA, and Sheinberg DL (1996) What is rivaling during rivalry? *Nature* 380:621–624.

Matsuura K, Zhang B, Smith EL III, and Chino YM (1999) Prolonged recovery following retinal injuries improves the responsiveness of newly activated units following cortical map reorganization. *Soc Neurosci Abstr* 29:1937.

Maunsell JHR, Nealey TA, and DePriest DD (1990) Magnocellular and parvocellular contributions to responses in the middle temporal area (MT) of the macaque monkey. *J Neurosci* 10:3323–3334.

McIlwain JT (1966) Some evidence concerning the physiological basis of the periphery effects in the cat's retina. *Exp Brain Res* 1:265–271.

McLean J and Palmer LA (1998) Plasticity of neuronal response properties in adult cat striate cortex. *Vis Neurosci* 15:177–196.

Merzenich MM, Kaas JH, Wall JT, Nelson JR, Sur M, and Felleman DJ (1983a) Topographic reorganization of somatosensory cortical areas 3b and 1 in adult monkeys following restricted deafferentation. *Neuroscience* 8:33–55.

Merzenich MM, Kaas JH, Wall JT, Sur M, Nelson RJ, and Felleman DJ (1983b) Progression of change following median nerve section in the cortical representation of the hand in areas 3b and 1 in adult owl and squirrel monkeys. *Neuroscience* 10:639–665.

Merzenich MM, Nelson RJ, Stryker MP, Cynader MS, Schoppmann A, and Zook JM (1984) Somatosensory cortical map changes following digit amputation in adult monkeys. *J Comp Neurol* 224:591–605.

Mori T, Zhang B, Smith EL III, and Chino YM (2000) Topographic map reorganization of visual cortex following unilateral retinal lesions in 8–week old cats. *Soc Neurosci Abstr* 26:2193.

Murakami I, Komatsu H, and Kinoshita M (1997) Perceptual filling-in at the scotoma following a monocular retinal lesion in the monkey. *Vis Neurosci* 14:89–101.

Obata S, Obata J, Das A, and Gilbert CD (1999) Molecular correlates of topographic reorganization in primary visual cortex following retinal lesions. *Cereb Cortex* 9:238–248.

Pettet MW and Gilbert CD (1992). Dynamic changes in receptive field size in cat primary visual cortex. *Proc Natl Acad Sci USA* 89:8366–8370.

Pons TP, Garraghty PE, and Mishkin M (1988) Lesion-induced plasticity in the second somatosensory cortex of adult macaques. *Proc Natl Acad Sci USA* 85:5279–5281.

Ramachandran VS (1992) Blind spots. *Sci Am* 266:86–91.

Ramachandran VS and Gregory TL (1991) Perceptual filling-in of artificially induced scotomas in human vision. *Nature* 350:699–702.

Rauschecker JP (1998) Mechanisms of visual plasticity: Hebb synapses, NMDA receptors, and beyond. *Physiol Rev* 71:587–615.

Rodman HR, Gross CG, and Albright TD (1989) Afferent basis of visual response properties in area MT of the macaque. I. Effects of striate cortex removal. *J Neurosci* 9:2033–2050.

Rodman HR, Gross CG, and Albright TD (1990) Afferent basis of visual response properties in area MT of the macaque. II: Effects of superior colliculus removal. *J Neurosci* 10:1154–1164.

Rosa MGP, Schmid LM, and Calford MD (1995) Responsiveness of cat area 17 after monocular inactivation: Limitation of topographic plasticity in adult cortex. *J Physiol* 482:589–608.

Rosa MGP, Tweedale R, and Elston GN (2000) Visual responses of neurons in the middle temporal area of New World monkeys after lesions of striate cortex. *J Neurosci* 20:5552–5563.

Rosier AM, Arckens L, Demeulemeester H, Orban GA, Eysel UT, Wu YJ, and Vandesande F (1995) Effect of sensory deafferentation on immunoreactivity of GABAergic cells and on GABA receptors in the adult cat visual cortex. *J Comp Neurol* 359:476–489.

Schiller PH and Malpeli JG (1977) The effect of striate cortex coding on area 18 cells the monkey. *Brain Res* 126:366–369.

Schmid LM, Rosa MGP, and Calford MB (1995) Retinal detachment induces massive immediate reorganization in visual cortex. *Neuroreport* 6:1349–1353.

Schmid LM, Rosa MGP, Calford MB, and Ambler JS (1996) Visuotopic reorganization in the primary visual cortex of adult cats following monocular and binocular retinal lesions. *Cereb Cortex* 6:388–405.

Sergent J (1988) An investigation into perceptual completion in blind areas of the visual field. *Brain* 111:347–373.

Stelzner DJ and Keating EG (1977) Lack of interlaminar sprouting of retinal axons in monkey LGN. *Brain Res* 126:201–210.

Stepniewska I, Qi H-X, and Kaas JH (1999) Do superior colliculus projection zones in the inferior pulvinar project to MT in primates? *Eur J Neurosci* 11:469–480.

Toth LJ, Rao SC, Kim DS, Somers D, and Sur M (1996) Subthreshold facilitation and suppression in primary visual cortex revealed by intensive signal imaging. *Proc Natl Acad Sci USA* 93:9869–9874

Tripathy SP and Levi DM (1999) Looking behind a pathological blind spot in human retina. *Vision Res* 39:1917–1925.

Volchan E and Gilbert CD (1995) Interocular transfer of receptive field expansion in cat visual cortex. *Vision Res* 35:1–6.

Weiskrantz L and Cowey A (1967) Comparison of the effects of striate cortex and retinal lesions in visual acuity in the monkey. *Science* 155:104–106.

# 11

## The Blind Leading the Mind:
## Pathological Visual Completion in Hemianopia and Spatial Neglect

JASON B. MATTINGLEY AND ROBIN WALKER

Acquired lesions of the occipital cortex in humans typically cause blindness in the region of space represented by the damaged tissue. In unilateral cases, the field defect is restricted to the hemifield contralateral to the lesion (hemianopia) and results in loss of subjective visual experience in that region. It is well known that some visual processing within the hemianopic field may proceed in the absence of subjective experience (so-called *blindsight*; Weiskrantz, 1986), supporting the notion that multiple parallel pathways subserve different aspects of visual functioning (Mishkin et al., 1983; Milner and Goodale, 1995). In contrast to these blindsight cases in which there is preserved vision without awareness, some patients seem entirely *unaware* of their visual loss. In rare instances of complete cortical blindness due to bilateral occipital damage, this may result in Anton's syndrome, in which patients deny their visual impairment despite compelling evidence to the contrary (Anton, 1899). Even in cases of unilateral damage, however, patients may remain unaware of their hemianopia or may deny having any visual loss (Bisiach et al., 1986).

In this chapter, we focus on a particular visual anomaly that arises after unilateral damage, in which patients claim to see a complete visual shape even though a substantial portion of the stimulus falls within an objectively blind region of their contralesional visual field. This phenomenon, known as *pathological visual completion* (Walker and Mattingley, 1997, 1998), was first described by Poppelreuter in 1917 (Poppelreuter, 1917/1990) and has been the subject of numerous investigations by psychologists and neuroscientists ever since. Recently, the phenomenon has received renewed attention due to advances in understanding the neurophysiological mechanisms underlying perceptual completion in the normal visual system (Pessoa et al., 1998). We provide a historical account of Poppelreuter's pioneering work and then critically review previous studies of pathological visual completion, highlighting some of their methodological and theoretical shortcomings. Finally, we propose a framework for understanding pathological visual completion and suggest possible avenues for future research.

## A Critical Investigation of Pathological Visual Completion

The first comprehensive description of pathological visual completion was published by the German psychologist and neurologist Walther Poppelreuter in 1917 (Poppelreuter, 1917/1990). He made painstaking and rigorous observations on several hundred soldiers who had suffered focal brain lesions due to shrapnel wounds sustained during the First World War. His particular interest was in disturbances of higher visual capacities following occipital damage. In his 1917 monograph, Poppelreuter outlined a paradoxical phenomenon that he called the *apperceptive completion of gestalt*. In several patients suffering from hemianopic field loss, he had noticed that geometric forms presented so that they overlapped the field defect were nevertheless reported as if they were complete shapes. He described his observations thus:

> If one were dealing with a complete, abrupt right hemianopia then one would expect that this hemianopic subject could only see a semicircle if a complete circle were presented to him while he fixated foveally. That this must always be the case was also my original assumption when I started to carry out more accurate determinations of the residual macular visual field by means of tachistoscopic experiments, in order to avoid artificial results due to gaze-shifts. I supposed that if one shifted the circle gradually from the left intact field towards the right hemianopic field it should be possible to determine the field position where the circle can no longer be seen as a complete figure. When I tried to verify this prediction the surprising result emerged that patients who had abrupt hemianopias by perimetry did not themselves behave in accordance with the postulate. Even though the hemianopic line of demarcation crosses the visual field nearly vertically, indicating that the right half is blind, the patient nevertheless reported seeing the centrally located black circle completely at the moment of presentation, and not as a black semicircle. It is thus a paradox that the patient can apparently "see" with his "blind" field.
> 
> Poppelreuter, 1917/1990, p. 132

An example of one of Poppelreuter's own cases of pathological visual completion is reproduced in Figure 11-1. It shows the right homonymous hemianopia of Patient SW (in addition to a small left-sided scotoma) and illustrates the tachistoscopic arrangement for presenting visual stimuli that either abutted the patient's hemianopic field defect or fell entirely within it. With the former arrangement, SW reported seeing a complete square and a "diffuse indefinable darkness on the right." In contrast, when the square was presented entirely within the field defect, SW reported only a "gleam of light."

In addition to presenting these cases of completion of geometric figures (what we call *whole shapes*), Poppelreuter observed that some individuals saw complete stimuli even though the portion of the shape falling within the blind hemifield had been cut away to leave a gap (what we call *partial shapes*). Thus, for

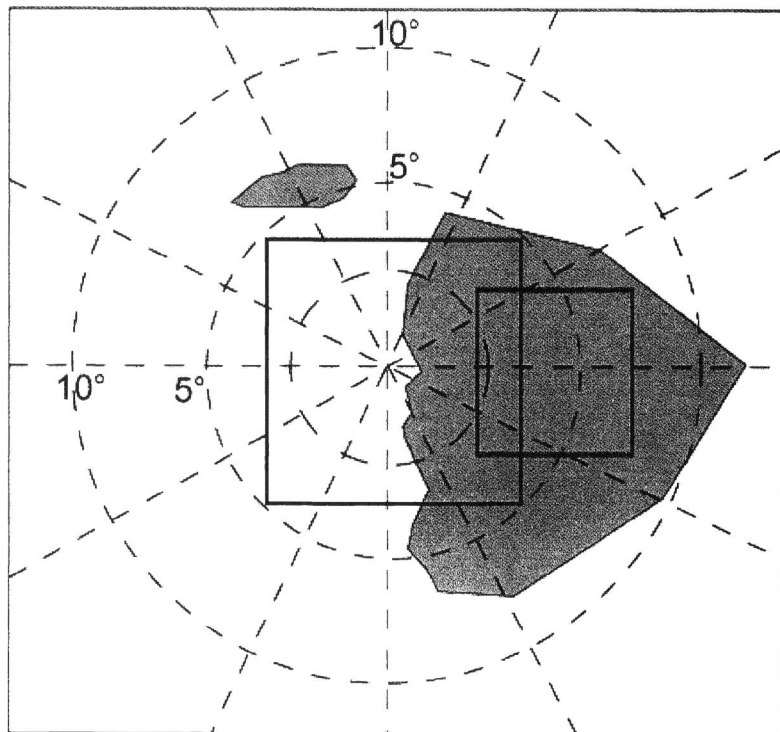

**Figure 11-1.** Perimetric visual field map for patient SW, reported by Poppelreuter (1917/1990). The irregularly shaped gray region on the right shows the spatial extent of the patient's hemianopic field defect, which resulted from a shrapnel injury affecting the medial region of the left occipital cortex. There is also a small scotoma on the left, presumably from more circumscribed damage to the right occipital cortex. The numbers on the vertical and horizontal axes represent eccentricities in degrees of visual angle. When a small square was presented tachistoscopically so that it fell entirely within the right-sided scotoma, SW reported a "gleam of light without any form." When a larger square was presented such that its right side fell within the scotoma, SW reported a "complete" square. (*Source:* Redrawn from Poppelreuter, 1917/1990)

example, patients were shown a semicircle with a single vertical edge and a curved segment lying to the left or right of it. When the shape was presented so that it fell entirely within the normally sighted field, patients correctly reported seeing a semicircle. However, when the same shape was presented so that the curved portion was in the sighted field and the vertical edge was just inside the blind field, some individuals reported a complete circle.

Because the phenomenon of pathological visual completion seemed to arise for both whole and partial shapes, Poppelreuter assumed that it was based on *completion by imagination*. In other words, he believed that the brain somehow fills in missing information from the blind field, and he drew an analogy with filling-in of the physiological blind spot in normal vision. Poppelreuter apparently made many such observations on a number of patients, and in the process he determined some of the boundary conditions for the phenomenon. For instance, he found that completed figures arose mainly for enclosed geometric forms, such as circles and squares, and only rarely for "contour figures (rings, etc.)." He also argued that pathological completion could play a beneficial role in cases of acquired visual loss after cortical lesioning by allowing object recognition to proceed despite the fragmentary afferent processing.

## *Why Study Pathological Visual Completion?*

The study of pathological visual completion is important for several reasons. First, it may provide important clues concerning the neural basis for visual completion in the normal human brain by revealing the nature of subjective visual experience in the absence of corresponding afferent inputs. In this sense, pathological completion is analogous to synesthesia, in which vivid sensations of color may be experienced in association with particular sounds or graphemic forms that do not themselves contain any chromatic information (Baron-Cohen and Harrison, 1997; Mattingley et al., 2001; Rich and Mattingley, 2002). Second, pathological visual completion may provide a potent basis for understanding the nature of neural plasticity and functional reorganization after acquired brain damage in humans. Finally, if it is proved to be a robust phenomenon, visual completion may offer new avenues for therapeutic interventions aimed at improving visual function following stroke.

Although Poppelreuter was at pains to point out that not all hemianopes he had seen exhibited pathological visual completion, his work led to a number of subsequent reports, all claiming to show such completion phenomena in patients with lesions in various regions of the cortical visual system. In this section, we summarize the evidence for perceptual completion in hemianopic patients and provide a critical appraisal of the techniques used to elicit the phenomenon. A more comprehensive review of the relevant literature has been published elsewhere (Walker and Mattingley, 1997).

Many studies of completion have employed tachistoscopic measures in which a visual stimulus is flashed briefly as patients fixate a central spot. Following exposure, patients are asked to indicate what they have seen, typically by verbal report or by drawing. Fuchs (1921/1938) reported a comprehensive investigation of completion in five hemianopic patients using tachistoscopic presentation of various simple and complex drawings. His patient "B" claimed to see complete symmetrical shapes for simple geometric forms (e.g., a disc, an outlined circle, a filled square) when the display was arranged so that the stimuli encircled the fixation point, thus encroaching on the hemianopic field. Interestingly, the same patient did not complete more complex visual stimuli, such as drawings of a dog, a face or a butterfly. Fuchs suggested that completion arose from a visual process that favored symmetrical or well-balanced forms, in keeping with Gestalt principles such as good continuation. The importance of global symmetry was also emphasized in a recent study by McCarthy et al. (1999). Their patient, with left occipital damage, showed a higher proportion of completion responses for upright face stimuli presented in the frontoparallel plane (i.e., front on) than for those rotated 90 degrees in the picture plane, which removed cues to vertical symmetry.

Williams and Gassel (1962) reported the occurrence of pathological visual completion even for rather complex stimuli such as faces under conditions of free viewing. For instance, several of their hemianopic patients claimed to see the whole of the examiner's face when fixating his nose (as in the standard confrontation technique for assessing visual fields), despite remaining unaware that a card had been moved into their hemianopic field. In her pioneering investigations of pathological visual completion, Warrington (1962, 1965) studied 26 hemianopic patients with striate and extrastriate lesions. She observed completion of both simple geometric forms and more complex drawings (e.g., house, face, flower, ship), but found that shapes that were unusual or more complex resulted in a lower incidence of pathological completion. She suggested that perceptual completion might be based upon patients' expectations, and on their knowledge that geometric forms and common objects typically appear as wholes when depicted in graphical form. In this context, it may be noteworthy that pathological completion is more common in patients with "mental disorientation" or "inattention" (Pollack et al., 1957), suggesting that failure to adopt a critical attitude when deciding whether a stimulus is complete may be an important contributing factor.

## *Methodological Considerations*

Recently, we reviewed the entire literature on pathological visual completion and compiled a list of the main features of these studies (see Table 11-1). Despite the compelling subjective reports, there are several methodological questions that need to be considered before accepting pathological visual completion as a genuine phenomenon. To what extent might residual vision within the blind hemifield account for completion responses? What techniques have been used to ensure that patients do not make eye movements to bring unseen stimuli into a region of normal vision? Can compensatory strategies such as eccentric fixation toward the affected hemifield account for some cases of pathological visual completion? These questions, which were also considered by Sergent (1988) in a landmark study, raise serious doubts about the validity of findings from many studies of pathological visual completion.

Perhaps the most important issue is the extent to which hemianopic patients who exhibit visual completion have residual visual sensitivity within their affected field. In order to understand pathological completion, it is necessary to decide whether such patients have *veridical* or *direct* perception of the portion of the visual stimulus that falls within their otherwise blind field or whether the identity of the unseen portion is somehow *inferred* (consciously or otherwise) from the fragment that is visible within the intact field. It is well known that there

**Table 11-1.** Summary of reported cases of pathological visual completion [Modified from Walker and Mattingley, 1997].

| Study | Lesion Localization | Veridical Perception of Whole Shapes | Completion of Partial Shapes | Neglect or Extinction? | Comments |
|---|---|---|---|---|---|
| Poppelreuter (1917/1990) | 6 cases; lesions not documented | 3 | Not reported | +dss 2 cases ? 4 cases | |
| Fuchs (1921/1938) | 5 cases; lesions not documented | 5 | 1 (4 not reported) | ? 5 cases | |
| Bender and Teuber (1946) | 1 thalamus<br>1 R posterior parietal<br>1 bilateral occipital | 1<br>1<br>1 | 1 (but "unsure")<br>1 not tested<br>1 (1 exposure) | ?<br>+dss<br>+dss | |
| Pollack et al. (1957) | 23 "hemianopes"; lesions not documented | not tested | 10 | † 8 cases | |
| Warrington (1962) | 13 parietal<br>5 occipital<br>1 frontal<br>1 temporal | 11<br>0<br>0<br>0 | 11<br>0<br>0<br>0 | + 8 cases<br>No neglect<br>No neglect<br>No neglect | |
| Warrington (1965) | ∗26 hemianopic | Not tested | 13 | ? | ∗ Same patients reported in Warrington (1962) + 6 additional cases |
| Williams and Gassel (1962); Gassel and Williams (1963) | 1 L parietal glioma<br>1 L occip. lobectomy<br>1 R hemispherectomy<br>1 L postartery<br>1 R third ventricle | 1<br>1<br>1<br>1<br>1 | 1<br>1<br>Not doc.<br>1<br>1 | +dss<br>+dss<br>?<br>?<br>? | 7-yr-old child<br><br>Mentally retarded<br><br>11-yr-old child |
| Torjussen (1978) | 1 vascular thrombosis<br>1 cerebral hemorrhage<br>1 cerebral tumor | 1<br>1<br>1 | 0<br>0<br>0 | ?<br>?<br>? | |
| Perenin et al. (1986) (see Weiskrantz, 1990) | 1 L hemispherectomy<br>1 L occipital | 1<br>1 | 0∗<br>0∗ | ?<br>? | ∗ Frequency of completion of partial circles <5% |

**Table 11-1.** (*Continued*)

| Study | Lesion Localization | Veridical Perception of Whole Shapes | Completion of Partial Shapes | Neglect or Extinction? | Comments |
|---|---|---|---|---|---|
| Sergent (1988) | 1 R occipital | 0 (0)[a] | 0 (0) | No neglect | |
| | 1 L occipital + parietal | — (1) | — (1) | + R neglect | |
| | 1 L occipital + parietal | 1 (0) | 1 (0) | + R neglect | |
| | 1 R temporo-parietal | — (1) | — (1) | + L neglect | |
| | 1 R parieto-occipital | 1 (0) | 1 (0) | No neglect | |
| | 1 R temporo-parietal | 1 (0) | 1 (0) | + L neglect | |
| Ramachandran (1993) | 2 occipital | Not tested | 2 (incomplete vertical lines)[b] | ? | Completion of bars with gaps over scotoma |
| Halligan and Marshall (1994) | 1 R middle cerebral artery territory | Not tested | 1 | + L neglect | 1 case of neglect |
| Hornak (1995) | 3 occipital | Not tested | 0 | No neglect | |
| | 1 optic radiation | Not tested | 0 | No neglect | |
| | 1 parieto-occipital | Not tested | 0 | No neglect | 5 cases of neglect; patients not hemianopic |
| | 5 R parietal | Not tested | 5 | + L neglect | |
| Walker and Young (1996) | 1 R middle cerebral artery territory | 1 | 1 | + L neglect | Not hemianopic |
| Marcel (1998) | 1 L occipital | 1 | 0 | No neglect | GY—blindsight patient |
| | 1 L occipital + temporoparietal | 1 | 0 | No neglect | |
| Jackson (1999) | 1 L occipital | Not tested | Not tested | No neglect | GY—blindsight patient |
| McCarthy and Plant (1999) | 1 L occipital | 1 | 1 | No neglect | |

Table Legend

+ = neglect revealed by suitable assessment.

+ dss = extinction revealed by double simultaneous stimulation (confrontation testing or testing with briefly presented stimuli).

† = neglect or extinction reported, but assessment procedure not described.

? = neglect or extinction not reported and may not have been assessed.

[a]Completion demonstrated in patients (drawing responses are shown in parentheses).

[b]Completion was of gaps between vertical lines and was not included in totals for partial figures.

can be significant recovery of visual sensitivity in the blind hemifield after injury (Zihl and von Cramon, 1985; Kolb, 1990). Moreover, in many cases the macular region may be spared, leaving the central few degrees of vision unaffected. Unless the visual fields are mapped carefully, hemianopic patients with loss of vision at the periphery may nevertheless perceive completed shapes presented within the foveal region.

Unfortunately, not even a painstaking objective assessment of the visual fields will guarantee an accurate measure of residual vision. Williams and Gassel (1962) found that the different techniques used to assess hemianopic field defects (e.g., confrontation, campimetry, perimetry) yielded conflicting estimates of visual thresholds. Mapping of the extent of visual loss was found to vary according to such factors as the color and luminance of the target stimuli and background, their size and shape, and whether the target was stationary or moving. Williams and Gassel also found that light scatter from targets presented in the hemianopic field could provide a cue to indicate the presence of unseen visual information, thus suggesting the presence of a complete shape. It seems likely that several early experiments suffered from this problem, including Poppelreuter's study of patient SW, as described above (Fig. 11-1).

A second methodological issue to be considered in interpreting studies of pathological visual completion concerns the possibility of unwanted (or undetected) eye movements into the affected hemifield. At least some studies used lengthy viewing durations so that patients could readily direct eye movements toward the affected side, thus bringing otherwise undetected portions of the stimulus into the intact field. For example, Bender and Teuber (1946) had their hemianopic patients stare at a display of the American flag and report the afterimage they experienced. They found that the reported afterimage was typically larger than would be expected based on patients' apparent field defect, and concluded that there must have been pathological completion of an unseen portion of the stimulus. The authors endeavored to rule out the potential contribution of eye movements by showing that a pencil moved in the region of the field defect during adaptation was not reported, but this crude test is not particularly convincing.

Williams and Gassel (1962; see also Gassel and Williams, 1963) used prolonged exposure to examine visual completion of the examiner's face during confrontation testing of the visual fields. They used a combination of direct observation and electro-oculographic recording to monitor eye movements. Unfortunately, the accuracy of these techniques is limited to a visual angle of 1 to 3 degrees, and so they are unlikely to have detected any small eye movements made by patients into the affected hemifield. Several studies have acknowledged the potential problem of unwanted eye movements and have adopted methodologies to circumvent them. In addition to the afterimage method described above, Bender and Teuber (1946) presented stimuli tachistoscopically for durations of 20–100 ms, too brief to allow effective saccades into the blind field. As outlined above, similar techniques have been adopted by other researchers (Warrington, 1962, 1965; Perenin et al., 1986; Sergent, 1988; Hornak, 1995; Walker and Young, 1996).

Eccentric fixation poses another problem for the interpretation of studies claiming to show pathological visual completion. Hemianopic patients may deviate their gaze toward the impaired hemifield to compensate for their visual loss (Williams and Gassel, 1962; Sergent, 1988). Sergent (1988) showed that even very small deviations of fixation could dramatically alter the frequency with which hemianopic patients gave responses suggestive of pathological completion. She included a *pre-exposure screen* in her tachistoscopic presentations, which effectively ensured that patients fixated centrally prior to exposure of the stimulus cards. Without this stringent fixation control, four of her six hemianopic patients showed responses consistent with visual completion. In contrast, with fixation controlled, only one patient showed completion. Moreover, Sergent found that the frequency of completion responses in the uncontrolled condition was positively correlated with the extent of the patients' eccentric fixation, suggesting that the perception of completed forms may be due to direct viewing in the intact hemifield.

To summarize, we have considered three possible confounding factors in interpreting cases of pathological visual completion: (1) residual vision in the affected hemifield; (2) eye movements toward the affected hemifield; and (3) eccentric fixation. We have shown that each of these factors can account for at least some of the reports of visual completion in neurological cases, a conclusion also reached by Sergent (1988) in her pioneering study. Any interpretation of pathological completion must take into account these limitations, and future studies will need to adopt appropriate techniques for circumventing them. We advocate an approach that incorporates thorough mapping of thresholds to a range of visual stimuli, together with careful monitoring of eye movements during stimulus presentation.

## Neuroanatomical Considerations

There is now substantial evidence concerning the neural locus of visual completion responses from animal neurophysiology (Von der Heydt et al., 1984; Fiorani et al., 1992; De Weerd et al., 1995). Unfortunately, although the visual pathways in humans have been extensively mapped, it has proved more difficult to determine the critical lesion locus that leads to pathological completion. In Table 11-1 we have provided information on lesion location (where available) in all reported cases of pathological visual completion. It is important to note that lesion localization is fairly imprecise in several of the early reports and so should be interpreted with caution. In some cases, the damage was quite extensive (e.g., following unilateral hemispherectomy: Williams and Gassel, 1962; Perenin et al., 1986), whereas in others the lesion was relatively small and circumscribed (e.g., Sergent, 1988). Perhaps the most striking feature of the lesion data shown in Table 11-1 is that very few patients had damage restricted to the occipital cortex or optic radiations, whereas most had lesions that involved extrastriate and association areas. These observations are summarized in Figure 11-2, which shows the percentage of all patients who completed either whole shapes (*veridical per-*

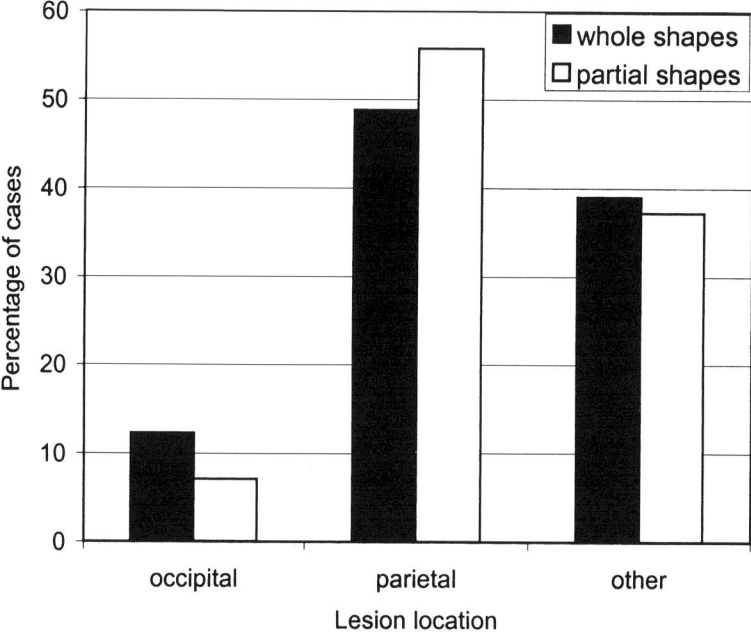

**Figure 11-2.** Percentage of cases showing pathological visual completion (or *veridical perception*) for partial and whole shapes as a function of lesion location. The "other" category represents patients in whom lesions either were not documented or involved regions beyond the parietal and occipital cortices.

*ception*; Walker and Mattingley, 1997) or partial shapes abutting the field defect (*pathological completion*). Only 12% of all patients with veridical perception of *whole shapes* had circumscribed occipital damage, whereas 49% had parietal damage. Similarly, just 7% of all patients with pathological completion of *partial shapes* had occipital lesions, whereas 56% had parietal lesions. Note that these percentages may underestimate the proportion of parietal cases showing completion, given that lesion data were not provided in several of the early reports. Based on this survey of the literature, we must conclude that pathological visual completion arises most frequently following parietal damage in humans and that cases due to circumscribed occipital damage are exceedingly rare.

Despite their apparent rarity, there are several important cases in which pathological completion has been observed in patients with restricted occipital damage. Marcel (1998), for example, tested the well-known occipital blindsight patient GY and observed completion for both whole and partial shapes. A more recent study by Jackson (1999), also in patient GY, has claimed to show completion effects in the control of reach-to-grasp movements. This innovative study revealed appropriate scaling of grip aperture to objects (rectangular blocks) situated across the vertical midline, despite impaired size judgments for the same objects based on perception alone. Though intriguing, these results seem more consistent with GY's preserved unconscious visual capacities (i.e., blindsight) than with conscious visual completion of the kind we have focused on here.

It is important to distinguish between pathological completion in patients with large occipital or parietal lesions and the filling-in of small scotomas that may occur following circumscribed damage within the visual cortex. For instance, Ramachandran (1993; see also Chapter 8 in this volume) described two occipital patients for whom simple shapes and textures appeared to fill in across their scotomas with prolonged viewing. Kamitani and Shimojo (1999) reported analogous effects in normals for scotomas induced by transcranial magnetic stimulation (TMS) over occipital cortex. They found that single TMS pulses delivered approximately 100 ms after presentation of a sinusoidal grating induced scotomas whose shape was compressed along the axis of the stripes. The authors suggested that this compression, which led to scotomas with an elliptical shape, may have been due to filling-in of part of the suppressed region induced by the TMS pulse. They suggested that such filling-in might be achieved via long-range facilitation among neurons with similar preferred orientations and collinear alignment, which could effectively reduce the inhibitory effect of the magnetic stimulation (Kamitani and Shimojo, 1999).

Changes in the perceived shape and size of objects seem to be characteristic of completion across scotomas, whether these are induced artificially (Kapadia et al., 1994), or by cortical lesions (Safran et al., 1999). For instance, Safran et al. (1999) found that patients with paracentral homonymous scotomas due to occipital damage showed systematic distortions of visual stimuli that fell across their field defects. This effect was particularly apparent when the patients were asked to stare at the face of the examiner. After several seconds, the patients reported that one of the examiner's shoulders (the one falling within the scotoma) appeared narrower than the other, a phenomenon the authors called the *thin man* phenomenon. These observations suggest that visual distortions due to filling-in may provide an important diagnostic sign in cases of cortical scotoma.

Another distinguishing feature of patients with small cortical scotomas is that the filling-in typically emerges gradually over several seconds (e.g., Ramachandran, 1993; Safran et al., 1999). This is in contrast with pathological completion in hemianopia, as originally described by Poppelreuter and subsequent investigators, which apparently occurs with stimuli presented for just a fraction of a second (typically <200 ms; see Walker and Mattingley, 1997). The delay for filling-in of cortical scotomas is similar to that observed for artificial scotomas in normals (Ramachandran and Gregory, 1991). It also fits with the time course of *climbing activity* in V2 and V3 neurons of the rhesus monkey, which has been interpreted as a neurophysiological analog of filling-in across artificial scotomas in humans (De Weerd et al., 1995).

Given the prolonged time course for pathological filling-in across small occipital scotomas, compared with the very brief exposures associated with pathological completion in most other cases, we suggest that distinct neural mechanisms underlie the two. It seems likely that completion across an occipital scotoma reflects preservation of mechanisms responsible for filling-in across artificial scotomas, such as dynamic changes in the receptive fields of neurons representing adjacent regions of the visual field (Fiorani et al., 1992; Chapter 9, this volume). Filling-in of cortical scotomas may also be due to an increase in the size of receptive fields of neurons near the border of the lesion. In support of this idea, Eysel and Schweigart (1999) found that small excitotoxic lesions of area 17 in cats led to substantial increases in the receptive field size of neurons adjacent to the lesion when examined at 2 months. These increases in size could not have been due simply to increased excitability of cells at the border of the lesion, since the receptive field changes were not apparent 2 days after lesioning. Nor could they have been due to horizontal intracortical connections from adjacent cells, since these were eliminated by the excitotoxic injection. Instead, the enlarged receptive fields must have arisen from *feedforward* connections from collaterals of intact geniculostriate afferents and/or from *feedback* connections from area 18, which receives direct geniculocortical inputs in the cat (Eysel and Schweigart, 1999). Functional brain imaging in humans with V1 damage has also demonstrated the importance of extrageniculostriate inputs, particularly from the superior colliculus and pulvinar, for residual vision within the blind hemifield (e.g., Ptito et al., 1999).

In contrast with the mechanisms underlying filling-in of small cortical scotomas, pathological completion in patients with complete homonymous hemianopia is typically instantaneous, and tends to involve stimuli that extend a considerable distance into the blind hemifield (Poppelreuter, 1917/1990; Fuchs, 1921/1938; Williams and Gassel, 1962; Gassel and Williams, 1963; Torjussen, 1978). It seems likely that such instantaneous completion across hemianopic field defects arises from mechanisms that are fundamentally different from those associated with filling-in of cortical scotomas. As we outline below, the fact that most hemianopic patients with completion have parietal damage may provide important clues in uncovering the neural basis of perceptual completion in these individuals.

## *Is Pathological Completion Due to Biased Spatial Attention?*

A significant problem in assessing the integrity of the visual fields arises in patients with extrastriate damage, particularly when this includes the parietal lobe. Such individuals frequently have unilateral spatial neglect, which manifests as a severe deficit of spatial attention in the context of preserved afferent inputs in most cases (for a review see Driver and Mattingley, 1998). Patients with neglect are typically unaware of visual stimuli on their contralesional side, and so can perform as if they have hemianopia. Silberpfennig (1941) reported two patients with *pseudohemianopsia* whose apparent field defects were overcome by boosting their sustained attention (or arousal), a manipulation that has since been found to improve contralesional awareness in patients with spatial neglect (Robertson et al., 1998). Kooistra and Heilman (1989) observed a patient with an apparent left hemianopia whose detection of visual targets in the affected hemifield improved when she deviated her gaze into the right (ipsilesional) hemispace, suggesting that visual space representations are updated by extraretinal information (Andersen et al., 1993). Even patients with the milder disorder of extinction (Mattingley, 2002), in which contralesional stimuli are detected normally when presented in isolation but are missed when shown concurrently with a stimulus on the ipsilesional side, may appear to have hemianopia on perimetric testing. Walker et al. (1991) showed that left hemianopia diagnosed by standard perimetry may be abolished in some cases when a temporal gap is introduced between the offset of the central fixation spot and the onset of a peripheral target. This simple manipulation reduces competition from the central spot and permits available attentional resources to be devoted to detection of the contralesional target events.

As Table 11-1 indicates, many patients described as showing pathological visual completion due to parietal lesions had attentional deficits such as neglect (Warrington, 1962; Gassel and Williams, 1963; Sergent, 1988; Halligan and Marshall, 1994) and extinction (Poppelreuter, 1917/1990; Pollack et al., 1957). Indeed, Poppelreuter himself noted that two of his patients exhibited *hemianopic weakness of attention* under conditions of concurrent bilateral stimulation (i.e., extinction), although he did not consider that this alone could account for their pathological completion. In her pioneering study, Warrington (1962) found that of 13 hemianopic patients showing visual completion phenomena, 11 had parietal lesions, and 8 of these showed clinical evidence of unilateral spatial neglect. Warrington was the first to suggest that (right) parietal damage is specifically related to the occurrence of pathological visual completion.

There is ample evidence that parietal lesion patients with spatial neglect have a striking deficit of awareness of contralesional visual stimuli, despite often showing intact implicit or unconscious processing of the neglected information (Driver and Mattingley, 1998). The deficit is not restricted to stimuli falling within the affected hemifield but may extend to the contralesional side of individual words (*neglect dyslexia*: Costello and Warrington, 1987; Behrmann et al., 1990) or objects (Driver, 1995). This profound impairment of visual awareness for the contralesional side of coherent objects is evident in the spontaneous drawings made by such patients (Fig. 11-3A) and in their perception of chimeric pictures in which the left and right halves differ (Fig. 11-3B). In a tachistoscopic investigation, Hornak (1995) found that right half-shapes were reported as complete by four out of five patients with spatial neglect but without hemianopia. Similarly, Walker et al. (1996) reported a right parietal patient who saw half-shapes as complete and who failed to identify the left side of chimeric faces (Fig. 11-3C) even when these were presented entirely within the right (ipsilesional) hemifield. It is therefore not surprising that so many cases of pathological visual completion involve parietal damage, in which the patient may simply remain unaware of the absence of visual information arising in the blind hemifield (Walker and Young, 1996; Walker and Mattingley, 1997). Thus, rather than actively filling in missing details, parietal patients may simply ignore the absence of information on the affected side, as has been suggested for the physiological blind spot in normals (Dennett, 1991; but see Durgin et al., 1995).

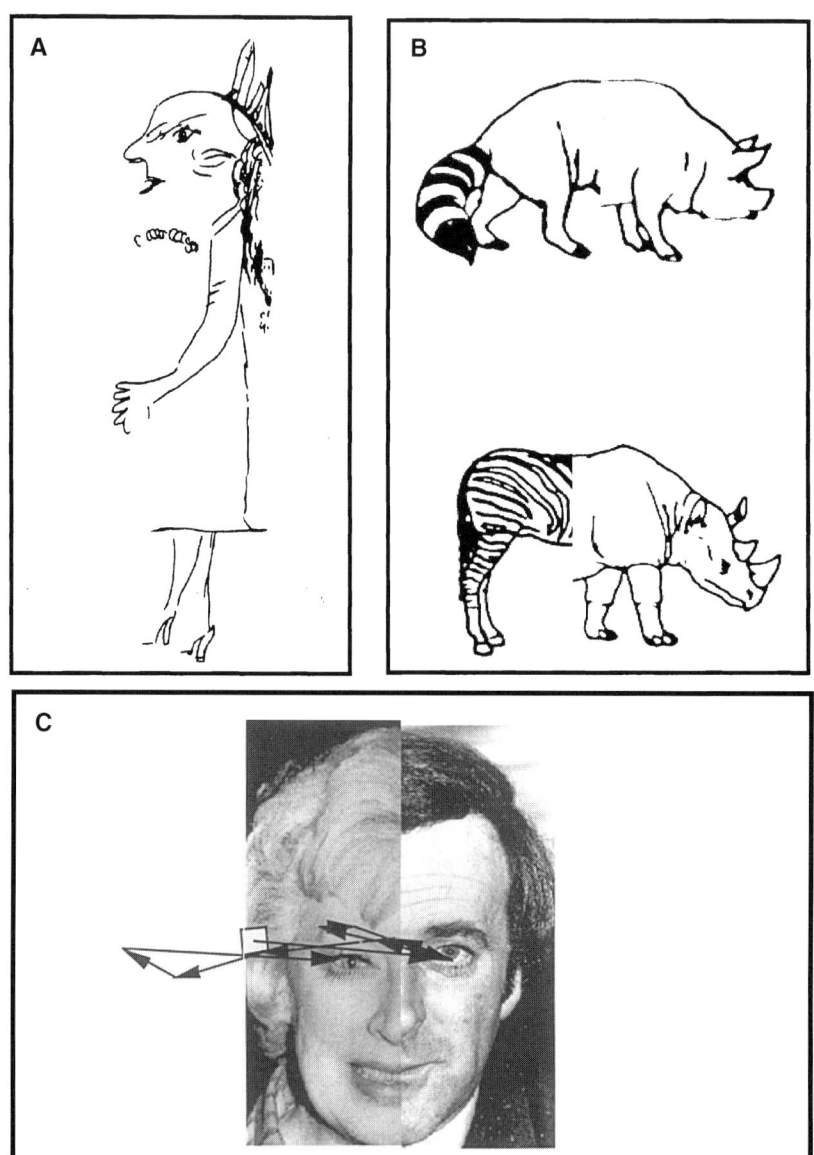

**Figure 11-3.** The effects of left spatial neglect on visual perception. (A) Spontaneous drawing of a woman made by a patient with right hemisphere damage. Note that a large part of the left side of the body is missing, as well as the left side of each of the woman's shoes. (B) Examples of chimeric stimuli used to reveal neglect of the left side of individual objects. The stimulus at the top is composed of the head of a pig and the hind end of a raccoon; the stimulus at the bottom is composed of the head of a rhinoceros and the hind end of a zebra. A right parietal patient with left-sided neglect failed to report the identity of the left side of either stimulus and did not notice that the stimuli were composed of two different halves. (C) Eye movement traces (black arrows) showing the scan path of a patient with left-sided neglect during examination of a face chimera presented to the right of fixation. The patient scanned both sides of the stimulus but reported the face on the right side only. (*Source:* Walker et al., 1996)

## Possible Explanations for Pathological Visual Completion

We have reviewed evidence suggesting that pathological visual completion is extremely rare in hemianopic patients with isolated occipital lesions. Where it has been reported, patients have typically shown veridical perception of whole figures positioned across the intact and hemianopic fields. In contrast, there have been very few cases of occipital damage leading to pathological completion of partial shapes abutting the hemianopic field (Perenin et al., 1986; Marcel, 1998). On the other hand, completion of partial shapes in patients with parietal damage has been reported by many investigators across a variety of behavioural paradigms (Warrington, 1962, 1965; Sergent, 1988; Halligan and Marshall, 1994; Hornak, 1995; Walker and Young, 1996). We have suggested that these parietal cases of pathological completion are due to impairments of spatial attention, most notably visual neglect, affecting the contralesional side of individual objects (see also Walker and Mattingley, 1997, 1998). Such patients tend to report partial shapes as complete because they remain unaware of the absence of visual information on the contralesional side, rather than actively filling in the missing information, as has been suggested elsewhere (e.g., Ishiai et al., 1989; Halligan and Marshall, 1994; Chatterjee, 1995; Hornak, 1995). We acknowledge, however, that there may be equally plausible alternative explanations, as we outline below.

It is possible that facilitatory interhemispheric interactions underlie some cases of pathological visual completion. For example, Torjussen (1978) proposed that veridical perception of whole shapes by hemianopes may arise from facilitation of visual sensitivity in the blind field by concurrent stimulation in the normally sighted field. Such interhemispheric interactions may be organized with mirror symmetric topography (Pöppel and Richards, 1974) and could be mediated by interactions between parieto-occipital cortex and midbrain structures such as the superior colliculus. This idea has received some support from the work of Sprague (1966), who showed that deficient contralesional orienting after unilateral ablation of occipital cortex in the cat is restored by a subsequent lesion of contralateral midbrain structures, including the superior colliculus and substantia nigra. The *Sprague effect* can be understood in terms of the pattern of facilitatory and inhibitory interactions that exist between relevant midbrain and cortical structures. Within each hemisphere, parieto-occipital projections to the ipsilateral colliculus are facilitatory. By contrast, the colliculi on the two sides are mutually inhibitory, as are the two parieto-occipital cortices. Following lesioning of occipital cortex in one hemisphere, facilitatory input to the colliculus on the same side is reduced, as is inhibitory input to the occipital cortex on the contralateral side. Thus, the net effect of unilateral occipital ablation is disinhibition of both the colliculus and the parieto-occipital cortex on the contralesional side. By lesioning the colliculus in the hemisphere opposite the cortical ablation, the balance of activity across the two hemispheres is restored and visual orienting becomes relatively symmetrical again. These findings demonstrate the functional significance of interhemispheric interactions in vision, though it should be noted that primary visual cortex lesions may have quite different consequences in cats and humans.

There is some evidence that perception of shapes in the blind field by hemianopes with occipital damage arises due to facilitatory interhemispheric interactions. In his study of occipital patients TP and GY, Marcel (1998) found stimuli in the blind hemifield that were not reported when presented in isolation, but were nevertheless perceived correctly when a similar shape appeared concurrently in the sighted field (veridical perception). Thus, for example, if the left half of a circle was flashed in the left hemifield together with the right half in the right hemifield, both patients reported the two shapes correctly, even though a single half-circle flashed in the blind field was never reported. Critically, the patients' perception of shapes in the blind hemifield occurred only when the two shapes fell close to the vertical midline (within 1 degree on either side) and when they occupied *homologous* locations in the two fields. The improved reporting of shapes in the blind hemifield under simultaneous bilateral stimulation is suggestive of facilitatory interactions between the two hemispheres. Interestingly, this pattern is the opposite of that encountered in parietal extinction, where reporting of contralesional targets is *worse* under conditions of bilateral stimulation due to competitive interactions between the two stimuli (Driver et al., 1997; Mattingley, 2002). In this context, however, we note that recent work has shown that in some cases of extrastriate damage, reporting of contralesional visual targets is better when these occur together with a stimulus on the ipsilesional side than when they appear in isolation, a phenomenon known as *antiextinction* (Goodrich and Ward, 1997). It remains for future studies to determine the extent to which completion and anti-extinction effects may be related.

At this stage, it is not clear precisely what mechanisms may underlie the putative facilitatory interactions observed in some occipital cases. One possibility is that undamaged extrastriate areas within the ipsilesional hemisphere may receive partial information from the damaged striate cortex, in addition to callosal inputs from homologous areas in the undamaged hemisphere signaling a visual stimulus in a mirror symmetric location of the sighted field. Such activation of extrastriate areas in the affected hemisphere may be particularly susceptible to modulation by inputs from the opposite hemisphere in the absence of inhibitory signals from damaged striate cortex on the same side. Thus, when a whole shape is presented centrally, the portion falling within the sighted field will activate stored shape descriptions, which in turn may reduce the threshold for detecting fragments of the stimulus that fall in the blind hemifield. Such interactions between *perceptual* and *conceptual* levels of visual representation have indeed been suggested to underlie some forms of pathological visual completion (Warrington, 1965; Halligan and Marshall, 1994).

## Conclusion

To summarize, there are several potential mechanisms that might lead to pathological visual completion. Our favored explanation for parietal patients, who constitute the majority of reported cases, is that they are simply unaware that stimulus information is missing from the affected hemifield due to deficits of spatial attention, and so respond as if they have seen a whole shape. For cases showing completion following circumscribed occipital damage, which is rare, there may be facilitatory interactions between brain regions representing homologous regions of the intact and affected fields. Where such interactions do arise, we speculate that the completion processes may be highly domain specific, so that elementary features such as color and form may be completed independently, with characteristic time courses and neural substrates.

One of the main shortcomings of previous studies of pathological visual completion has been their reliance upon direct measures of performance, which rely on patients' subjective reports of their visual experience. As in other areas of neuropsychology, it seems likely that significant advances in understanding visual completion could be made by employing *indirect* measures of performance in order to determine the effects of any pathological completion on responses in a separate task. For example, partial shapes abutting the blind field could be used as primes to either facilitate or interfere with processing of a subsequent target event presented entirely within the normally sighted field. Our idea is to arrange the primes so that if they are seen as partial shapes they will be congruent with the target stimulus, but if they are completed they will be incongruent with the target, thereby inducing interference. Patients can thus be instructed to ignore any primes, since they are irrelevant to the primary task of responding to a visual target in the sighted field. This indirect method has the additional advantage of reducing the confounding effects of eccentric fixation or eye movements toward the affected hemifield, since patients are no longer being asked to report what they cannot see. The advantages of this general approach have been shown repeatedly in neuropsychological patients, including those with blindsight (e.g., Marcel, 1998; de Gelder et al., 1999) and spatial neglect (e.g., McGlinchey-Berroth et al., 1993).

Recent advances in functional brain imaging techniques could also be fruitfully applied to the problem of pathological completion, perhaps in conjunction with the indirect behavioral methods we have advocated here. In this context, event-related functional magnetic resonance imaging or event-related potentials could be used to measure differences in the location, timing, and extent of neural activity associated with perception of complete versus incomplete stimuli. This general approach has recently yielded important insights into the neural substrates of unconscious processing in blindsight and extinction (Weiskrantz et al., 1995; Rees et al., 2000). Finally, it would be useful to test whether completion phenomena similar to those reported in patients can also be elicited in normals using TMS (cf. Kamitani and Shimojo, 1999). A comparison of the effects of focal TMS at occipital versus parietal sites could elucidate the neural basis for the completion phenomena seen in patients with damage to these distinct areas.

In conclusion, we suggest that pathological visual completion is an important phenomenon to be addressed by contemporary cognitive neuroscience. There is much intriguing data in the various historical accounts and some tantalizing results based on direct methods of investigation. However, we know little about the underlying neural or perceptual basis for its occurrence. Most cases arise from extrastriate (especially parietal) lesions, suggesting an attentional basis to the phenomenon. We have advocated a new approach to the study of pathological completion, which involves the kinds of indirect measures that have been applied so successfully to other neuropsychological disorders of visual function. Coupled with functional brain imaging methods and TMS, we believe that a coherent account of pathological visual completion is not far away.

*Acknowledgments*

This work was supported by grants from the Australian Research Council and the University of Arizona (Center for Consciousness Studies) to JBM and by the Wellcome Trust (U.K.) to RW. Parts of this work appeared in R. Walker and J.B. Mattingley (1997). Ghosts in the machine? Pathological visual completion phenomena in the damaged brain. *Neurocase* 3:313–335.

## References

Andersen RA, Snyder LH, Li C-S, and Stricanne B (1993) Coordinate transformations in the representation of spatial information. *Curr Opin Neurobiol* 3:171–176.

Anton G (1899) Ueber die Selbstwahrnehmungen der Herderkrankungen des Gehirns durch den Kranken bei Rindenblindheit und Rindentaubheit. *Arch Psychiatry* 32:86–127.

Baron-Cohen S and Harrison JE (1997) *Synaesthesia: Classic and Contemporary Readings*. Cambridge: Blackwell.

Behrmann M, Moscovitch M, Black SE, and Mozer M (1990) Perceptual and conceptual mechanisms in neglect dyslexia: Two contrasting case studies. *Brain* 113:1163–1183.

Bender MB and Teuber HL (1946) Phenomena of fluctuation, extinction and completion in visual perception. *Arch Neurol Psychiatry* 55:627–658.

Bisiach E, Vallar G, Perani D, Papagno C, and Berti A (1986) Unawareness of disease following lesions of the right hemisphere: Anosognosia for hemiplegia and anosognosia for hemianopia. *Neuropsychologia* 24:471–482.

Chatterjee A (1995) Cross-over, completion and confabulation in unilateral spatial neglect. *Brain* 118:455–465.

Costello AD and Warrington EK (1987) The dissociation of visuospatial neglect and neglect dyslexia. *J Neurol Neurosurg Psychiatry* 50:1110–1116.

de Gelder B, Vroomen J, Pourtois G, and Weiskrantz L (1999) Non-conscious recognition of affect in the absence of striate cortex. *Neuroreport* 10:3759–3763.

De Weerd P, Gattass R, Desimone R, and Ungerleider LG (1995) Responses of cells in monkey visual cortex during perceptual filling in of an artificial scotoma. *Nature* 377:731–734.

Dennett DC (1991) *Consciousness Explained*. Boston: Little, Brown and Company.

Driver J (1995) Object segmentation and visual neglect. *Behav Brain Res* 71(1–2):135–146.

Driver J and Mattingley JB (1998) Parietal neglect and visual awareness. *Nat Neurosci* 1:17–22.

Driver J, Mattingley JB, Rorden CR, and Davis G (1997) Extinction as a paradigm measure of attentional bias and restricted capacity following brain injury. In: Thier P and Karnath H-O (eds), *Parietal Lobe Contributions to Orientation in 3D Space*. Heidelberg: Springer-Verlag, pp 401–430.

Durgin FH, Tripathy SP, and Levi DM (1995) On the filling in of the visual blindspot: Some rules of thumb. *Perception* 24:827–840.

Eysel UT and Schweigart G (1999) Increased receptive field size in the surround of chronic lesions in the adult cat visual cortex. *Cereb Cortex* 9:101–109.

Fiorani M, Rosa MGP, Gattass R, and Rocha-Miranda CE (1992) Dynamic surrounds of receptive-fields in primate striate cortex: A physiological basis for perceptual completion. *Proc Natl Acad Sci, USA* 89:8547–8551.

Fuchs W (1921/1938) Completion phenomena in hemianopic vision. Translated by Ellis WD. *A Source Book of Gestalt Psychology*. London: Kegan Paul, pp 344–356.

Gassel MM and Williams D (1963) Visual functions in patients with homonymous hemianopia. II. *Brain* 86:229–260.

Goodrich SJ and Ward R (1997) Anti-extinction following unilateral parietal damage. *Cogn Neuropsychol* 14:595–612.

Halligan PW and Marshall JC (1994) Completion in visuo-spatial neglect: A case study. *Cortex* 30:685–694.

Hornak J (1995) Perceptual completion in patients with drawing neglect: Eye-movement and tachistoscopic investigation. *Neuropsychologia* 33:305–325.

Ishiai S, Furukawa T, and Tsukagoshi H (1989) Visuospatial processes of line bisection and the mechanisms underlying unilateral spatial neglect. *Brain* 112:1485–1502.

Jackson SR (1999) Pathological perceptual completion in hemianopia extends to the control of reach-to-grasp movements. *Neuroreport* 10:2461–2466.

Kamitani Y and Shimojo S (1999) Manifestation of scotomas created by transcranial magnetic stimulation of human visual cortex. *Nat Neurosci* 2:767–771.

Kapadia MK, Gilbert CD, and Westheimer G (1994) A quantitative measure for short-term cortical plasticity in human vision. *J Neurosci* 14:451–457.

Kolb B (1990) Recovery from occipital stroke: A self report and an inquiry into visual processes. *Can J Psychol* 44:130–147.

Kooistra CA and Heilman KM (1989) Hemispatial visual inattention masquerading as hemianopia. *Neurology* 39:1125–1127.

Marcel AJ (1998) Blindsight and shape perception: Deficit of visual consciousness or of visual function? *Brain* 121:1565–1588.

Mattingley JB (2002) Spatial extinction and its relation to normal attention. In: Karnath H-O, Milner AD, and Vallar G (eds), The Cognitive and Neural Bases of Spatial Neglect. Oxford: Oxford University Press, pp 293–316.

Mattingley JB, Rich AN, Yelland G, and Bradshaw JL (2001) Unconscious priming eliminates automatic binding of color and alphanumeric form in synaesthesia. *Nature* 410:580–582.

McCarthy RA, James-Galton M, and Plant GT (1999) Making faces: Constraints on visual completion in a case of hemianopia (ARVO abstract). *Invest Ophthalmol Vis Sci* 40:S352.

McGlinchey-Berroth R, Milberg WP, Verfaellie M, Alexander MP, and Kilduff PT (1993) Semantic processing in the neglected visual field: Evidence from a lexical decision task. *Cogn Neuropsychol* 10:79–108.

Milner AD and Goodale MA (1995) *The Visual Brain in Action*. Oxford: Oxford University Press.

Mishkin M, Ungerleider LG, and Macko KA (1983) Object vision and spatial vision: Two cortical pathways. *Trends Neurosci* 6:414–417.

Perenin MT, Girard-Madoux P, and Jeannerod M (1986) From completion to residual vision in hemianopic patients (abstract). *Behav Brain Res* 20:130.

Pessoa L, Thompson E, and Noë A (1998) Finding out about filling in: A guide to perceptual completion for visual science and the philosophy of perception. *Behav Brain Sci* 21:723–802.

Pollack M, Battersby WS, and Bender MB (1957) Tachistoscopic identification of contour in patients with brain damage. *J Comp Physiol Psychol* 50:220–227.

Pöppel E and Richards W (1974) Light sensitivity in cortical scotomata contralateral to small islands of blindness. *Exp Brain Res* 21:125–130.

Poppelreuter W (1917/1990) *Disturbances of Lower and Higher Visual Capacities Caused by Occipital Damage: With Special Reference to the Psychopathological, Pedagogical, Industrial, and Social Implications* (trans J Zihl). Oxford: Clarendon Press.

Ptito M, Johannsen P, Faubert J, and Gjedde A (1999) Activation of extrageniculostriate pathways after damage to area V1. *Neuroimage* 9:97–107.

Ramachandran VS (1993) Filling in gaps in perception: Part II. Scotomas and phantom limbs. *Curr Directions Psychol Sci* 2:56–65.

Ramachandran VS and Gregory RL (1991) Perceptual filling in of artifically induced scotomas in human vision. *Nature* 350:699–702.

Rees G, Wojciulik E, Clarke K, Husain M, Frith C, and Driver J (2000) Unconscious activation of visual cortex in the damaged right hemisphere of a parietal patient with extinction. *Brain* 123:1624–1633.

Rich AN and Mattingley JB (2002) Anomalous perception in synaesthesia: A cognitive neuroscience perspective. *Nat Rev Neurosci* 3:43–52.

Robertson IH, Mattingley JB, Rorden C, and Driver J (1998) Phasic alerting of neglect patients overcomes their spatial deficit in visual awareness. *Nature* 395:169–172.

Safran AB, Achard O, Duret F, and Landis T (1999) The "thin man" phenomenon: A sign of cortical plasticity following inferior homonymous paracentral scotomas. *Br J Ophthalmol* 83:137–142.

Sergent J (1988) An investigation into visual completion in blind areas of the visual field. *Brain* 111:347–373.

Silberpfennig J (1941) Contributions to the problem of eye movements. III. Disturbances of ocular movements with pseudohemianopsia in frontal lobe tumours. *Confinia Neurol* 4(1–2):1–13.

Sprague JM (1966) Interaction of cortex and superior colliculus in mediation of visually guided behaviour in the cat. *Science* 153:1544–1547.

Torjussen T (1978) Visual processing in cortically blind hemifields. *Neuropsychologia* 16:15–21.

Von der Heydt R, Peterhans E, and Baumgartner G (1984) Illusory contours and cortical neuron responses. *Science* 224:1260–1262.

Walker R, Findlay JM, Young AW, and Lincoln NB (1996) Saccadic eye movements in object-based neglect. *Cogn Neuropsychol* 13:569–615.

Walker R, Findlay JM, Young AW, and Welch J (1991) Disentangling neglect and hemianopia. *Neuropsychologia* 29:1019–1027.

Walker R and Mattingley JB (1997) Ghosts in the machine? Pathological visual completion phenomena in the damaged brain. *Neurocase* 3:313–335.

Walker R and Mattingley JB (1998) Pathological completion: The blind leading the mind? *Behav Brain Sci* 21:778–779.

Walker R and Young AW (1996) Object-based neglect: An investigation of the contributions of eye movements and perceptual completion. *Cortex* 32:279–295.

Warrington EK (1962) The completion of visual forms across hemianopic field defects. *J Neurol Neurosurg Psychiatry* 25:208–217.

Warrington EK (1965) The effect of stimulus configuration on the incidence of the completion phenomenon. *Br J Psychol* 56:447–454.

Weiskrantz L (1986) *Blindsight. A Case Study and Implications.* Oxford: Oxford University Press.

Weiskrantz L (1990) Outlooks for blindsight: explicit methodologies for implicit processes. [The Ferrier Lecture, 1989]. *Proc R Soc Lond* B(239):247–278.

Weiskrantz L, Barbur JL, and Sahraie A (1995) Parameters affecting conscious versus unconscious visual discrimination without V1. *Proc Natl Acad Sci USA* 92:6122–6126.

Williams D and Gassel MM (1962) Visual functions in patients with homonymous hemianopia. I. *Brain* 85:175–250.

Zihl J and von Cramon D (1985) Visual field recovery from scotoma in patients with postgeniculate damage. *Brain* 108:335–365.

# III

# LONG-TERM CORTICAL REMAPPING

# 12

# Plasticity of the Human Auditory Cortex

CHRISTO PANTEV, NATHAN WEISZ,
MICHAEL SCHULTE, AND THOMAS ELBERT

The perception of timbre, pitch, and sound localization relies on the temporal characteristics of the stimulus. The auditory system accomplishes this partly through the cochlea that transforms sound into spatiotemporal response patterns (Shamma, 2001). A fundamental characteristic of the central auditory processing that already results from stimulus coding in the cochlea is the tonotopic organization of main-line auditory nuclei and fields. Several cortical areas with tonotopic characteristics have been identified in animals (Merzenich et al., 1973, 1975, 1976; Schreiner, 1991; Rauschecker et al., 1995). Tonotopic organization of the human auditory cortex has been demonstrated with magnetic source imaging and other magnetoencephalographic (MEG) techniques (Elberling et al., 1982; Romani et al., 1982; Pantev et al., 1988, 1989, 1995, 1996; Yamamoto et al., 1988; Tiitinen et al., 1993; Cansino et al., 1994). Although there are a few studies that indicate tonotopy by means of hemodynamic patterns, MEG-based techniques have produced the most detailed picture of the functional organization of the human auditory cortex (for review, see Hari, 1990; Jacobson, 1994; Elbert, 1998; Pantev and Lütkenhöner, 2000). The main sources of cortical auditory evoked magnetic fields (AEF) are the intracellular currents that flow when pyramidal cells are depolarized, in the case of auditory stimulation, mostly in the walls of the Sylvian fissure and the superior temporal sulcus (STS).[1]

Research, particularly in the past two decades, revealed that the functional organization of the mammalian cortex, even when mature, is not statically fixed but adjusts in response to alteration of behaviorally relevant input and processing. Injuries like deafferentation through damage of a section of hair cells in the cochlea also remodel the respective cortical representation. With a focus on work in humans, this chapter presents examples of cortical reorganization and describes the principles underlying the plastic capacity of the cortical auditory system and its perceptual alterations.

## Principles of Cortical Reorganization

The knowledge that cortical representations are dynamic and continuously modified by experience is based on a series of classical animal studies, in particular those conducted over the past two decades by M. Merzenich, N. Weinberger, G. Recanzone, J. Rauschecker, C. Gilbert, and others. Studies in humans support and complement these findings. Following Elbert and Heim (2001), the underlying principles are summarized in Table 12-1.

The first example of cortical reorganization following increased and behaviorally relevant stimulation has been provided by studying string players (Elbert et al., 1995). Musicians are usually motivated to practice for hours each day over many years to develop their specific skills. During their performance, the digits of the left hand are continuously engaged in fingering the strings, while the right-hand task of manipulating the bow involves much less individual finger stimulation. A reconstruction of the cortical somatosensory hand regions revealed an expansion of the representational zones of the left hand compared to those of the right hand in string players relative to nonmusicians.

Thus, musicians stimulate their fingers with increasing frequency, and at the same time, their auditory system processes motivationally relevant sounds. What holds for the somatosensory cortex also goes for auditory processing: High-amplitude responses of the auditory cortex were elicited when the musicians listened to their own instrument, whereas tones from other instruments evoked smaller responses (Pantev et al., 2001).

Inactivation of peripheral sensory nerves (e.g., by amputation of a limb) leads to a lack of stimulation of the respective cortical representational zone. The malstimulated area—for instance, the arm region—remains not inactive but engages in information processing of nearby zones. As a consequence, the adjacent face

**Table 12-1.** The principles of cortical reorganization

- Increased use or behaviorally relevant stimulation of a receptor pool leads to an expansion of the respective cortical representation.
- Reduced use or deafferentation causes invasion of the representational zone from sites nearby on the map. Topographically distorted representations may be accompanied by unpleasant phenomena such as phantom limb pain or tinnitus.
- Synchronous, behaviorally relevant stimulation at nearby sites results in a fusion of the representations, that is, temporally correlated activities shape cortical representations.
- Asynchronous stimulation of two different receptor pools tends to segregate the representational zones. In this way, separate finger regions or categorical perception of phonemes emerge.
- Cortical reorganization requires a heavy training schedule and a high motivational drive in a behaviorally relevant context.
- Cortical reorganization can be evoked in response to a lesion of cortical tissue in closely related cortical regions. After stroke, nonlesioned but deafferented brain regions alter their organization.

and shoulder areas move into the *vacant* arm territory (equal to invasion). This means that tactile stimulation of the face or shoulder in people with arm amputation activates not only neurons of the face and shoulder regions, but also the cortical representational area of the amputated arm. Studies in humans demonstrated a close association between invasion and pathological symptoms, in particular with phantom limb pain and—in the auditory sensory modality—with tinnitus. These examples illustrate that cortical reorganization is not necessarily adaptive, but can lead to a maladaptive disaster.

As an alternative to the mechanisms of cortical reorganization, one may suppose that a relatively small reorganization along the sensory pathway could affect the subsequent cortical area on a macroscopic scale. However, it was demonstrated that thalamic organization changed dramatically, when the cortical efferents projecting to the thalamus were inactivated (Ergenzinger et al., 1998). Thus, reorganization in earlier synaptic stages of the sensory pathway is influenced by top-down processing (Braun et al., 2000). The functional organization of one level is governed by the interplay of earlier and later representational stages.

## Plasticity of the Human Auditory Cortex

### *Plasticity Following Deafferentation*

In adult animals, after restricted monaural lesioning of the cochlear epithelium, the tonotopic cortical map can reorganize (Robertson and Irvine, 1989; Rajan et al., 1993) such that cortical neurons deprived of their usual most-sensitive afferent input now respond to tone frequencies adjacent to the frequency range damaged by the lesion (lesion-edge frequencies). Further, the new responses occur with intensity thresholds similar to those recorded in the cortical regions normally representing the lesion-edge frequencies. This results in an expanded map representation of the lesion-edge frequencies. The findings demonstrated that cortical regions that have lost their normal input take over and serve functions found in adjacent cortical areas (Stanton and Harrison, 1996; Rajan, 1998).

Studies in humans may to some extent allow determination of whether the conditions found to apply in the animal studies also produce reorganizational changes in the human auditory cortical maps. One constraint, however, is that observations in humans are restricted to natural lesions, and there is no control of the technique used to produce the lesion, its extent, or the exact mechanism of the consequent pathology. Nevertheless, humans with lesions induced by acoustic trauma or by sudden hearing loss of unknown etiology are suitable for studies of lesion-induced changes in the auditory pathway and cortex.

One such study examined the functional reorganization of auditory cortical structures in humans as a response to the deafferentation caused by cochlear damage in the high-frequency range (Dietrich et al., 2001). Eight right-handed patients (age range, 20–58 years; mean age, 38 years) with steep high-frequency cochlear hearing loss and a lesion existing for more than 6 months were compared to 12 right-handed, normally hearing controls (age range, 22–30 years; mean age, 25 years). Auditory stimuli consisted of tone bursts of three different frequencies in the frequency range with no hearing loss. One frequency was defined as the lesion-edge frequency, and two frequencies were chosen in the intact range (Fig. 12-1). Randomized tone bursts with carrier frequencies of 500, 1000, 2000, and 4000 Hz were used in the control group. In order to assess the cortical reorganization consequent to the deafferentation due to cochlear damage in the high-frequency range, the corresponding dipole moments of the underlying cortical sources were estimated. This measure indicates the total number of neurons involved during a cortical response (Williamson and Kaufman, 1990). Figure 12-1 shows the results for a single patient, comparing the strength of the cortical areas corresponding to the lesion-edge frequency with the cortical strength of the two frequencies in the intact frequency range. In addition, the corresponding audiogram is presented. The results demonstrate that in seven out of eight patients, the cortical strength evoked by a stimulus with lesion-edge frequency is larger than the one that results from stimulation in the intact frequency range. The data indicate that the cortical strength for stimuli in the lesion edge is significantly larger than for those in the intact frequency range ($F(1,6) > 5.6$; $P < .05$). No significant difference was found in the comparison of the dipole moments for the two intact-range frequencies. The specificity of the result, suggesting enhanced cortical representation near the lesion edge, is further supported by the observation that control subjects did not show a significant difference in dipole moments between any of the four different frequencies, chosen in the range of the intact and lesion edges of the patient population. The variation in dipole moment was equally small for the right and left hemispheres.

The significant increase in dipole moment value for the lesion-edge frequency compared to the frequencies in the intact range suggests an expansion of the cortical representation of the lesion-edge frequency. This expansion probably reflects the recruitment of deafferented cortical neurons into cortical networks, representing intact cochlear regions. The data from 12 subjects with normal hearing indicate that the dipole moments in these regions do not vary systematically with the investigated frequencies. Therefore, it is likely that the distortion of dipole moments in the range of the lesion edge indicates a distortion of the tonotopic map in this region. These findings indicate an invasion of the cortical representation of the lesion-edge frequency into the partially deafferented region, corresponding to the principles formulated in Table 12-1, and they are consistent with the observations in animals where cochlear lesion have been induced operatively (Robertson and Irvine, 1989; Rajan et al., 1993; Irvine et al., 2000; Salvi et al., 2000). In the present study, neurons in the deprived regions of cortex appeared to respond to tone frequencies adjacent to the frequency range damaged by the lesion, as indicated by the increase in the cortical strength. From these results, it seems likely that the increase in cortical strength represents an expansion of the frequency representation of cortical areas adjacent to the deprived area. An al-

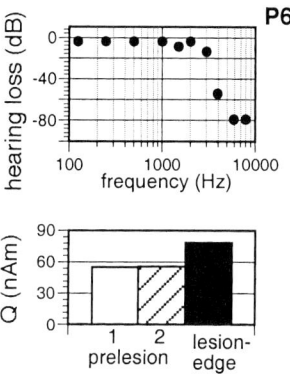
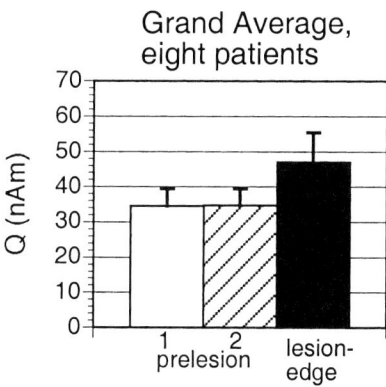

**Figure 12-1.** Individual cortical strength values (dipole moments in nAm) and corresponding audiogram of a representative patient for two prelesion frequencies and the lesion-edge frequency (top). The cross-averaged cortical strength values with the standard error of the mean, calculated over all patients, are shown at the bottom. Six of the patients showed a unilateral high-frequency hearing loss with normal hearing of the other side (hearing loss less than 15 dB within the frequency range from 125 to 8000 Hz). The other two patients revealed a bilateral high-frequency hearing loss. The tested side was the one with the steeper slope on the audiogram. Audiological examinations, including brainstem electric response audiometry (BERA), did not reveal retrocochlear hearing loss in any of the patients. Tinnitus, including the evaluation of tinnitus pitch and loudness, was assessed by the tinnitus questionnaire of Goebel and Hiller (1998). The time between the magnetoencephalographic (MEG) assessment and the onset of the lesion for the eight patients was as follows: 7, 39, 43, 76, 11, 15, 23, and 9 months. The lesion-edge frequency was determined individually with respect to the patient's steep high-frequency hearing loss, and it was located adjacent to the sharp deterioration in thresholds at higher frequencies. The two frequencies in the intact region were located next to the lesion-edge frequency. The intensity of each tone burst was set at 60 dB above the individually assessed hearing threshold.

ternative explanation is that the same neurons are activated by the lesion-edge frequency as prior to the lesion, but that there is now increased neuronal synchronicity. This explanation, however, is less likely because not just the peak, but the total area of the N1m component of the stimulus-evoked magnetic field, became enlarged. Recruitment of a larger neuronal population may occur through a decrease in cortical lateral inhibition, although a recent study (Rajan and Irvine, 1998) shows that loss of lateral inhibition alone does not produce cortical map reorganization or synaptic and dendritic changes within existing terminal arbors (Darian-Smith and Gilbert, 1995). It has been suggested that effects observed in cortical organization may be secondary to subcortical changes (e.g., Rajan et al., 1993). While subcortical reorganization has been demonstrated in the auditory (Willott, 1986) and somatosensory (Garraghty and Kaas, 1991) systems after damage of respective receptor surfaces, it should be noted that subcortical changes can also be secondary to cortical reorganization as fibers project back top-down to each relay in the sensory pathway. In the thalamocortical network, for instance, there are 10 times more fibers projecting from cortex to thalamus than bottom-up from thalamus to cortex (Ergenzinger et al., 1998). Generally, the cortical changes that result from nervous system injury or from increased use cannot be explained by thalamic reorganization only (e.g., Florence et al., 2001), although thalamic drive of cortical reorganization of ventral posterior (VP) thalamic nuclei after rhizotomy has been found (Jones and Pons, 1998; Woods et al., 2000).

## Reorganization in Tinnitus

Patients with subjective tinnitus perceive auditory signals (mostly a whistle or noise) in the absence of any internal or external source of sound. The exact pathophysiological mechanisms leading to this disturbing symptom are mostly unknown, although the high prevalence of tinnitus in subjects with damage or degeneration of the internal ear suggests that it might be cochlear in origin. However, the fact that tinnitus is consciously perceived, and that a transection of the auditory nerve does not lead to amelioration (Douek, 1987); suggests that a central nervous system phenomenon must underlie tinnitus generation. A recent postron emission tomography (PET) study (Lockwood et al., 1998) showed altered activation in the primary auditory cortex contralateral to the ear in which the tinnitus was perceived in patients who are able to modulate the tinnitus loudness via oral-facial movements. This finding was confirmed in another study (Wallhausser-Franke et al., 1996) performed to objectify tinnitus using the 2-deoxyglucose method. After creating salicylate-induced tinnitus in gerbils, they observed increased activation in the auditory cortex and contrary to previous reports (Jastreboff et al., 1987; Brummet, 1995) a reduction of neuronal activity in the inferior colliculus.

Work on tinnitus in humans (Muhlnickel et al., 1998) is based on an analogy that we drew to our findings in patients with phantom limb pain. These patients report sensations from their phantom limb, including phantom limb pain in the majority of cases. In patients with upper-limb amputation, we found that regions of the somatosensory cortex formerly responding to stimulation of the arm responded to stimulation of the mouth and chin; that is, the deafferented region was *invaded* by adjacent regions of the somatotopic map (Elbert et al., 1994, 1997). Moreover, the amount of reorganization was almost perfectly ($r = .93$) correlated with the strength of the phantom limb pain (Flor et al., 1995). Parallels were drawn between phantom limb pain, a feeling present despite lack of sensory input, and tinnitus, an auditory phenomenon with no objective sound source. Based on this parallel, we hypothesized that tinnitus might be a phantom phenomenon of the auditory modality related to distortions of the tonotopic map, just as phantom limb pain seems related to sensorimotor map distortion.

To test this hypothesis, 10 subjects (mean age, 32.4 years) with tonal tinnitus between 2000 and 8000 Hz and a maximal hearing loss of 25 dB participated in a study using magnetic source imaging to determine the tonotopic organization of the auditory cortex. Four of the patients had right-ear, two had left-ear, and four had bilateral tinnitus. The experienced strength of the tinnitus was assessed with a modified German version of the West Haven–Yale Multidimensional Pain Inventory (Flor et al., 1990), in which pain was substituted for by sounds. Fifteen subjects, matched for age and gender, without tinnitus and with normal hearing served as controls. Each ear was sequentially stimulated with four sets of 200 pure tone pulses of 500 ms duration and 70 dB above the individual hearing level. Standard carrier frequencies for healthy controls were set at 1000, 2000, 4000, and 8000 Hz. For the tinnitus subjects, three standard frequencies that were most distant from the tinnitus frequency were used in addition to a tone that matched the tinnitus frequency (mean, 4500 Hz; SD, 1100). The standard tone closest to the tinnitus frequency was deleted from the tone series (4000 Hz in all cases).

Neuromagnetic recordings were taken during the auditory stimulation. A single equivalent current dipole (ECD) model was used to identify the source of the N1m component. In most subjects, the N1m dipole locations form a linear function with the logarithm of the stimulus frequency in the medial-lateral direction along Heschl's gyrus, with higher frequencies being located more medial (Pantev et al., 1995). In three-dimensional space, the N1m dipole locations form a trajectory representing the tonotopic map.

The tonotopic map was reconstructed in the tinnitus group using the three standard frequencies that differed most from the tinnitus frequency. The Euclidean distance between this trajectory and the dipole location for the tinnitus frequency was calculated to obtain a measure for the amount of deviation of the tinnitus frequency from the tonotopic organization. For the purpose of comparison, a representative tinnitus frequency of 4000 Hz was defined for the control group. The average distance was significantly larger in the contralateral hemisphere (mean of both contralateral hemispheres in the bilateral tinnitus subjects) for the tinnitus group (5.3 mm, SD $= 3.1$) than for the healthy controls (2.5 mm, SD $= 1.3$; $t = 3.13$, $p < .01$). Figure 12-2 exemplifies this difference, depicting the tonotopic map of one tinnitus subject and one healthy control by superimposing the equivalent current dipole sources on an axial magnetic resonance imaging (MRI) slice of the auditory cortex. This result indicates an expansion of the tono-

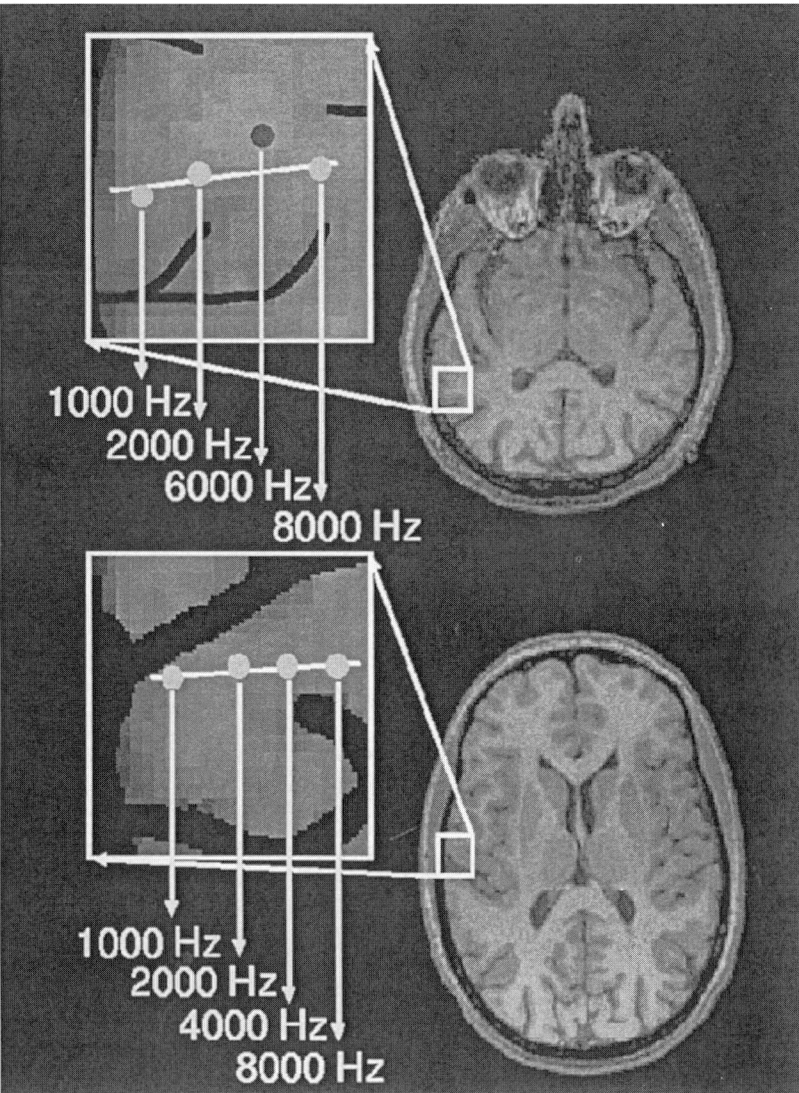

**Figure 12-2.** A tonotopic map is depicted for one tinnitus subject (top) and one healthy control (bottom). The dark circle in the upper portion of the figure represents the location of the tinnitus frequency. Note that whereas the four standard frequencies form a linear trajectory in the healthy control, the tinnitus frequency clearly deviates from the linear trajectory in the tinnitus subject. (From Mühlnickel et al., 1998 with permission)

topic map at the tinnitus frequency into neighboring regions. The distortion of the tonotopic map is furthermore suggested by the regression coefficient of the four log-transformed frequencies and their location in the medial-lateral dimension, reaching only .29 for the contralateral and .45 for the ipsilateral hemisphere. Normal values usually lie above .90 (here: .92).

Interestingly, the amount of reorganization of the tonotopic map and the subjective strength of tinnitus showed a strong positive correlation (Spearman's $r =$ .82). This result suggests that neuroplastic alterations contribute to the aversion symptomatic in tinnitus. Although no conclusion about the cause(s) of the plastic changes can be derived from this study, it seems appropriate to speculate that in most cases of tinnitus the initial event might be an event that caused cochlear damage, which has been shown to be related to an enlargement of the lesion-edge frequency (see the previous section). Clues for this hypothesis stem from the frequent occurrence of tinnitus in persons with (especially high-frequency) hearing loss (Lenarz, 1992) and from the fact that the tinnitus frequency commonly lies between the frequency normally represented in the deafferented region and the frequency represented at lesion-edge (Feldmann, 1992). Regardless of the initial cause, however, this study opens up exciting vistas about the treatability of tinnitus using methods aimed at altering cortical reorganization. For example, previous studies on animals (Recanzone et al., 1993) and humans (Menning et al., 2000) demonstrated that plastic changes in the auditory cortex could be induced by intensive frequency discrimination training. On a more general level, promising results come from various pathologies related to cortical reorganization such as writer's cramp or phantom limb pain by special training aimed at stimulating the deafferented cortical region (Elbert and Rockstroh, 2001).

## Short-Term Plasticity

All of the studies reported above investigated cortical reorganization on a time scale of weeks to years. But changes in cortical dynamics occur rapidly following deafferentation. Studies have shown that neurons broaden and shift their receptive fields to sensory surfaces near or beyond the edge of the lesioned zone within a few minutes after deafferentation in the somatosensory (Krubitzer et al., 1995; Doetsch et al., 1996) and visual (Gilbert, 1998) systems, and within hours in the auditory system (Robertson and Irvine, 1989). Rapid retuning has also been observed after *functional deafferentation* of visual neurons by artificial scotomas (Gilbert et al., 1996) and of somatosensory representations in humans as a form of task and context dependency (Braun et al., 2000). Rapid expansion of receptive fields appears to be due in part to an unmasking of existing excitatory connections through a reduction of intracortical inhibition by the functional lesion (Ziemann et al., 1998). However, because rapid changes in receptive field properties continue to develop for an hour or more and are sensitive to N-methyl-D-aspartate (NMDA) (receptor for neurotransmitter glutamate) receptor blockade, plastic changes in synaptic efficacy have also been implicated. If so, rapid changes in cortical dynamics induced by deafferentation may have mechanisms in common with changes induced by behavioral training that has been found to alter the tuning of somatosensory (Diamond et al., 1994) and auditory (Weinberger, 1995; Weinberger and Bakin, 1998) cortical neurons within minutes to hours.

We used MEG measurements to examine the effect of functional deafferentation in the human auditory system (Pantev et al., 1999). Subjects listened for 3 hours on 3 consecutive days to music notched at a narrow frequency band centered on 1 kHz. Immediately before and after listening to the notched music, auditory cortical representations were measured neuromagnetically for a "test" stimulus of 1 kHz bandpassed noise centered on the notched region and a "control" stimulus of 0.5 kHz bandpassed noise centered one octave below this region. If cortical neurons deprived of their afferent input were recruited into the function of closely adjacent cortical regions, it could be expected that the neural representation of the test stimulus would diminish after listening to the notched music, whereas the neural representation of the control stimulus (which was distant from the region of the functional deafferentation) would not change. In order to address the time course and reversibility of cortical remodeling induced by this procedure, the experiment was repeated on 3 consecutive days. The comparison of the field amplitudes of selected MEG channels or of the calculated root mean squared (RMS) values for the whole sensor array before and after 3 hours of listening to notched music is acceptable only if the position of the head with respect to the sensor array is more or less constant between the two measurement periods. Therefore, special efforts (retention of the evacuated vacuum cushion between measurements and photographs of head position) were made to achieve this relative constancy. Ten normally hearing, right-handed subjects were investigated. They were asked to listen attentively to music of their choice for continuous periods of 3 hours. The music was manipulated in such a way that a notch between 0.7 and 1.3 kHz, centered on 1 kHz, was produced using a band rejection filter. Music was presented binaurally at a moderate loudness of about 60–70 dB sound pressure level (SPL) through earphones. During the listening period, the subjects were allowed to read a book or surf the Internet. Owing to the presence of the notch, for this period of time the afferent input to cortical neurons tuned to frequencies around 1 kHz was abolished. MEG measurements were taken before and after the period of listening to the notched music.

Figure 12-3 demonstrates how the dipole moment of the equivalent cortical source and the RMS field value, respectively, changed after listening to notched music. "Before" minus "after" differences are shown separately for the test and control stimuli averaged over all subjects and days. The figure shows that for the test stimulus, these values decrease after listening to notched music, whereas for the control stimulus, they remain almost constant. This short-term plasticity effect reversed within 24 hours, as neural indicators (dipole moments and signal power) derived from measurements prior to the intervention were not different from those taken on 3 subsequent days. In conclusion, the results provide evidence that different organizational structures of cortical representational maps can occur or develop within a time frame as short as a few hours, in this case following functional deafferentation of the adult human auditory cortex. A particular cortical map can appear within 3 hours of deafferentation and then persist for hours.

The temporal properties of the notching effect are consistent with animal studies in which selected regions of the cochlea have been deafferented by electrolytic lesions. Cortical neurons deprived of their afferent input initially show elevated response thresholds and then shift their tuning preferences away from the le-

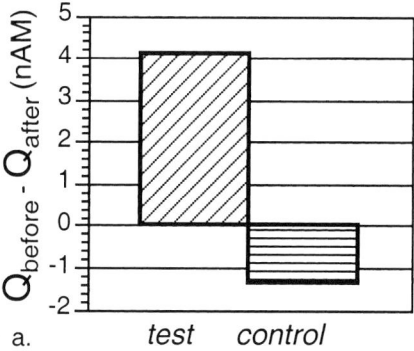

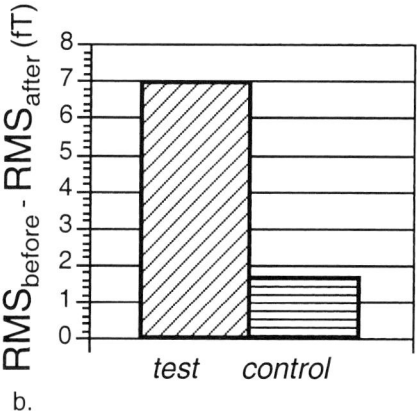

**Figure 12-3.** (a) Change in the strength of the cortical source calculated as the equivalent current dipole moment (Q, nAm) fitted to the N1m component for test and control stimuli averaged over subjects and days of "before" minus "after" measurements. (b) Change in the root mean square (RMS, fT) of the N1m component for test and control stimuli averaged over subjects and days of "before" minus "after" measurements.

sioned area to frequencies near the edge of the deafferented region over a period of 1–3 hours or more (Robertson and Irvine, 1989). While the reduction of responsiveness at the 1 kHz functional deafferentation is expected, the temporal dynamics of remodeling (including persistence during the measurement of neural representations and recovery of the 1 kHz representation within 24 hours) point to modification of synaptic efficacy by a plastic mechanism. It should be noted that the 0.5 kHz control stimulus was placed some distance away from the site of the functional deafferentation (one octave), because the precise border of the lesioned area and the sensitivity of MEG measurements to dynamics occurring in this area are unknown. Whether augmentation of the cortical representation at edge frequencies can be probed by test stimuli placed closer to the site of the functional lesion remains to be determined.

Growing evidence from animal studies as well as the results presented here suggest that the functional organization of the adult auditory cortex appears to be dynamic and modifiable by plastic mechanisms over relatively brief time frames. The rapidity of the observed neuronal changes argues against synaptogenesis, although such a process appears to underlie alterations of sensory maps that result from years of deafferentation and often extend across large regions of the cortical surface. Long-term potentiation and long-term depression appear to be better models, since these phenomena are properties of neocortical synapses and can occur roughly within the time frame investigated by this study.

## *Plasticity Induced by Learning in Discrimination of Virtual Auditory Objects*

The short-term plastic behavior of the auditory cortex due to learned recognition of an auditory Gestalt was investigated in the following study. In this study, we created a short melody composed of eight harmonic complex tones. A harmonic complex tone is the sum of sinusoidal sound waves with frequencies that are integer multiples of a certain fundamental frequency ($f_0$). The perceived pitch of such complex tones corresponds to the $f_0$ even when the $f_0$ is absent (*pitch of the missing fundamental* or *virtual pitch*; Terhardt, 1974). In the case of virtual pitch perception, the information from the different harmonics must be bound together in order to perceive the virtual pitch, also known as an *auditory illusion*. This auditory binding becomes more difficult when few and/or higher harmonics are present. The design of this experiment has been inspired by the results of an earlier MEG study (Knief et al., 2000) in which functional differences of evoked gamma band activity due to the perception of coherent versus noncoherent auditory stimuli were observed. Here, we constructed a melody consisting of eight complex tones, which were composed of three harmonics (see Fig. 12-4a). Each complex tone of the melody could be perceived according to either the spectrum frequencies (spectral pitch) or the virtual pitch corresponding to the missing fundamental frequency.

The missing fundamental frequencies of the eight complex tones followed the beginning of the tune "Frère Jacques" (virtual melody), whereas the harmonics were chosen so that the spectral melody had an inverse contour to the virtual one. Thus, the melody was used as an indicator of whether subjects perceived the spectral pitch or the virtual pitch of the complex tones. Ten subjects, who were only able to perceive the spectral pitch melody, were investigated. Then they were trained intensively until they learned to perceive the virtual pitch melody. Thus, we were able to investigate the involvement of plastic reorganizational processes in virtual pitch formation of the human auditory cortex. The magnetic AEFs were recorded contralateral to the ear of presentation over both

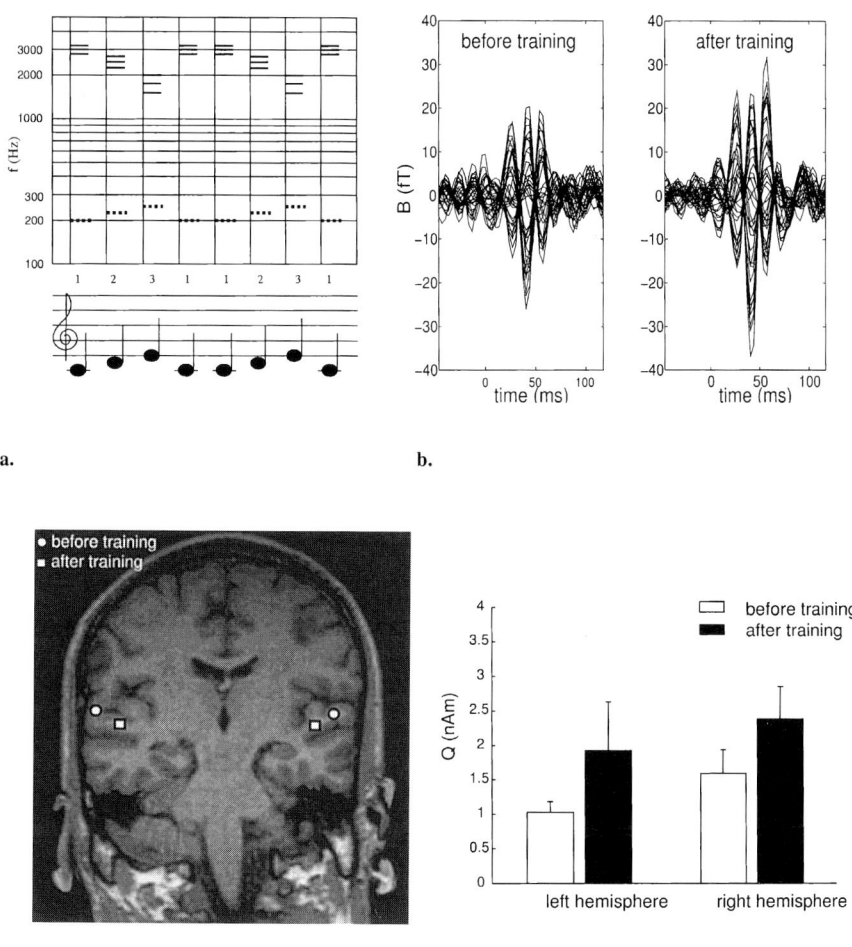

**Figure 12-4.** (a) Stimulus sequence of the virtual melody. The sequence consists of three different complex tones played in the order 12311231. The fundamental frequencies ($f_{0i}$) were chosen as follow: $f_{01}$, 200 Hz; $f_{02}$, 225 Hz; and $f_{03}$, 250 Hz. The virtual melody follows the tune "Frere Jacques," whereas the spectral melody given by the central frequencies of three harmonics has an inverse pitch contour. (b) Averaged gamma band responses of about 600 epochs of one representative subject to tone 1 (bandpass filtered: 24–48 Hz). Data for all 37 measurement channels are plotted together for the session before (left) and after training (right). (c) Location of estimated current dipoles for gamma band responses integrated into the magnetic resonance imaging (MRI) overlay of one subject. Circles denote the source location before training, and squares denote the estimated location after training. (d) Estimated dipole moments of the gamma band activity for the left and right hemispheres, cross-averaged over all subjects. Black bars show the values after training and white bars before training. Error bars indicate the standard error of the mean.

hemispheres before and after training in a passive listening paradigm by means of MEG.

In all 10 test subjects, the training resulted in a sudden switch from the spectral to the virtual mode of pitch perception. Group results were determined in seven subjects who trained for about 1 week (two subjects perceived the virtual melody during the first measurement, and one subject trained over 7 weeks). The clear change in perception was accompanied by a distinct increase in the transient gamma-band evoked field, which has often been found to be associated with integrative cognitive functions such as the binding process during object recognition. During the perception of a Gestalt, the different characteristics of an object are combined into a coherent percept, and the oscillatory neural discharges in the gamma frequency range have been proposed to be a representation of this binding process (Singer and Gray, 1995; Tallon-Baudry and Bertrand, 1999). A strong increase was found for the evoked gamma band field and for the corresponding estimated cortical strength (cf. Figs. 12-4b and 12-4d). RMS values averaged across subjects increased significantly from 6.2 to 7.9 fT for the left hemisphere and from 4.96 to 6.38 fT for the right hemisphere (ANOVA: $F = 7.3; p = .031$). Similar behavior was observed for the estimated cortical strength (dipole moment) of the gamma band response. The estimated cortical strength of the corresponding sources increased significantly from $1.03 \pm 0.16$ nAm to $1.92 \pm 0.71$ nAm in the left hemisphere and from $1.59 \pm 0.35$ nAm to $2.38 \pm 0.47$ nAm in the right hemisphere between the two corresponding sessions ($F = 6.46, p = .039$). However, between the hemispheres, no significant differences were observed ($F = 0.84, p = .39$).

The estimated equivalent cortical sources were significantly displaced toward the midline, by about 6.6 mm and 5.1 mm in the left and right hemispheres, respectively. An additional analysis was performed by means of independent component analysis (ICA). The number of independent components in which the evoked gamma band response could be separated is related to its spatiotemporal variability. After training, fewer independent components were needed to explain the gamma band responses than before. The obtained ICA results can be explained by a higher synchronization of the cortical networks involved in the generation of the evoked gamma band activity.

In this study, the question of learning-induced plasticity in the perception of the virtual pitch of complex tones was directly addressed. The auditory Gestalt recognition was associated with plastic reorganizational processes expressed as an increase in RMS value, cortical strength, shift in source location, and lower spatiotemporal variability. Together, these results suggest that the integration of different spectral pitches into a single coherent percept is associated with a convergence of harmonically related information. The enhancement of RMS and cortical strength values may be explained either by higher synchronization (already suggested by ICA), by enlargement of the involved cortical networks, or most probably by both. As the latency of the evoked gamma band is about 30–70 ms, the plastic reorganization of neural networks is likely to take place at the level of the primary auditory cortex.

## Reorganization After Long Lasting, Intensive Training (Long-Term Plasticity)

The following MEG study was carried out to evaluate the cortical representations in highly skilled musicians in comparison with nonmusicians (Pantev et al., 1998). The group of 20 musicians consisted of music students with absolute pitch ($n = 9$) as well as musical students with relative pitch ($n = 11$), who had played their instruments for a mean period of $21 \pm 6$ and $15 \pm 3$ years, respectively. The control group ($n = 13$) consisted of students who had never played an instrument. The auditory evoked fields with the major component N1m were elicited by a semirandomized blockwise presentation of four piano tones, C4, C5, C6, and C7 (American notation, having the first harmonics at 262, 523, 1046, and 2093 Hz, respectively), and four pure tones corresponding to the fundamental frequencies of the piano tones. Each tone was presented 128 times while subjects watched cartoon videos intended to fixate their attention.

A highly significant difference between the musicians and controls was found in the strength of the cortical sources activated by the piano tones compared to the pure tones (Fig. 12-5). The two types of tones were matched for loudness. For both groups of musicians with absolute or relative pitch, the equivalent dipole moment was 21%–28% larger for piano tones than for pure tones. For the control group, no significant difference was found in dipole moment between the piano and pure tones. The observed increase in dipole moment reflects an expansion of the cortical representation areas involved in processing of the piano tones. This expansion may have occurred either because more neurons were engaged in the processing of these tones in skilled musicians or because the synchrony of neural activity was greater as a consequence of their musical training.

Prior to the experiment, the musicians were interviewed to determine the age at which their musical training had commenced. The observed functional expansion was correlated with the age at which the musicians began to practice. In this respect, no difference was found between musicians with absolute and relative pitch. A significant linear correlation was obtained between the mean dipole moment for the piano tones and the age of inception of musical training. This result indicates that the younger the age at which the subjects started playing their instrument, the larger the cortical representation of the tones of the musical scale. The observed relationship, that is, the enlargement of cortical representation for subjects who began to practice prior to the age of 9 years, is similar to that reported in a previous study of the somatosensory representations of fingering digits in highly skilled string players (Elbert et al., 1995). In that study, expansion of the somatosensory representation was most evident in musicians whose practice had commenced before the age of 10 years. The similar dependence of auditory and somatosensory representations on practice commencing prior to the age of about 10 years suggests that cortical reorganization induced by training of a musical skill conforms to the pattern of sensory input experienced during practice. Although we cannot completely separate the effects due to the duration of training from the effects consequent on the age at which train-

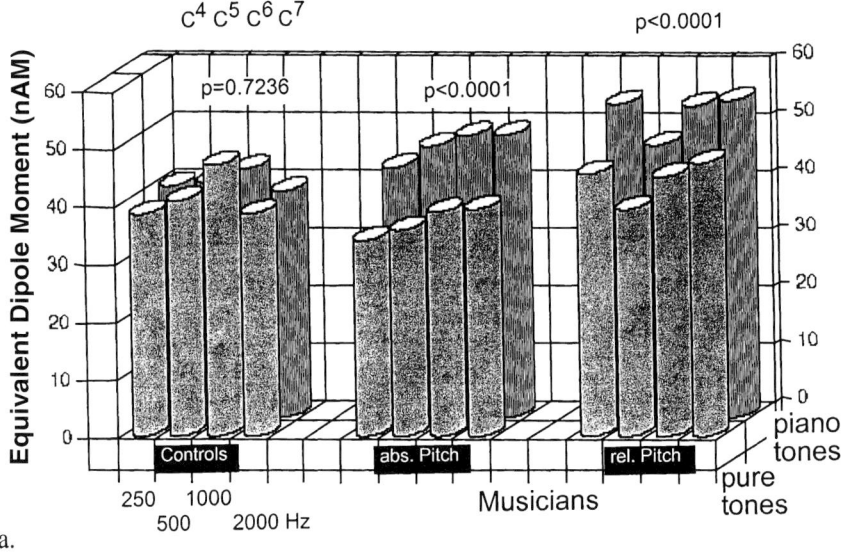

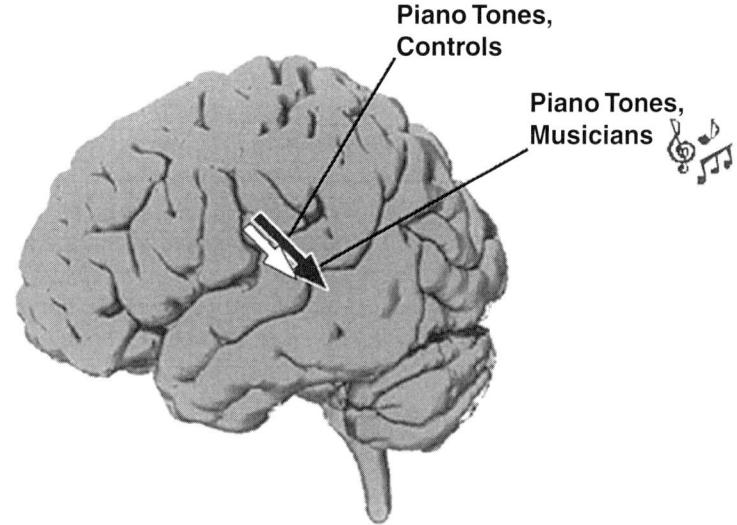

**Figure 12-5.** (a) Equivalent dipole moment amplitude (strength of neuronal activation during the auditory N1m peak of the auditory evoked field) shown for pure tones and piano tones in control subjects and musicians with absolute or relative pitch. (b) Mean values of the strength of cortical activation during the auditory N1m evoked field for piano tones in control subjects and musicians with absolute or relative pitch.

ing commenced, it seems unlikely that duration was the critical variable because, at the time of our measurements, the musicians had practiced their skill for an average of 18 ± 5 years.

The significant expansion of the cortical representation observed in musicians for tones of the musical scale corresponds to the results of an earlier MRI study (Schlaug et al., 1995) and also to those of a recent study (Schlaug, 2001), which describe a structural enlargement of the planum temporale of the left hemisphere in musicians with absolute pitch compared to nonmusicians. Our data thus associate a use-correlated functional property with cortical architectonics and raise the further possibility that musical experience during childhood may have influenced the structural development of the auditory cortex. A special role for early experience is compatible with evidence for maturation of fiber tracts and the presence of intracortical neuropil persisting up to the age of 7 years (Yakovlev and Lecours, 1967). These results, when interpreted in the context of previously reported evidence for expansion of somatosensory representations of the fingering digits in skilled violinists (Elbert et al., 1995), suggest that use-dependent functional reorganization extends across the sensory cortices to reflect the pattern of sensory input processed by the subject during musical skill development.

## Conclusion

This chapter's aim was to point out the relationship between neuroplastic changes in the auditory cortex and its perceptual manifestations. The long- and short-term plastic behavior of the human auditory cortex was examined in different studies. It was shown that deafferentation due to cochlear damage in patients with high-frequency hearing loss goes along with an enlargement of the lesion-edge frequency. Plastic modifications of the tonotopic map following deafferentation may also underlie the expanded representation of the tinnitus frequency found in tinnitus patients. Thus, a mechanism designed to adjust cortical organization to the individual's needs and environment may have maladaptive consequences. In the intact organism, cortical reorganization is an essential basis for training and adaptive responses, like the ability to acquire motor or perceptual skills and to model the environment in the form of context-dependent cortical representational maps.

## Notes

1. During MEG recordings, the recording place is so far away from the source that microscopic details of the source current density distribution are irrelevant. It follows the important model simplification of an ECD. Such a current dipole is unequivocally defined by the three-dimensional space coordinates as well as the orientation and amplitude of the dipole moment. Given a constant direction of the ECD, the dipole moment indicates the total strength of cortical activation, that is, the number of neurons involved during a cortical response. If this number increases, the dipole moment also increases. Any active focal area can be modeled by an ECD. Williamson and Kaufman (1990) estimate that each

dendritic current flow contributes to the dipole moment according to the formula dipole moment = (conductivity) × (cross section of the dendrite) × (potential difference along the dendrite). If the diameter of an apical dendrite is assumed to be 4 $\mu$m with a intracellular conductivity of about .25/$\Omega$m and a potential difference of 10 mV, about 30,000 dendrites would be necessary to produce a dipole moment of 10 nAm. Only currents flowing tangentially with respect to the magnetic sensors are detected. Magnetic fields generated by axonal currents are assumed to be quadrupolar and are neglected in the calculation.

## References

Braun C, Schweizer R, Elbert T, Birbaumer N, and Taub E (2000) Differential activation in somatosensory cortex for different discrimination tasks. *J Neurosci* 20:446–450.

Brummet RE (1995) A mechanism for tinnitus? In: Vernon JA and Moller AR (eds), *Mechanisms of Tinnitus.* Boston: Allyn and Bacon, pp 7–10.

Cansino S, Williamson S, and Karron D (1994) Tonotopic organization of the human auditor association cortex. *Brain Res* 663:38–50.

Darian-Smith C and Gilbert CD (1995) Topographic reorganization in the striate cortex of the adult cat and monkey is cortically mediated. *J Neurosci* 15:1631–1647.

Diamond ME, Huang W, and Ebner FF (1994) Laminar comparison of somatosensory cortical plasticity. *Science* 265:1885–1888.

Dietrich V, Nieschalk M, Stoll W, Rajan R, and Pantev C (2001) Cortical reorganization in patients with high frequency cochlear hearing loss. *Hear Res* 158:95–101.

Doetsch GS, Harrison TA, MacDonald AC, and Litaker MS (1996) Short-term plasticity in primary somatosensory cortex of the rat: Rapid changes in magnitudes and latencies of neuronal responses following digit denervation. *Exp Brain Res* 112:505–512.

Douek E (1987) Tinnitus following surgery. *Proc III Int Tinnitus Semin,* Karlsruhe: Harsch, pp 64–69.

Elberling C, Bak C, Kofoed B, Lebech J, and Saermark K (1982) Auditory magnetic fields. Source localization and "tonotopical organization" in the right hemisphere of the human brain. *Scand Audiol* 11:61–65.

Elbert T (1998) Neuromagnetism. In: Andrä WA and Nowak H (eds), *Magnetism in Medicine: A Handbook.* Berlin: John Wiley & Sons, 190–261.

Elbert T, Flor H, Birbaumer N, Knecht S, Hampson S, and Taub E (1994) Extensive reorganization of the somatosensory cortex in adult humans after nervous system injury. *NeuroReport* 5:2593–2597.

Elbert T and Heim S (2001) A light and a dark side. *Nature* 411:139.

Elbert T, Pantev C, Wienbruch C, Rockstroh B, and Taub E (1995) Increased cortical representation of the fingers of the left hand in string players. *Science* 270:305–307.

Elbert T and Rockstroh B (in press) Corticale Reorganisation: Von der Neuroplastizität zur Neurorehabilitation. In: Karnath O and Thier P (eds), *Neuropsychologie.* Berlin: Springer.

Elbert T, Sterr A, Flor H, Rockstroh B, Knecht S, Pantev C, Wienbruch C, and Taub E (1997) Input-increase and input-decrease types of cortical reorganization after upper extremity amputation in humans. *Exp Brain Res* 117:161–164.

Ergenzinger ER, Glasier MM, Hahm JO, and Pons TP (1998) Cortically induced thalamic plasticity in the primate somatosensory system. *Nat Neurosci* 1:226–229.

Feldmann H (1992) *Epidemiologie.* Stuttgart: Thieme.
Flor H, Elbert T, Knecht S, Wienbruch C, Pantev C, Birbaumer N, Larbig W, and Taub E (1995) Phantom limb pain as a perceptual correlate of massive cortical reorganization in upper limp amputees. *Nature* 375:482–484.
Flor H, Rudy TE, Birbaumer N, Streit B, and Schugens MM (1990) Zur Anwendbarkeit des West Haven-Yale Multidimensional Pain Inventory im deutschen Sprachraum. *Der Schmerz* 4:82–87.
Florence SL, Boydston LA, Hackett TA, Lachoff HT, Strata F, and Niblock MM (2001) Sensory enrichment after peripheral nerve injury restores cortical, not thalamic, receptive field organization. *Eur J Neurosci* 13:1755–1766.
Garraghty PE and Kaas JH (1991) Functional reorganization in adult monkey thalamus after peripheral nerve injury. *NeuroReport* 2:747–750.
Gilbert CD (1998) Adult cortical dynamics. *Physiol Rev* 78:467–485.
Gilbert CD, Das A, Ito M, Kapadia M, and Westheimer G (1996) Spatial integration and cortical dynamics. *Proc Natl Acad Sci USA* 93:615–622.
Göbel G and Hiller W (1998) *Tinnitus Fragelogen.* Hogrefe, Göttingen.
Hari R (1990) The neuromagnetic method in the study of the human auditory cortex. In: Grandori F, Hoke M, and Romani GL (eds), *Auditory Evoked Magnetic Fields and Electric Potentials.* Basel: Karger Verlag, pp 222–282.
Irvine DRF, Rajan R, and McDermott HJ (2000) Injury-induced reorganization in adult auditory cortex and its perceptual consequences. *Hear Res* 147:188–199.
Jacobson GP (1994) Magnetoencephalographic studies of auditory system function. *J Clin Neurophysiol* 11:343–364.
Jastreboff PJ, Brennan JF, and Sasaki CT (1987) Behavioral and electrophysiological model of tinnitus. *Proc III Int Tinnitus Seminar, Karlsruhe* 95–99.
Jones EG and Pons TP (1998) Thalamic and brainstem contributions to large-scale plasticity of primate somatosensory cortex. *Science* 282:1121–1125.
Krubitzer L, Clarey J, Tweedale R, Elston G, and Calford M (1995) A redefinition of somatosensory areas in the lateral sulcus of macaque monkeys. *J Neurosci* 15:3821–3839.
Lenarz T (1992) *Epidemiologie.* Stuttgart: Thieme.
Lockwood AH, Salvi RJ, Coad ML, Towsley ML, Wack DS, and Murphy BW (1998) The functional neuroanatomy of tinnitus: Evidence for limbic system links and neural plasticity. *Neurology* 50:114–120.
Menning H, Roberts LE, and Pantev C (2000) Plastic changes in the auditory cortex induced by intensive frequency discrimination training. *NeuroReport* 11:817–822.
Merzenich MM, Kaas JH, and Roth GL (1976) Comparison of tonotopic maps in animals. *J Comp Neurol* 166:387–402.
Merzenich MM, Knight PL, and Roth GL (1975) Representation of cochlea within primary auditory cortex in the cat. *J Neurophysiol* 38:231–249.
Merzenich MM, Knight PL, and Roth GL (1973) Cochleotopic organization of primary auditory cortex in the cat. *Brain Res* 63:343–346.
Muhlnickel W, Elbert T, Taub E, and Flor H (1998) Reorganization of auditory cortex in tinnitus. *Proc Natl Acad Sci USA* 95:10340–10343.
Pantev C, Bertrand O, Eulitz C, Verkindt C, Hampson S, Schuierer G, and Elbert T (1995) Specific tonotopic organizations of different areas of the human auditory cortex revealed by simultaneous magnetic and electric recordings. *Electroencephalogr Clin Neurophysiol* 94:26–40.
Pantev C, Hoke M, Lehnertz K, Lütkenhöner B, Anogianakis G, and Wittkowski W (1988)

Tonotopic organization of the human auditory cortex revealed by transient auditory evoked magnetic fields. *Elecroencepalogr Clin Neurophysiol* 69:160–170.

Pantev C, Hoke M, Lutkenhoner B, and Lehnertz K (1989) Tonotopic organization of the auditory cortex: Pitch versus frequency representation. *Science* 246:486–488.

Pantev C and Lütkenhöner B (2000) Magnetoencephalographic studies of functional organization and plasticity of the human auditory cortex. *J Clin Neurophysiol* 17:130–142.

Pantev C, Oostenveld R, Engelien A, Ross B, Roberts LE, and Hoke M (1998) Increased auditory cortical representation in musicians. *Nature* 392:811–814.

Pantev C, Roberts LE, Elbert T, Ross B, and Wienbruch C (1996) Tonotopic organization of the sources of human auditory steady-state responses. *Hear Res* 101:62–74.

Pantev C, Roberts LE, Schulz M, Engelien A, and Ross B (2001) Timbre-specific enhancement of auditory cortical representations in musicians. *NeuroReport* 12:169–174.

Pantev C, Wollbrink A, Roberts LE, Engelien A, and Lutkenhoner B (1999) Short-term plasticity of the human auditory cortex. *Brain Res* 842:192–199.

Rajan R (1998) Receptor organ damage causes loss of cortical surround inhibition without topographic map plasticity. *Nat Neurosci* 1:138–143.

Rajan R and Irvine DRF (1998) Neuronal responses across cortical field A1 in plasticity induced by peripheral auditory organ demage. *Audiol Neuro-Otol* 3:123–145.

Rajan R, Irvine DR, Wise LZ, and Heil P (1993) Effect of unilateral partial cochlear lesions in adult cats on the representation of lesioned and unlesioned cochleas in primary auditory cortex. *J Comp Neurol* 338:17–49.

Rauschecker JP, Tian B, and Hauser M (1995) Processing of complex sounds in the macaque nonprimary auditory cortex. *Science* 268:111–114.

Recanzone G, Schreiner C, and Merzenich M (1993) Plasticity in the frequency representation of primary auditory cortex following discrimination training in adult owl monkeys. *J Neurosci* 13:87–103.

Robertson D and Irvine DR (1989) Plasticity of frequency organization in auditory cortex of guinea pigs with partial unilateral deafness. *J Comp Neurol* 282:456–471.

Romani GL, Williamson SJ, Kaufman L, and Brenner D (1982) Characterization of the human auditory cortex by the neuromagnetic method. *Exp Brain Res* 47:381–393.

Salvi RJ, Wang J, and Ding D (2000) Auditory plasticity and hyperactivity following cochlear damage. *Hear Res* 147:261–274.

Schlaug G (2001) The brain of musicians. A model for functional and structural adaptation. *Ann NY Acad Sci* 930:281–299.

Schlaug G, Jancke L, Huang Y, and Steinmetz H (1995) In vivo evidence of structural brain asymmetry in musicians. *Science* 267:699–701.

Schreiner CE (1991) Functional topographies in the primary auditory cortex of the cat. *Acta Otolaryngol Suppl (Stockh)* 491:7–15.

Shamma S (2001) On the role of space and time in auditory processing. *Trends Cogn Sci* 5:340–348.

Stanton SG and Harrison RV (1996) Abnormal cochleotopic organization in the auditory cortex of cats reared in a frequency augmented environment. *Auditory Neuroscience* 7:97–107.

Terhardt E (1974) Pitch, consonance, and harmony. *J Acoust Soc Am* 55:1061–1069.

Tiitinen H, Alho K, Huotilainen M, Ilmoniemi RJ, Simola J, and Näätänen R (1993) Tonotopic auditory cortex and the magnetoencephalographic (MEG) equivalent of the mismatch negativity. *Psychophysiology* 30:537–540.

Wallhausser-Franke E, Braun S, and Langner G (1996) Salicylate alters 2–DG uptake in the auditory system: A model for tinnitus? *NeuroReport* 7:1585–1588.

Weinberger NM (1995) Dynamic regulation of receptive fields and maps in adult sensory cortex. *Annu Rev Neurosci* 18:129–158.

Weinberger NM and Bakin JS (1998) Learning-induced physiological memory in adult primary auditory cortex: Receptive field plasticity, model and mechanisms. *Audiol Neuro-Otol* 3:145–167.

Williamson SJ and Kaufman L (1990) Theory of neuroelectric and neuromagnetic fields. In: Grandori F, Hoke M, and Romani GL (eds), *Auditory Evoked Magnetic Fields and Electric Potentials*. Basel: Karger, pp 1–39.

Willott JF (1986) Effects of aging, hearing loss, and anatomical location on thresholds of inferior colliculus neurons in C57BL/6 and CBA mice. *J Neurophysiol* 56:391–408.

Woods TM, Cusick CG, Pons TP, Taub E, and Jones EG (2000) Progressive transneuronal changes in the brainstem and thalamus after long-term dorsal rhizotomies in adult macaque monkeys. *J Neurosci* 20:3884–3899.

Yakovlev PI and Lecours A (1967) In: Minkowski A (ed), *Regional Development of the Brain in Early Life*. Oxford: Blackwell, pp 3–70.

Yamamoto T, Williamson SJ, Kaufman L, Nicholson C, and Llinas R (1988) Magnetic localization of neural activity in the human brain. *Proc Natl Acad Sci USA* 85:8732–8736.

Ziemann U, Hallett M, and Cohen LG (1998) Mechanisms of deafferentation-induced plasticity in human motor cortex. *J Neurosci* 18:7000–7007.

# 13

# Plasticity in Adult M1 Cortex During Motor Skill Learning

## JULIEN DOYON AND LESLIE G. UNGERLEIDER

There is ample evidence indicating that the brain is malleable well into adulthood. Studies conducted in animals have demonstrated that, like cortical sensory areas, representational maps in the primary motor cortex (M1) can be altered using electrical stimulation, pharmacological manipulation, and injuries to the peripheral and central nervous systems, as well as behavioral experience through repeated practice of a motor task (e.g., Nudo et al., 1997; Sanes and Donoghue, 2000). Recent studies in humans have also shown that functional motor representations in M1 undergo considerable plasticity following damage to the brain or practice of a specific motor ability. In this chapter, we concentrate on the results of a large body of studies that examined the cerebral plasticity in M1 using neurophysiological approaches in monkeys and rodents, or behavioral experiments using modern brain mapping techniques such as positron emission tomography (PET), functional magnetic resonance imaging (fMRI) and transcranial magnetic stimulation (TMS) in human adults. More specifically, we describe the plastic changes that occur within M1 over the course of learning in order to determine their role in the acquisition, consolidation, and long-term retention of new motor skilled behaviors. The physiological and neurobiological correlates of such plasticity are also discussed to give insights into the underlying mechanisms for the representational functional changes associated with the learning and retention of a motor skill.

## Plasticity in Adult M1 Cortex Associated with Motor Learning

### Motor Skill Learning: Definition

In our daily life activities, we use a variety of motor skills that have been acquired incrementally through repeated practice and interactions with our environment. These include, for example, the use of smooth coarticulation of finger movements into a specific sequence (e.g., when playing the piano), of regular multijoint movement synergies (e.g., during reaching for and grasping of small objects), and of a smoothly executed eye–body coordinated action (e.g., hitting a golf ball with a club). To study the cognitive processes and the neural substrates mediating our ability to learn such skilled behaviors in the laboratory, investigators have used experimental paradigms that fall into two categories. The first measures the incremental blending of movements into a well-executed behavior (motor sequence learning). The second tests our capacity to compensate for environmental changes (motor adaptation) (Grafton et al., 1994, 1995; Karni et al., 1995, 1998; Flament et al., 1996; Doyon et al., 1996, 2002a; Shadmehr and Brashers-Krug, 1997; Shadmehr and Holcomb, 1997). Operationally defined, these two forms of motor skills refer to the process by which movements, produced alone or in a sequence, come to be performed effortlessly through repeated practice (Willingham, 1998).

In both animals and humans, motor skill learning is usually measured by a reduction in reaction time and in the number of errors, and/or by a change in movement synergy and kinematics (Hikosaka et al., 1995; Karni, 1996; Doyon, 1997; Doyon et al., 1997, 1998; Shadmehr and Brashers-Krug, 1997; Doyon and Ungerleider, 2002b; see Squire, 1992, for reviews). With some skills, such as learning to play a new melody on a musical instrument, early learning can be facilitated by using explicit knowledge (i.e., requiring thought). For most motor skills, however, performance is ultimately overlearned to a point where it can be performed implicitly (i.e., without thought). Compared to other forms of memory (e.g., episodic memory), these changes in performance are known to evolve slowly, requiring many repetitions over several training sessions (Karni, 1996; Squire, 1992). Indeed, psychophysical studies have demonstrated that the incremental acquisition of motor skills follows two distinct stages: first, an early, fast learning stage in which considerable improvement in performance can be seen within a single training session; and second, a later, slow stage in which further gains can be observed across several sessions (and even weeks) of practice (Brashers-Krug et al., 1996; Nudo et al., 1996; Karni et al., 1998). In addition to these two stages, an intermediate phase corresponding to a consolidation period of the motor routine has recently been proposed, as spontaneous gains in performance have been reported following a latent period of more than 6 hours after the first training session without additional practice on the task (Karni and Sagi, 1993; Jackson et al., 1997). Additionally, little or no interference from a competing task has been reported, provided that it is performed beyond a critical time window of about 4–6 hours (Brashers-Krug et al., 1996; Rey-Hipolito et al., 1997; Shadmehr et al., 1997a). Finally, with extended practice, the skilled behavior is thought to become resistant to both interference and the simple passage of time. Once overlearned, a motor skill can thus be readily retrieved with reasonable performance despite long periods without practice.

## Functional Anatomy of Motor Skill Learning

Based on a plethora of animal and human studies, several brain structures, including the striatum, cerebellum, and motor-related cortical regions, have been thought to be critical for the acquisition and/or retention of motor skilled behaviors (Bloedel, 1992; Graybiel, 1995; Ungerleider, 1995; Karni, 1996; Doyon, 1997; Thach, 1997; Doyon et al., 2002b; Georgopoulos, 2000; Sanes et al., 2000; see Van Mier, 2000, for reviews). Anatomical studies have demonstrated that these structures form two distinct cortical-subcortical circuits: a cortico-basal ganglia-thalamo-cortical loop and a cortico-cerebello-thalamo-cortical loop (Picard and Strick, 1996; Tanji, 1996; Middleton and Strick, 1997). Evidence supporting the role of these cortical-subcortical systems in motor skill learning has come from impairments found in patients with striatal dysfunction (e.g., in Parkinson's or Huntington's disease), with damage to the cerebellum, or with a circumscribed lesion involving the frontal motor areas (Harrington et al., 1990; Sanes et al., 1990; Pascual-Leone et al., 1993; Willingham and Koroshetz, 1993; Ackermann et al., 1996; Doyon et al., 1997, 1998; Gabrieli et al., 1997). Further support has come from neurophysiological studies (Graybiel et al., 1994; Nudo et al., 1996; Tanji, 1996), as well as from lesion experiments in rodents (McDonald and White, 1993; see White, 1997, for a review) and in nonhuman primates (Milak et al., 1997; Lu et al., 1998). More recently, however, modern brain imaging techniques have also allowed us not only to confirm the functional contribution of both cortico-striatal and cortico-cerebellar systems in motor skill learning, but also to identify in vivo the neural substrates mediating this type of memory and the functional dynamic changes that occur over the entire course of the acquisition process (Karni, 1996; Doyon, 1997; Doyon et al., 2002b; Van Mier, 2000; see Ungerleider, 1995, for reviews).

Based on a recent review of imaging studies, we have proposed that representational changes within the cortico-striatal and cortico-cerebellar systems depend not only on the stage of learning, but also on whether subjects are required to learn a new sequence of movements or learn to adapt to environmental perturbations (Doyon et al., 2002b). Specifically, we have proposed that early in learning, during the fast learning phase, both motor sequence and motor adaptation tasks recruit similar cerebral structures: the striatum, cerebellum, and motor cortical regions (e.g., premotor cortex, supplementary motor area [SMA], pre-SMA, anterior cingulate), as well as prefrontal and parietal areas. During this phase, dynamic interactions between these structures are thought to be critical for establishing the motor routines necessary to learn the skilled motor behavior. When a task is well learned, such that there has been some consolidation of the skill, asymptotic performance has been achieved and performance of the skill has become automatic. However, the neural representation of the motor skill is then thought to be distributed in a network of structures that involves either the cortico-cerebellar or the cortico-striatal circuit, depending on the type of motor learning acquired. At this stage, we have suggested that for motor adaptation, the striatum is no longer necessary for the retention and execution of the acquired skill; regions representing the skill now involve the cerebellum and related cortical regions. By contrast, we have proposed a reverse pattern of plasticity in motor sequence learning, such that with extended practice the cerebellum is no longer essential, and the long-lasting retention of the skill now involves representational changes in the striatum and its associated motor cortical regions.

Although this new model helps us understand the possible functional reorganization that occurs at the system level during the different phases of motor learning, several questions remain regarding the role of the cortical regions, and of M1 in particular, in this form of memory. For example, what is the role of M1 in the early acquisition process of a motor skill? Is the activity often seen in M1 during learning associated only with motor performance (force, direction of movements, etc.) or with skill learning as well? Does M1 contribute to the neural substrate mediating the consolidation, long-term representation, and retention of a motor skilled behavior? Finally, what are the possible physiological and neurobiological mechanisms underlying the representational changes in M1 observed over the course of learning? These questions are addressed in the following sections of this chapter, using animal neurophysiological data and brain imaging results in human adults.

## Rapid Functional Reorganization in M1: Animal Data

In the past decade, rapid plastic changes in M1 architecture have often been reported in animal studies using several methodological approaches (see Sanes et al., 2000, for a review). For example, reorganization of movement representations in this cortical region has been demonstrated in electrical stimulation mapping experiments in which the facial motor nerve was sectioned (Donoghue et al., 1990; Sanes et al., 1992), as well as in studies that looked at the effects of circumscribed lesions in M1 (Nudo and Milliken, 1996), repetitive M1 stimulation (Nudo et al., 1990), changes in posture (Sanes et al., 1992), lesions to peripheral nerves (Donoghue et al., 1990), and pharmacological manipulations involving focal blocking of the inhibitory neurotransmitter $\gamma$-amino butyric acid (GABA) (Jacobs and Donoghue, 1991).

In addition, dynamic transformations in M1 representations have been inferred based on cell recording studies that examined changes in neuronal activity as animals acquire a new motor skill (Wise et al., 1998; Li et al., 2001). For instance, Wise and colleagues (1998) compared the pattern of neural activity in either the caudal portion of the dorsal premotor cortex (PMdc), the SMA, or M1, while monkeys adapted to different visuomotor transforms of the relationship between the movements of a joystick and those of a cursor that appeared in one of eight positions arranged in a circle around a target stimulus located at the center of a screen. Of the 209 neurons that showed learning-related activity, 89 were located in the PMdc, 32 were found in the SMA, and the others (88) belonged to M1. Interestingly, the activity in these motor regions was not only modulated during motor adaptation, but also continued for dozens of trials after performance reached a plateau. Furthermore, there was no clear asymptote of this activity change up to the 30-minute limit of the monitoring time, suggesting that the continued modification in the pattern and magnitude of the activity in motor cortices reflected the early stages of consolidation.

In another important neurophysiological study, Gandolfo et al. (2000) also demonstrated the existence of rapid single-cell plasticity in M1 as monkeys learned a motor skill. In this study, two monkeys were required to make visually guided reaching movements in an eight-target task while holding a robot manipulandum with the right hand. They were tested in three experimental conditions: in a no–force field (baseline) condition, in a force field (learning) condition that interfered with the execution of the reaching movements, and in a washout (aftereffect) condition during which the force field was removed. The directional tuning activity of 143 neurons located in the shoulder region of the contralateral M1 cortex was recorded as the monkeys performed movements in these three experimental conditions. Two cell types of interest were found. The first type consisted of cells that displayed transient changes in their tuning properties in the force-field (learning) condition. These cells, however, quickly returned to their baseline level of activity in the washout condition, suggesting that they were involved in motor adaptation but not in the retention of this new skill. By contrast, the second group of cells, called *memory cells*, also changed their activity in the force-field (learning) condition, but these cells maintained this pattern of activity even after several washout periods. The latter findings suggest that cells in M1 can contribute not only to the incremental acquisition of a motor skill but also to its retention.

## Rapid Functional Reorganization in M1: Human Data

In humans, rapid modifications in M1 functional representations, similar to the ones described above in animals following alterations in sensory experience, have also been reported using brain mapping techniques. For example, changes in M1 maps have been described in TMS studies after limb amputations (Hall et al., 1990; Cohen et al., 1991), forced immobilization (Liepert et al., 1995), injury to the spinal cord (Topka et al., 1991), transient deafferentation of the forearm (Brasil-Neto et al., 1992), and repeated cortical stimulation of M1 cortex (Berardelli et al., 1998). However, evidence of plasticity in the human adult M1 cortex associated with early motor learning remains scarce and controversial.

Stimulation studies with TMS in healthy volunteers have demonstrated that repeated practice of simple or complex sequential movements produces rapid cortical representational changes in M1 cortex (Pascual-Leone et al., 1994; Classen et al., 1998; Muellbacher et al., 2001). For example, Classen and his coworkers (1998) have recently used focal TMS and transcranial electrical brain stimulation (TES) of M1 cortex in normal control subjects to examine whether repetition of simple thumb movements during a short period of time can cause representational changes in the direction of TMS-evoked movements. After identifying the optimal scalp position for eliciting isolated movements of the thumb and their vector directions, these investigators asked their subjects to repeat paced (1 Hz), brisk voluntary thumb movements in the direction opposite to that of the predetermined TMS-evoked movements for up to 30 minutes (see Fig. 13-1). Following practice, TMS came to evoke movement-vector changes toward the direction of training. This change in direction was transient, however; the movement vector returned to its baseline direction level approximately 15–20 minutes after training stopped. Interestingly, other control experiments showed that this effect was specific to the training direction. TMS alone, tonic isometric contractions in the direction opposite to the baseline condition, and training with randomly determined directional movements did not elicit any direction change in TMS-pro-

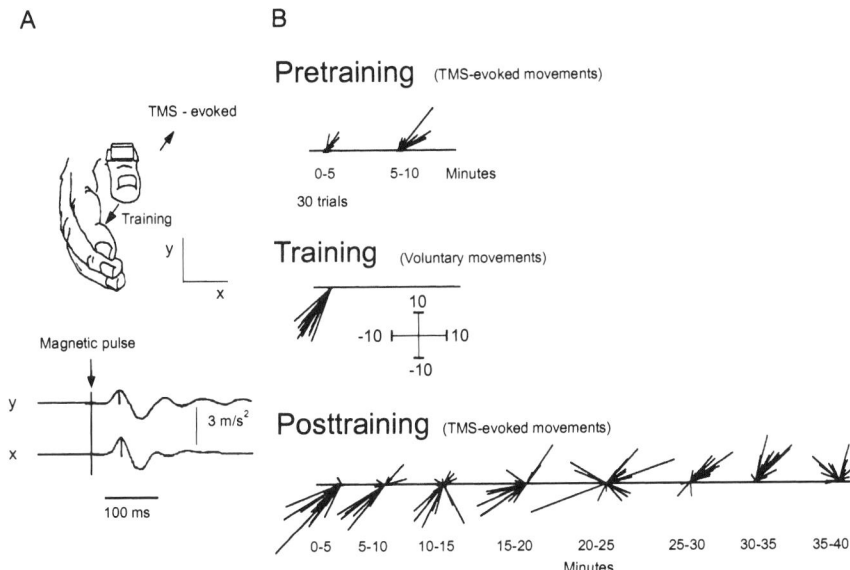

**Figure 13-1.** (A) Principles of movement recording used by Classen and colleagues (1998). Original acceleration signals in the horizontal (abduction and adduction) and vertical (extension and flexion) axes of thumb movements. The direction of transcranial magnetic stimulation (TMS)–evoked or voluntary movement was derived from the first-peak acceleration in the two major axes of the movement. (B) Directional change of the first-peak-acceleration vector of movements evoked by TMS after 30 minutes of training in a representative subject. Pretraining, TMS evoked extension and abduction thumb movements were measured. Training consisted of repetitive, stereotyped, brisk thumb movements in a flexion and adduction direction. TMS-derived vectors are grouped into intervals of 5 minutes. For clarity, vectors representing only the last 3 minutes of training are shown for training movements. After training, the direction of TMS-evoked thumb movements changed from the pretraining direction to the trained direction. The movement angle gradually changed back toward the pretraining direction after approximately 15–25 minutes. (Reprinted from Journal of Neurophysiology, 79, Classen et al., Rapid plasticity of human cortical movement representation induced by practice, pp. 1117–1123, Copyright (1998), with permission from the American Physiological Society.)

duced movements. In addition, the results revealed that the plastic changes in M1 depended upon the amount of training, as short (i.e., 5 minutes) periods of practice led to a significant M1 representational change in a limited number of subjects only, whereas 30 minutes of training was enough to evoke maximal effects in all subjects. Finally, TES stimulation before and after training produced a similar (albeit not as strong) pattern of results, suggesting that the physiological mechanism for these plastic changes was located at the cortical rather than at the subcortical level. Based on their findings, Classen et al. (1998) suggested that single-joint movements, repeated over a short period of time, were effective in producing rapid plasticity in human cortical movement representations.

In another TMS study, Pascual-Leone and colleagues (1994) have demonstrated that M1 activity can also be modulated through learning of a complex sequence of movements. Using a version of the serial reaction time (SRT) task first developed by Nissen and Bullemer (1987), they measured motor cortical output maps of muscles involved in the task while groups of subjects were either acquiring implicitly a 12-item sequence of movements or were asked to respond to randomly presented stimuli. Importantly, the subjects were tested on their explicit knowledge of the sequence after each block until they were able to generate it entirely without making any errors. TMS mapping was carried out every two blocks, allowing comparisons between the subjects' performance on the task and its effect on the modulation of M1 output maps. At the behavioral level, subjects showed evidence of implicit learning at the beginning of the learning process but then developed gradual explicit knowledge of the sequence with practice. Motor cortical mapping revealed that the output maps of the subjects in the random group did not differ over time. However, representational maps of those in the learning group increased significantly until they attained full explicit knowledge of the motor sequence, but then returned to their baseline topography afterward. Furthermore, this progressive enlargement of the cortical output maps during implicit learning was specific to the muscles involved in the task, and not to other muscles known to be inactive in these types of sequential movements. Pascual-Leone et al. (1994) concluded that M1 cortex shows rapid functional plasticity with learning, and that its activity is sensitive to the transfer from the implicit to the explicit learning state.

Although evidence from the TMS studies reviewed above supports the view that M1 activity is modulated during the early acquisition process of a new motor skill, findings based on other imaging techniques such as PET and fMRI do not yet provide a clear and easily interpretable picture. Indeed, while several investigators have reported that M1 plays a role in the initial learning phase of a motor skill (Seitz et al., 1990; Grafton et al., 1992, 1994, 1995; Schlaug et al., 1994; Hazeltine et al., 1997; Shadmehr and Holcomb, 1997; Honda et al., 1998; Van Mier et al., 1998), other groups of researchers failed to observe changes in M1 activity at this stage of the acquisition process (Jenkins et al., 1994; Rauch et al., 1995; Doyon et al., 1996; Jueptner et al., 1997a, 1997b; Krebs et al., 1998). For example, using the rotor pursuit test and an activation paradigm with PET, Grafton and his colleagues (1992, 1994) have reported learning-related activity in M1 (as well as in the SMA and pulvinar) when subjects were acquiring the kinematic movements necessary to keep a stylus on a disk that was set to rotate at 60 rotations per minute. However, other investigators did not find any dynamic functional changes in M1 cortex during implicit learning of a repeating sequence of movements that were externally triggered through visual stimulation (Doyon et al., 1996; Rauch et al., 1997), and others failed to report functional plasticity in M1 during learning of an internal model necessary to adapt to perturbation forces applied to a subject's arm when pointing to circularly arranged targets (Krebs et al., 1998).

The lack of consistency in the pattern of results with imaging techniques like PET and fMRI is due, in part, to the control conditions that investigators have used to contrast with the motor skill learning condition. For example, significant activity in M1 cortex was consistently reported in previous studies when the control condition did not exclude the contributions of increases in the number of movements produced in the experimental scanning conditions (Seitz et al., 1990; Schlaug et al., 1994) or the contributions of disparities in movement kinematics like changes in speed, force, coordination, and/or somatosensory feedback (see Van Mier, 2000, for a review). Thus, in such studies, changes related to motor learning have been confounded with those related to motor performance. By contrast, when investigators have used control conditions that allow better identification of the neural substrates mediating the process of learning a motor skill, unconfounded by the subject's execution of discrete movements (Doyon et al., 1996; Rauch et al., 1997; Krebs et al., 1998), or have compared directly the patterns of activity obtained in both early and advanced phases of learning (Doyon et al., 1996; Jenkins et al., 1994; Jueptner et al., 1997a), opposite patterns of results have been obtained. For instance, in a PET study designed to investigate the neuroanatomical systems involved in both early and advanced phases of implicit motor learning using a touch-screen version of the serial reaction time task, Doyon and colleagues (1996) compared the subjects' level of regional cerebral blood flow (rCBF) activity measured while they were performing a newly learned sequence of finger and arm movements to that of two control conditions: a random and a perceptual condition. In the learning condition, subjects were given only one block of trials during which they were asked to react to visual stimuli that were presented in a recurring 10-item sequence of which the subjects were not aware. By contrast, in the random control condition, subjects were exposed to the same visual stimuli and were required to produce the same motor response as in the motor learning condition, except that stimuli were presented at random instead of in a fixed repeating, embedded sequence. Finally, in the perceptual control condition, they were simply asked to look at the stimuli that appeared in a random order and to stay motionless. Interestingly, when the early learning condition was compared to the perceptual condition, significant peaks of activity were observed in motor-related regions, like M1 and primary somatosensory cortex, SMA and thalamus contralaterally, as well as the cerebellum ipsilaterally. Subtraction of the random condition from this experimental learning condition revealed a single activation in the posterior occipito-temporal region, but not in the motor regions mentioned above (Fig. 13-2). This finding suggests that, at this stage of the implicit learning process, activity in M1 was related to the subject's motor performance, but not to learning per se.

Apart from the effects of the control condition noted above, a detailed analysis of imaging studies looking at the early phase of motor skill learning has not

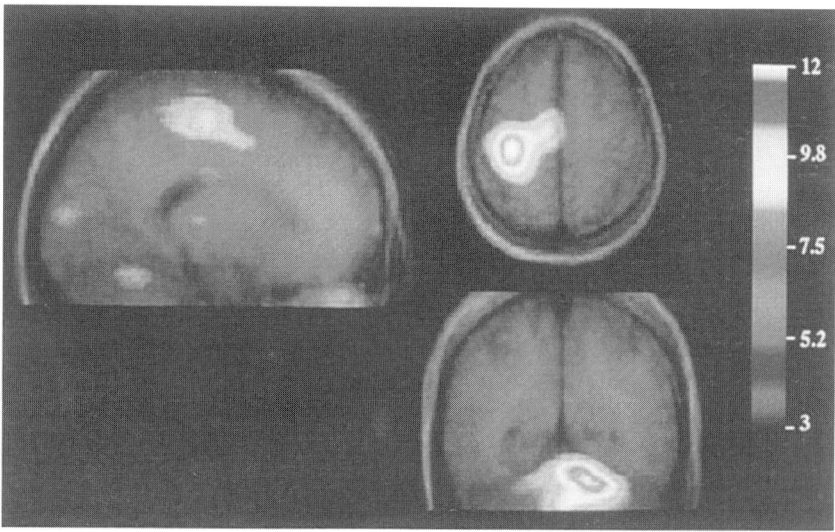

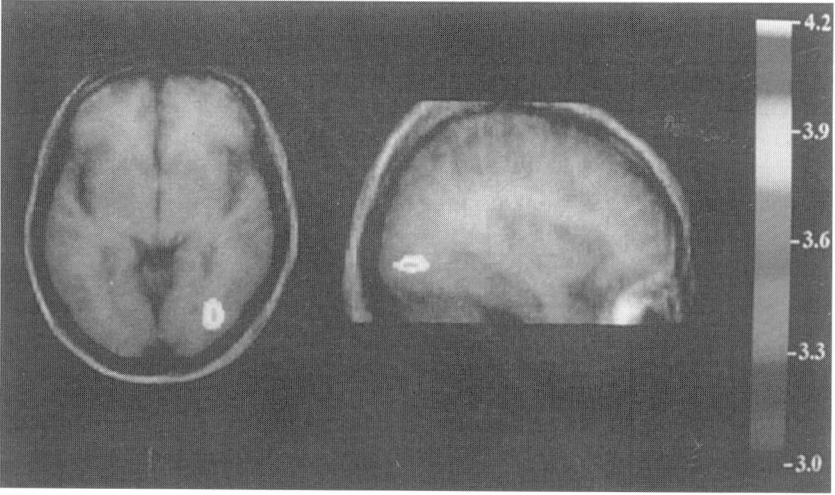

**Figure 13-2.** Merged PET-MRI sections illustrating cerebral blood flow increases averaged over 14 subjects in the experiment of Doyon and colleagues (1996). Top: Newly learned sequence minus perceptual condition; bottom: newly learned sequence minus random condition. Each subtraction yielded focal changes in blood flow shown as $t$-statistic images. The subject's left is on the left side in these sections. Note the difference in the patterns of findings based merely on the control condition used for the subtraction.

yet provided other easily identifiable reasons for the inconsistencies in M1 activation. First, the presence or absence of nonconfounded, use-dependent activity in M1 cannot be related to the imaging technique itself because both patterns of findings have been reported in previous PET studies: the presence of M1 plasticity (e.g., Seitz et al., 1990; Grafton et al., 1992, 1994; Schlaug et al., 1994) and the absence of M1 plasticity (e.g., Doyon et al., 1996; Krebs et al., 1998). Second, the lack of consistency in activating M1 cannot be due to the nature of the task. While some groups of investigators have reported implicit, learning-related plastic changes in M1 using the serial reaction time task (Grafton et al., 1995; Hazeltine et al., 1997; Honda et al., 1998), other investigators have not (Doyon et al., 1996; Rauch et al., 1997). Third, the inconsistency cannot result simply from the statistical approach (e.g., repeated measures analysis of variance [ANOVA], regression analysis, subtraction analysis) used in analyzing the functional data. Indeed, Grafton et al. (1995) have demonstrated the existence of M1 activity during implicit but not during explicit learning of a motor sequence using the same ANOVA method. Finally, this inconsistent pattern of results cannot be related to the type of learning process (implicit, explicit) or to the type of motor learning (sequence learning, motor adaptation) under which the skill is acquired. While Grafton and colleagues (Grafton et al., 1995; Hazeltine et al., 1997) have seen M1 activation, particularly during implicit (but not during explicit) learning of a sequence of movements with the serial reaction time task, Krebs and coworkers (1998) did not observe any plastic changes in this area using the forced-field, pointing target task, a motor adaptation paradigm that also relies on implicit motor learning.

In conclusion, contrary to studies using TMS, the results of PET and fMRI studies reported above do not yet allow one to decide whether or not M1 cortex is involved in the early learning process of a motor skill, that is, in the building up of motor routines necessary to execute the motor action. Although it is difficult to pin down the reasons for this incongruent pattern of findings between imaging techniques, it is possible to identify some of the methodological factors that should help researchers to solve this issue in future research. Apart from the experimental considerations mentioned above, such as the nature of the task (motor sequence vs. motor adaptation), the learning process (implicit vs. explicit), the experimental design (subtraction vs. parametric approach), the statistical approach (subtraction vs. regression vs. ANOVA) and the control condition (rest vs. active control condition), other methodological aspects will also need to be considered. As suggested by Frutiger and colleagues (2000), it will be important to consider the fact that (1) subjects differ substantially in their level of cognitive, perceptual, motoric, and learning abilities, and these individual differences can interact with task demands, producing considerable variability in both functional and behavioral data; (2) the subject's performance during skill learning can vary across the entire course of learning such that different temporal patterns of activation can be seen within related brain areas (Grafton et al., 1998; Sakai et al., 1998; Toni et al., 1998); (3) most imaging experiments have relied only on global behavioral measures with broad sensitivity and poor specificity (such as reaction times and number of errors made over practice trials), and thus little is known about the dynamic brain activity associated with changes in more specific aspects of kinematic control (see Flament et al., 1996; Shadmehr and Holcomb, 1997; Shadmehr and Holcomb, 1999, for exceptions); and (4) there may be no causal link between the imaging and behavioral data, even though the same experimental paradigm was used to collect both types of measures. In fact, because imaging and behavioral measures are known to reflect multiple parallel processes that vary dynamically over time, between individuals and with information processing levels, establishing links between imaging data and behavior may require the development of more specific performance measures.

Thus, in order to clarify the role of M1 in early motor learning, more studies using a subject-tailored approach will be required in which the amount of practice given to a subject on a particular task is dependent upon its level of performance and not on a fixed, predetermined number of trials. The use of precise kinematic measures that are better tuned to known physiological properties of M1 cortex (e.g., velocity, force, direction of movements) instead of global measures of learning (e.g., reaction time) will also be essential. Data-driven instead of a priori design-based, statistical methods with multivariate and multiple regression techniques may prove to be more sensitive for picking up changes of activity in M1, and for determining how these changes correlate with kinematic correlates of motor learning. Designs that allow one to scan subjects over the entire course of the fast learning phase (e.g., until subjects have reached asymptotic performance in the first training session) should be helpful in identifying the dynamic changes in activation within this phase. Finally, methods to measure functional and effective connectivity over time may also be valuable in identifying whether or not M1 cortex is involved in the learning of a motor skill, as there is now evidence that activity in areas that do not reach statistical significance may co-occur with other cerebral structures that are known to contribute to the acquisition process (Buchel and Friston, 2001). Because TMS studies have shown correlates of early phases of motor learning, it can be expected that with improved design and sensitivity, imaging studies will start to produce comparable data.

## *Contribution of M1 to the Consolidation of Skilled Motor Behaviors*

The conditions under which consolidation of new motor skilled behaviors occurs have been the focus of an increasing number of recent investigations (Brashers-Krug et al., 1996; Jackson et al., 1997; Rey-Hipolito et al., 1997; Shadmehr and Brashers-Krug, 1997; Karni et al., 1998). Nevertheless, the neural network supporting this phase of the acquisition process remains ill-defined. Previous work with PET has revealed that the consolidated representation of an internal model following practice on a force-field motor adaptation task depends on a network that includes the cerebellum, the dorsal premotor cortex and posterior parietal regions (Shadmehr and Holcomb, 1997). Additionally, a recent study by Muellbacher and collaborators (2002) has demonstrated that M1 cortex is also important for the early stage of motor memory consolidation. These investigators used a metronome-paced ballistic pinch task in which healthy subjects were required to practice fast pinching movements of the left index finger and thumb (Muellbacher et al., 2001) during two 5-minute periods (Practice 1 and Practice 2) and one 10-minute period (Practice 3). The periods of practice were separated by a 15-minute rest period during which low-frequency repeated TMS (rTMS) was applied. Under these conditions, the subjects rapidly learned to optimize their performance, as measured by a positive change in peak pinch force and peak pinch acceleration during the Practice 1 period, and then showed both retention of this new skill and further improvement in performance following additional practice (Fig. 13-3). Interestingly, however, rTMS applied over the M1 cortex after both Practice 1 and Practice 2 periods canceled the retention of the behavioral improvement, suggesting that rTMS had disrupted the early consolidation process. Moreover, subsequent experiments revealed that this disruption effect was specific to the memory consolidation process. First, the investigators showed that rTMS applied to subjects who had not practiced the task did not produce any change in both peak force and peak acceleration, suggesting that stimulation of M1 cortex did not interfere with basic motor behavior per se. Second, rTMS applied 6 hours after a 5-minute period of practice had no effect on retention of the improved performance, indicating that stimulating M1 did not hinder the recall of the new skilled behavior. Finally, rTMS over the occipital or the dorsolateral prefrontal cortex did not affect the subjects' retention of the new skill, supporting the role of M1 cortex in early memory consolidation of an elementary motor skill.

## *Functional Reorganization in M1 After Extensive Practice: Animal Data*

In animals, the role of M1 cortex in motor learning has repeatedly been demonstrated in awake, behaving animals using physiological investigations of neuronal properties after the animals have received extended practice, that is, after they have been overtrained on a particular motor task (e.g., Georgopoulos and Pellizzer, 1995; Carpenter et al., 1999; for reviews, see Georgopoulos et al., 1993; Georgopoulos, 2000; Sanes et al., 2000). Under such conditions, it has been shown that M1 cortex contributes to complex behaviors engaging both motor and cognitive dimensions (e.g., Georgopoulos, 2000). In addition, other investigators have reported the existence of experience-dependent representational changes within M1 after extended practice on motor learning tasks in both rodents (e.g., Kleim et al., 1998, 2002) and monkeys (Nudo et al., 1996; Plautz et al., 2000), which can persist in the absence of continued practice (Kleim et al., 1998; Plautz et al., 2000).

For example, in a study designed to investigate the dynamic plastic changes in M1 cortex following motor skill learning, Nudo and colleagues (1996) used intracortical microstimulation mapping techniques in normal monkeys to derive detailed maps of the representation of distal forelimb movements. These

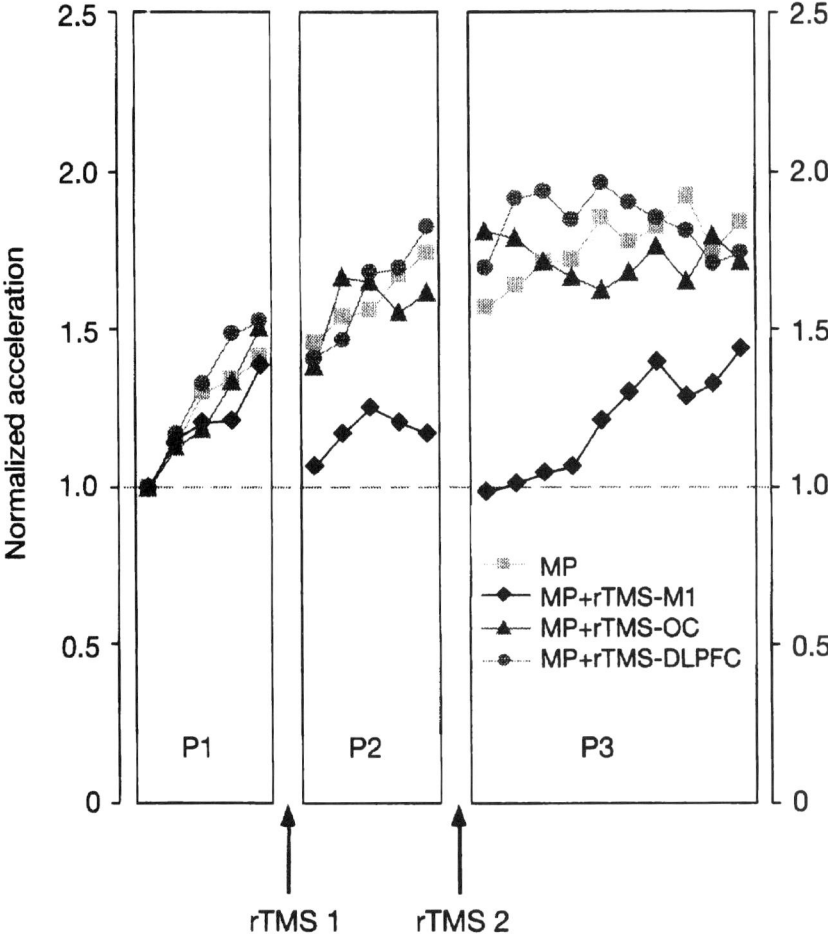

**Figure 13-3.** Effects of motor practice and repetitive transcranial magnetic stimulation (rTMS) on motor learning and early motor consolidation: acceleration data (Muellbacher et al., 2002). Each symbol represents the (normalized) mean peak acceleration for each practice condition. During Practice 1 (P1) there was an increase in peak pinch acceleration under all conditions. rTMS of M1 canceled the retention of the behavioral improvement of Practices 1 and 2 (P2). The ability to improve behavior by subsequent practice (P3) was unimpaired, but the final improvement was less marked than in the subjects who did not receive rTMS of M1. rTMS of the occipital cortex or dorsolateral prefrontal cortex had no impact on early motor consolidation. MP, motor practice; OC, occipital cortex; DLPFC, dorsolateral prefrontal cortex. (Reprinted from Nature, 415, Muellbacher et al., Early consolidation in human primary motor cortex, pp 620–644, Copyright (2002), with permission from Nature Publishing Group.)

maps were generated after either extended practice on a digit or forearm training task, or after a nonspecific behavioral training condition. In the digit training task, monkeys were required to retrieve food pellets from wells that decreased in size, necessitating increasingly fine skilled finger manipulations to grasp the pellets. By contrast, in the forearm training task, monkeys were required to make alternating clockwise and counterclockwise rotations of an eyebolt by producing repetitive cycles of supination and pronation of the forearm. The results (Fig. 13-4) revealed that, compared to maps derived before training (baseline), digit representations in M1 cortex expanded following practice on the reach-and-grasp pellet task, whereas the representational zones for the wrist/forearm movements contracted. Interestingly, a reverse pattern of findings was observed after training on the eyebolt turning task: Maps representing the forearm expanded in M1, while those of the digits contracted. Based on this study, Nudo et al. (1996) have argued that repeated cocontraction of muscles necessary to execute the motor behavior comes to be represented together in the cortex during learning, and that this temporal contiguity of inputs is essential in driving the dynamic changes in M1 cortex. In subsequent studies using a similar behavioral paradigm, Plautz and colleagues (2000) found that simple repetitive motor activity of the hand alone was not sufficient to produce changes in representational maps in M1 cortex of adult monkeys. Taken together, these findings constitute further evidence that motor cortical maps are alterable in adult life, and indicate that the learning of a motor skill is a prerequisite for representational plasticity to occur in M1.

Similar experience-dependent expansion of movement representations in M1 cortex after motor skill learning has also been reported in rodents (e.g., Kleim et al., 1998, 2002). In their most recent study, Kleim and his collaborators (2002) used the standard intracortical microstimulation technique to derive cortical representational maps in M1 cortex before and after rats were trained to either reach and grasp for food through a slot (skilled reaching condition) or to obtain food pellets by simply pressing on a lever (unskilled reaching condition). The extent of the cortical maps was calculated for the rostral forelimb area (RFA), the caudal forelimb area (CFA) and the hindlimb area (HLA) of M1 cortex. As expected, the topography of movement representations for both the digits and wrist was greater for the trained than the untrained animals in the CFA region. Again, this change in motor representation was specific to the training condition, as a greater representation of elbow/shoulder movements in the CFA region was observed in the unskilled than in the skilled reaching condition. This pattern of plastic change was also restricted to the CFA (a region known to contribute to skilled distal forelimb movements [Whishaw and Pellis, 1990]), because no significant difference in the area of digit, wrist, and elbow/shoulder representational movements was observed in the RFA or in the HLA region. These findings support those of Nudo and colleagues (Nudo et al., 1996; Plautz et al., 2000), indicating that movement representations within M1 cortex are malleable and can be modified by extended practice on a task.

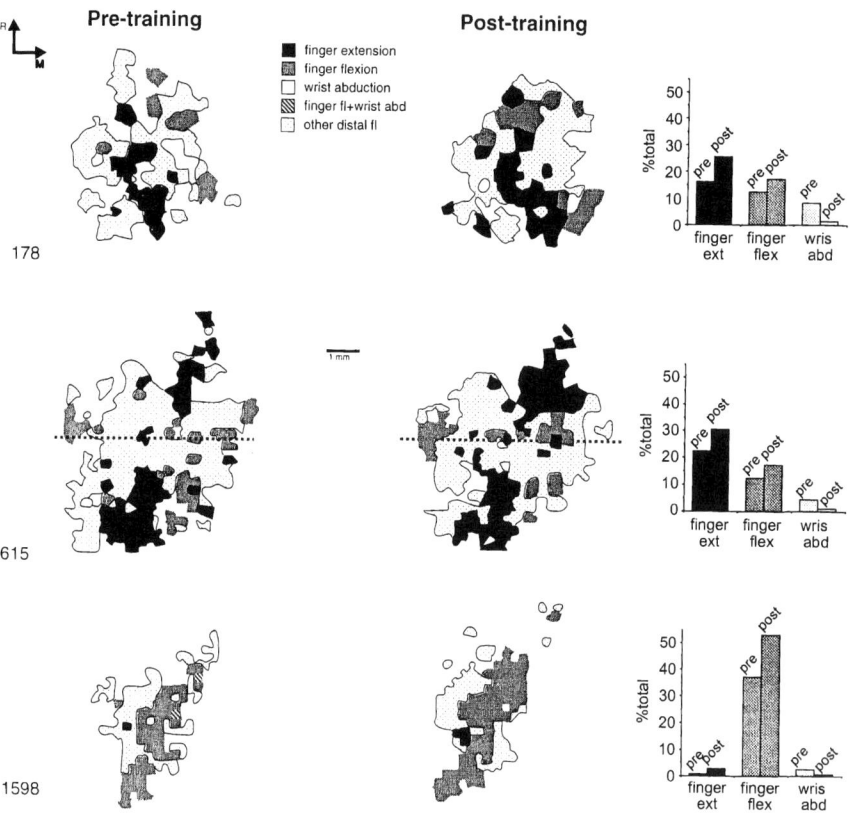

**Figure 13-4.** Representation of finger extension, finger flexion, and wrist movements in cortical area 4, as presented in Nudo et al. (1996). These data are derived from pre- and posttraining mapping procedures. In this illustration, finger extension movements are shown in *black*, thumb flexion movements are shown in *dark gray*, wrist abduction movements are shown in *light gray*, and finger flexion + wrist abduction dual responses are indicated by *diagonal lines*. For simplification, other dual responses are included in single-movement categories. In *bar graphs*, finger flexion + wrist abduction dual responses are included in each of the individual movement categories. Despite large variation in movement representations among individuals, similar changes were evident in each of the three cases. That is, the relative area devoted to both finger extension and finger flexion movements increased in each of the three cases; the relative area devoted to wrist abduction movements decreased in each of the three cases. The *dotted line* in case 615 denotes division of distal forelimb representation into caudal and rostral sectors. fl = flexion; ext = extension; flex = flexion; abd = abduction. [*Source:* © Society for Neuroscience, 1996.) (Reprinted from the Journal of Neuroscience, 16, Nudo et al., Use-dependent alterations of movement representations in primary motor cortex of adult squirrel monkeys, pp. 785–807, Copyright (1996), with permission from the Society of Neuroscience.)

## Functional Reorganization in M1 After Extensive Practice: Human Data

Few studies have investigated the neural substrate associated with the slow learning phase in humans, that is, when subjects have achieved asymptotic performance and some level of automatization of the motor skill. In one study, Karni and collaborators (1995, 1998) used a simple finger-opposition task in which normal, healthy subjects were trained and tested over the course of several weeks, and were scanned using fMRI at weekly intervals to image their brains. In this task, subjects were instructed to oppose the fingers of the nondominant hand to the thumb in one of two given sequences (Fig. 13-5A). The sequences were composed of five component movements or their mirror-reversed counterparts. Subjects were required to tap each sequence, with no visual feedback, as accurately and rapidly as possible. Initial performance of the two sequences, in terms of speed and accuracy, did not differ (see Figs. 13-5B and 13-5C). However, large gains in performance were induced by daily practice sessions of 10–20 minutes, during which subjects were instructed to repeatedly tap a given sequence in a rapid, self-paced, and accurate manner. Another sequence served as the unpracticed control sequence. Performance improvement reached asymptote after about 3 weeks of training with more than a doubling of the initial rate (Fig. 13-5B). The improvement was specific to the trained hand and did not generalize to the performance of the control sequence (Fig. 13-5C). These behavioral results suggest that a specific representation of the trained sequence of movements (rather than a representation of the individual component opposition movements) had developed as a function of training.

In the scanning sessions, Karni et al. (1995, 1998) measured motor-activity evoked signal changes at weekly intervals using a 4Tesla MRI system and a surface coil placed over M1's hand representation in the central sulcus of the contralateral hemisphere. During scanning, both the trained and the untrained control sequence were performed at a fixed, comfortable rate of 2 Hz, paced by the magnetic field gradient switch noise. Thus, both rate and component movements were matched, and the only difference between the two sequences during scanning was the difference in practice histories. The results showed that in the first scan session, performed before any training was given, a comparable extent of the contralateral M1 was activated by the execution of both sequences. However, by Session 4, which corresponded to 3 weeks of daily practice on the designated training sequence, and in all subsequent sessions, the extent of activation evoked by the trained sequence in M1 was significantly larger than the extent of activation evoked by the control, untrained sequence (Fig. 13-5D).

It is important to note that in the initial naive state, the activation in M1 was somewhat patchy; it remained so by Session 4, but to a lesser degree. Control experiments showed that it did not extend beyond the hand representation itself, indicating that an expansion of the total hand representation area had not occurred. Thus, the differential activation was accounted for by a subpopulation of pixels, in the hand area, that showed a significant response to performance of the

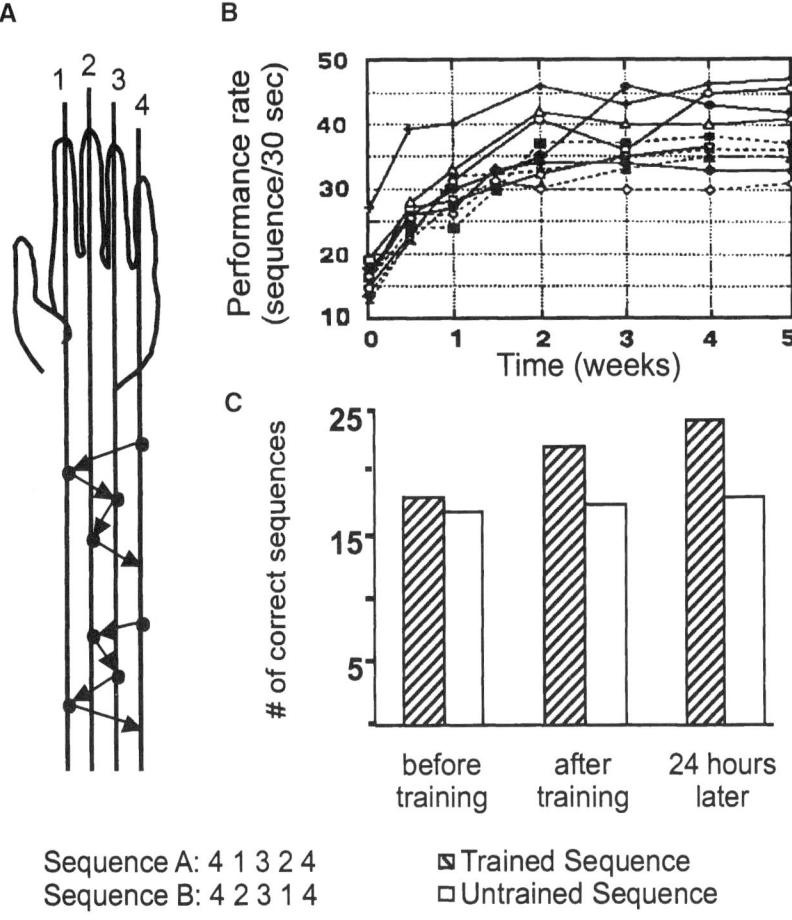

Sequence A: 4 1 3 2 4
Sequence B: 4 2 3 1 4

◪ Trained Sequence
☐ Untrained Sequence

**Figure 13-5.** The effects of long-term practice of a motor sequence. (A) The two sequences of finger-to-thumb opposition movements used in the study by Karni and colleagues (1995). In Sequence A the order of finger movements was 4, 1, 3, 2, 4 (numbering the fingers from index to little), and in Sequence B the order was 4, 2, 3, 1, 4, as indicated by the arrows (matched, mirror-reversed sequences). (B) Learning curves. Each curve depicts the performance of a single subject as a function of time. Pretraining is time point 0. Subjects reached asymptotic performance after about 3 weeks of training, at which point they had doubled the rate at which they could perform the trained sequence. (C) Behavioral evidence for consolidation of the motor sequence. Number of correct sequences performed during a test interval of 30 seconds for the two sequences (subjects randomly assigned to be the trained or the untrained control); before training, after a few minutes of externally paced performance of the randomly assigned trained sequence; and 24 hours later, with no additional training in the interval (overnight). (D) Emergence of differential activation in M1 evoked by the trained compared to the untrained (control) sequence following 2 weeks of daily practice on the designated trained sequence. Data are from a single subject. (E) Maintained differential activation 8 weeks later with no additional training in the interval. Sagittal sections in (D) and (E) are through the right hemisphere centered approximately 35 mm from midline. (Reprinted from Nature, 377, Karni et al., Functional MRI evidence for adult motor cortex plasticity during motor skill learning, pp. 155–158, Copyright (1995), with permission from Nature Publishing Group.)

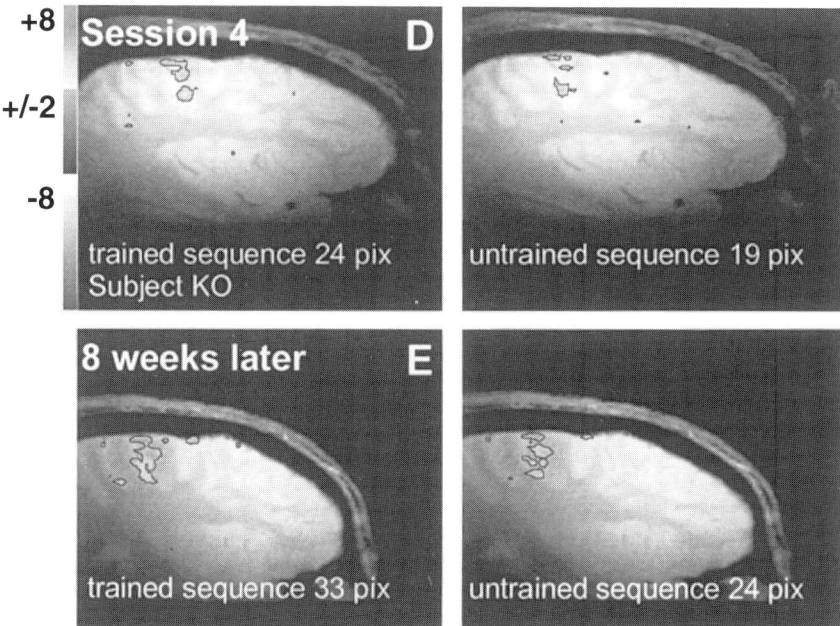

**Figure 13-5.** (*Continued*)

trained sequence, but little or no response to the performance of the untrained sequence. The more extensive activation evoked by the trained compared to the untrained sequence persisted in M1 weeks after training was discontinued (Fig. 13-5E). There was also no significant decrease in performance and, in fact, 1 year after training was stopped, there was still significant retention of the skill (results not shown here).

These imaging data suggest that long-term practice results in a gradually evolving, specific, and more extensive representation of the trained sequence of movements in M1. The results are compatible with the idea that motor practice induces the recruitment of additional M1 units into a local network specifically representing the trained motor sequence. This interpretation is in agreement with the work of Nudo et al. (1996) described above, who found that following a few weeks of training on the reach-and-grasp task, the evoked-movement digit representation as well as the representation of task-related movement combinations in M1 were gradually expanded. Thus, M1 may code not just single movements, but also complex movement sequences. This too is supported by the finding in monkeys that, following long-term practice, cocontracting muscles used in the task come to be represented together in M1 cortex (Nudo et al., 1996).

The effects of long-term training have been examined in only a few other studies. When this question has been addressed via imaging techniques using sequence learning tasks (Grafton et al., 1994; Elbert et al., 1995; Karni et al., 1995, 1998; Gordon et al., 1998; Toni et al., 1998; Hund-Georgiadis and von Cramon,

1999), the results have typically demonstrated that the creation of a long-term representation of sequence learning tasks necessitates, at the very least, the contribution not only of M1 but also of SMA (Karni et al., 1995, 1998; Classen et al., 1998; Gordon et al., 1998; Hund-Georgiadis et al., 1999).

## *Functional Reorganization in M1 and Retention of Motor Skill Learning*

Humans learn a wide variety of complex motor skills and retain them over long periods of time. Although robust long-term retention is a hallmark of motor learning, the neural structures involved in maintaining long-term representations of motor skills remain practically unknown. To address this question, Penhune and Doyon (2002) have recently used PET to compare brain regions active during recall of a timed motor sequence with those active during learning of this skill. Subjects were scanned during early learning (Day 1), late learning (Day 5: after 5 days of practice), and retention (after a 4-week delay with no additional practice) of a temporal motor sequence. In this task, subjects were required to reproduce a complex timed motor sequence by tapping in synchrony with a visual stimulus using a single key of the computer mouse. Stimuli were 10-element visual sequences made up of a series of white squares presented sequentially in the center of the computer screen. In the learned condition (LRN), the sequence was made up of five long (750 ms) and five short (250 ms) elements with a constant interstimulus interval (ISI) (500 ms). This sequence was taught explicitly to the subjects prior to scanning until they reached a criterion of three consecutive correct repetitions. Brain activations measured in this condition were compared to activations in an isochronous baseline condition (ISO), in which the sequence was made up of either all short or all long elements. Subjects' key-press and release durations were recorded by a computer and used to calculate the three indices of learning: accuracy, response variance, and response asynchrony.

On each scanning day, blood flow changes were measured in two scans while subjects performed either the LRN or the ISO condition. On Days 2–4, subjects returned to the laboratory to practice the sequences without scanning. Across these days, subjects performed 20 blocks (240 trials) of the LRN sequence and three blocks (36 trials) of the ISO sequences. After a 4-week delay with no additional practice, subjects again returned to the laboratory, and were scanned while performing a single block of the learned sequence (REC) and the ISO baseline condition. The subjects were specifically instructed not to practice the learned sequence during the 4-week delay and were debriefed on the final day of scanning to be sure that they had complied with that instruction.

Overall, the results revealed a network of cortical and subcortical structures that contributed differentially to the early and late phases of motor learning and to delayed recall. Early learning showed extensive activation of the cerebellar cortex. After 5 days of practice, cerebellar activity decreased and greater activity was observed in the putamen and frontal lobe. Most important, however, at delayed recall, significantly greater activation was seen in M1 cortex (as well as

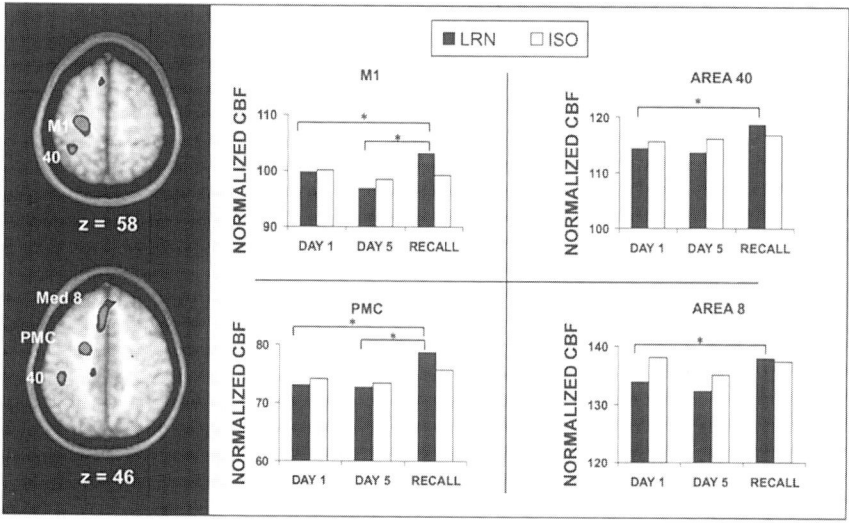

**Figure 13-6.** Results of the study by Penhune and Doyon (2002). The left panel presents z-statistic maps showing significant regions of activation in M1, premotor cortex (PMC), parietal cortex, and medial area 8 (Med 8) observed at recall (REC-LRN2). PET data are coregistered with the average magnetic resonance imaging (MRI) images of the nine subjects, and slice levels are given in the standardized space of Talairach and Tournoux (t-value range: 2.5 to 4.8). The right panel graphs changes in normalicized cerebral blood flow (CBF) values extracted from each voxel of interest (VOI) showing significant increases in activity between Day 5 and recall (significant differences are indicated with an asterisk). (Reprinted from the Journal of Neuroscience, 22, Penhune & Doyon, Dynamic cortical and subcortical networks in learning and delayed recall of timed motor sequences, pp. 1397–1406, Copyright (2002), with permission from the Society for Neuroscience.)

in the premotor cortex and parietal lobe), with no significant activity in the cerebellum or basal ganglia (Fig 13-6). Consistent with Doyon and Ungerleider's (2002b) model of cerebral plasticity associated with learning and retention of a skilled sequence of movements, these findings revealed that the cerebellum is primarily involved in the early phase of temporal motor sequence learning, with the basal ganglia possibly contributing to a later, automatization phase. Furthermore, this experiment demonstrated that relative to learning, delayed recall of a motor sequence appears to be mediated predominantly by a cortical network, including M1 cortex.

## Physiological and Neurobiological Correlates of Functional Reorganization in M1

The results of both animal and human studies reviewed thus far indicate that rapid and slow alterations in M1 representational maps can take place as a consequence not only of cortical stimulation and of central or peripheral damage, but of motor learning as well. Subcortical mechanisms thought to be responsible for this type of plasticity in M1 were proposed earlier (e.g., Randic et al., 1993), but recent evidence points to M1 cortex itself as a possible site for the reorganization. Indeed, animal work by Donoghue and colleagues (e.g., 1995, 1996) as well as several other investigators, have demonstrated that M1 plasticity depends upon the integrity of the horizontal connections that span the entire region, and that this cortical substrate works by combining M1 neurons into functional assemblies, which are then involved in constructing new motor maps (Donoghue, 1995; Donoghue et al., 1996; Huntley, 1997; Sanes et al., 2000).

Evidence supporting the role of the horizontal connections as a substrate for cortical plasticity comes from several sources. First, intracellular analyses and field-potential recordings of in vitro slice preparations have revealed the existence of horizontal connections throughout M1 cortex, especially in superficial layers II and III and in the deep layer V (Donoghue et al., 1996; see Sanes et al., 2000, for reviews). Second, Jacobs and Donoghue (1991) have shown that local blockade of GABAergic inhibition in one part of M1 unmasks existing horizontal connections that then reveal the existence of hidden representations of limb movements in other parts of M1. Third, Huntley (1997) has demonstrated that the extent of early M1 reorganization is related to the distribution of the intrinsic horizontal connections within M1. This author showed that cutting the motor nerve of rats' whiskers produced significant expansions of the forelimb area into the former vibrissa territory; however, this reorganization was apparent only in areas that contained strong horizontal connections between the whiskers and forelimb areas. Importantly, no change in movement representation was observed in regions in which these connections were either absent or sparse.

It has been proposed that rapid cortical plasticity can occur through synaptic modification of the local horizontal circuitry, which is modulated by $N$-methyl-D-aspartate receptors (Nudo et al., 1997; Sanes et al., 2000). However, persistent changes in the efficacy of this horizontal circuit have been proposed to result from synaptic modifications through mechanisms like long-term potentiation (LTP) and long-term depression (LTD). These mechanisms are believed to up- or downregulate the strength of the horizontal connections, depending on the pattern of activity (context) (Hess et al., 1996; Hess and Donoghue, 1996a, 1996b).

Along with these physiological changes in the horizontal circuit, neurobiological alterations have also been reported following motor learning. Indeed, behavioral training is known to induce changes in gene expression (Kleim et al., 1996), protein synthesis (Hyden and Lange, 1983) and neuron morphology, as measured by dendritic density (Greenough et al., 1985; Withers and Greenough, 1989; Kolb et al., 1994). Interestingly, Kleim and colleagues (2002) have demonstrated not only that motor learning produces changes in synaptogenesis, but also that these structural changes are colocalized to the region within which alterations in learning-dependent representational maps are observed following extended practice. These researchers have demonstrated that, compared to control animals, rats trained to reach for and grasp food pellets through a slot have significantly more synapses per neuron within layer V, specifically in the CFA. Such findings indicate, for the first time, that both functional and structural plasticity occur simultaneously within the same cortical region, and thus provide strong evidence that morphological changes contribute to the slow learning phase of a motor skilled behavior.

Although details of the physiological and neurobiological mechanisms supporting motor learning in humans are not available, recent investigations have shed some light on the neurotransmitters involved in use-dependent M1 plasticity. Work by Bütefisch and collaborators (2000) with the repetitive, directional thumb movements' task (developed by Classen et al., (1998) has demonstrated that plastic changes in M1 are dependent upon a physiological mechanism similar to LTP. Using a double-blind counterbalanced design, healthy subjects were tested in a baseline (drug naive) session, followed by three drug sessions separated by at least 72 hours each, in which they were given either dextromethorphan (DM), which blocks $N$-methyl-D-aspartate (NMDA) receptor activity, lorazepam (LZ), which enhances $\gamma$-aminobutyric acid type A (GABA$_A$) receptor function, or lamotrigine (LG), which changes the gating of voltage-activated Na$^+$ and Ca$^{2+}$ channels without affecting LTP induction. Evoked movement directions were measured using single-pulse TMS. The results revealed that plasticity in M1 cortex following training of thumb movements in a specific direction was reduced substantially by blocking the NMDA receptors with DM and by enhancing GABAergic receptor activity with LZ. Together, these results demonstrate the critical role of NMDA receptor activation and GABAergic inhibition in cortical plasticity in humans following motor learning.

In a follow-up double-blind, placebo-controlled, randomized study in which the directional thumb-movements' task and a similar TMS paradigm were used, Sawaki et al. (2002) have shown that use-dependent M1 cortex plasticity following practice of brisk thumb movements is cholinergic-dependent as well. Indeed, these authors reported that, compared to placebo, use-dependent TMS-evoked movement directions following training were significantly reduced following administration of scopolamine (a blocker of cholinergic muscarinic receptors), without affecting corticomotor excitability in M1 cortex. These findings support the notion that cortical plasticity is also influenced by central cholinergic neurotransmission through muscarinic receptor activation.

## Conclusion

Based on the body of animal and human work reviewed above, it appears that M1 cortex participates in the building up, consolidation, automatization, and retention phases of new motor skills learning. Controversy still exists with regard to its contribution to the fast changes in behavioral performance observed early in the acquisition process of a motor task. Indeed, demonstrations of rapid learning-dependent dynamic changes in M1 cortex have been less successful than those seen after extended practice. Early changes in M1 appear to be more sensitive to differences in imaging techniques (e.g., TMS vs. PET and fMRI) as well as to the methodological and statistical approaches used by the different groups of researchers. Furthermore, the functional role of M1 in the consolidation process and the long-term retention of motor skills will need to be confirmed using a variety of paradigms in both electrophysiological and imaging studies. However, the evidence gathered to date supports the notion that M1 cortex (in concert with other cortical and subcortical structures) constitutes one of the main nodes of the neural network involved in the different learning phases and recall of new motor skilled behaviors.

To further extend our knowledge of the role that M1 cortex may play in motor learning, future research will need to differentiate between the various forms of motor learning. Indeed, most of the published work conducted so far has used sequence learning tasks, and thus very little is known with respect to M1 participation in the acquisition, consolidation, and retention of skills based on motor adaptation paradigms. In a recent model, we have proposed that the cortico-cerebellar and cortico-striatal systems contribute differentially to motor adaptation and motor sequence learning, respectively, and that this is most apparent at the end of the training period (i.e., during slow learning) when subjects achieve asymptotic performance (Doyon et al., 2002b). According to this model, one would predict that the relative contribution of M1 cortex in building up motor routines, and in consolidating and storing memory traces of new motor skills, may differ between these two experimental paradigms. Moreover, better insights would be gained if future work correlated physiological changes with more precise kinematic measures of behavioral performance. Finally, examination of the interactions between M1 cortex and the other motor-related structures over time, using such holistic methodological approaches as functional and effective connectivity models, should provide a more complete understanding of the neural substrate mediating the acquisition, consolidation, and retention of motor skills.

*Acknowledgments*
We wish to thank Katherine Hanratty for her technical assistance in preparing the manuscript. This work was supported, in part, by grants from the Natural Sciences and Engineering Research Council of Canada, the Canadian Institutes of Health Research, and the National Center for Excellence-Stroke to JD and by funding from the NIMH-IRP to LGU.

## References

Ackermann H, Daum I, Schugens MM, and Grodd W (1996) Impaired procedural learning after damage to the left supplementary motor area (SMA). *J Neurol Neurosurg Psychiatry* 60:94–97.

Berardelli A, Inghilleri M, Rothwell JC, Romeo S, Curra A, Gilio F, Modugno N, and Manfredi M (1998) Facilitation of muscle evoked responses after repetitive cortical stimulation in man. *Exp Brain Res* 122:79–84.

Bloedel JR (1992) Functional heterogeneity with structural homogeneity: How does the cerebellum operate? *Behav Brain Sci* 15:666–678.

Brashers-Krug T, Shadmehr R, and Bizzi E (1996) Consolidation in human motor memory. *Nature* 382:252–255.

Brasil-Neto JP, Cohen LG, Pascual-Leone A, Jabir FK, Wall RT, and Hallett M (1992) Rapid reversible modulation of human motor outputs after transient deafferentation of the forearm: A study with transcranial magnetic stimulation. *Neurology* 42:1302–1306.

Buchel C and Friston K (2001) Interactions among neuronal systems assessed with functional neuroimaging. *Rev Neurol (Paris)* 157:807–815.

Butefisch CM, Davis BC, Wise SP, Sawaki L, Kopylev L, Classen J, and Cohen LG (2000) Mechanisms of use-dependent plasticity in the human motor cortex. *Proc Natl Acad Sci USA* 97:3661–3665.

Carpenter AF, Georgopoulos AP, and Pellizzer G (1999) Motor cortical encoding of serial order in a context-recall task. *Science* 283:1752–1757.

Classen J, Liepert J, Wise SP, Hallett M, and Cohen LG (1998) Rapid plasticity of human cortical movement representation induced by practice. *J Neurophysiol* 79:1117–1123.

Cohen LG, Bandinelli S, Findley TW, and Hallett M (1991) Motor reorganization after upper limb amputation in man. A study with focal magnetic stimulation. *Brain* 114:615–627.

Donoghue JP (1995) Plasticity of adult sensorimotor representations. *Curr Opin Neurobiol* 5:749–754.

Donoghue JP, Hess G, and Sanes JN (1996) Motor cortical substrates and mechanisms for learning. In: Bloedel JR, Ebner TJ, and Wise SP (eds), *Acquisition of Motor Behavior in Vertebrates* Cambridge, MA: MIT Press, pp 363–386.

Donoghue JP, Suner S, and Sanes JN (1990) Dynamic organization of primary motor cortex output to target muscles in adult rats. II. Rapid reorganization following motor nerve lesions. *Exp Brain Res* 79:492–503.

Doyon J (1997) Skill learning. In: Schmahmann JD (ed), *The Cerebellum and Cognition.* San Diego: Academic Press, pp 273–294.

Doyon J, Gaudreau D, Laforce RJ, Castonguay M, Bedard PJ, Bedard F, and Bouchard JP (1997) Role of the striatum, cerebellum, and frontal lobes in the learning of a visuomotor sequence. *Brain Cognition* 34:218–245.

Doyon J, Laforce RJ, Bouchard JP, Gaudreau D, Roy J, Poirier M, Bédard PJ, Bédard F, and Bouchard J-P (1998) Role of the striatum, cerebellum and frontal lobes in the automatization of a repeated visuomotor sequence of movements. *Neuropsychologia* 36:625–641.

Doyon J, Owen AM, Petrides M, Sziklas V, and Evans AC (1996) Functional anatomy of visuomotor skill learning in human subjects examined with positron emission tomography. *Eur J Neurosci* 8:637–648.

Doyon J, Song AW, Karni A, Lalonde F, Adams MM, and Ungerleider LG (2002a) Experience-dependent changes in cerebellar contributions to motor sequence learning. *Proc Natl Acad Sci USA* 99:1017–1022.

Doyon J and Ungerleider LG (2002b) Functional anatomy of motor skill learning. In: Squire LR and Schacter DL (eds), *Neuropsychology of Memory* (3rd ed.). New York: Guilford Press, pp 225–238.

Elbert T, Pantev C, Wienbruch C, Rockstroh B, and Taub E (1995) Increased cortical representation of the fingers of the left hand in string players. *Science* 270:305–307.

Flament D, Ellermann JM, Kim SG, Ugurbil K, and Ebner TJ (1996) Functional magnetic resonance imaging of cerebellar activation during the learning of a visuomotor dissociation task. *Hum Brain Mapp* 4:210–226.

Frutiger SA, Strother SC, Anderson JR, Sidtis JJ, Arnold JB, and Rottenberg DA (2000) Multivariate predictive relationship between kinematic and functional activation patterns in a PET study of visuomotor learning. *Neuroimage* 12:515–527.

Gabrieli JD, Stebbins GT, Singh J, Willingham DB, and Goetz CG (1997) Intact mirror-tracing and impaired rotary-pursuit skill learning in patients with Huntington's disease: Evidence for dissociable memory systems in skill learning. *Neuropsychology* 11:272–281.

Gandolfo F, Li C, Benda BJ, Schioppa CP, and Bizzi E (2000) Cortical correlates of learning in monkeys adapting to a new dynamical environment. *Proc Natl Acad Sci USA* 97:2259–2263.

Georgopoulos AP (2000) Neural aspects of cognitive motor control. *Curr Opin Neurobiol* 10:238–241.

Georgopoulos AP and Pellizzer G (1995) The mental and the neural: Psychological and neural studies of mental rotation and memory scanning. *Neuropsychologia* 33:1531–1547.

Georgopoulos AP, Taira M, and Lukashin A (1993) Cognitive neurophysiology of the motor cortex. *Science* 260:47–52.

Gordon AM, Lee JH, Flament D, Ugurbil K, and Ebner TJ (1998) Functional magnetic resonance imaging of motor, sensory, and posterior parietal cortical areas during performance of sequential typing movements. *Exp Brain Res* 121:153–166.

Grafton ST, Hazeltine E, and Ivry R (1995) Functional mapping of sequence learning in normal humans. *J Cogn Neurosci* 7:497–510.

Grafton ST, Hazeltine E, and Ivry RB (1998) Abstract and effector-specific representations of motor sequences identified with PET. *J Neurosci* 18:9420–9428.

Grafton ST, Mazziotta JC, Presty S, Friston KJ, Frackowiak RS, and Phelps ME (1992) Functional anatomy of human procedural learning determined with regional cerebral blood flow and PET. *J Neurosci* 12:2542–2548.

Grafton ST, Woods RP, and Mike T (1994) Functional imaging of procedural motor learning: Relating cerebral blood flow with individual subject performance. *Hum Brain Mapp* 1:221–234.

Graybiel AM (1995) Building action repertoires: Memory and learning functions of the basal ganglia. *Curr Opin Neurobiol* 5:733–741.

Graybiel AM, Aosaki T, Flaherty AW, and Kimura M (1994) The basal ganglia and adaptive motor control. *Science* 265:1826–1831.

Greenough WT, Larson JR, and Withers GS (1985) Effects of unilateral and bilateral training in a reaching task on dendritic branching of neurons in the rat motor-sensory forelimb cortex. *Behav Neural Biol* 44:301–314.

Hall EJ, Flament D, Fraser C, and Lemon RN (1990) Non-invasive brain stimulation reveals reorganized cortical outputs in amputees. *Neurosci Lett* 116:379–386.

Harrington DL, Haaland KY, Yeo RA, and Marder E (1990) Procedural memory in Parkinson's disease: Impaired motor but not visuoperceptual learning. *J Clin Exp Neuropsychol* 12:323–339.

Hazeltine E, Grafton ST, and Ivry R (1997) Attention and stimulus characteristics determine the locus of motor-sequence encoding. A PET study. *Brain* 120:123–140.

Hess G, Aizenman CD, and Donoghue JP (1996) Conditions for the induction of long-term potentiation in layer II/III horizontal connections of the rat motor cortex. *J Neurophysiol* 75:1765–1778.

Hess G and Donoghue JP (1996a) Long-term depression of horizontal connections in rat motor cortex. *Eur J Neurosci* 8:658–665.

Hess G and Donoghue JP (1996b) Long-term potentiation and long-term depression of horizontal connections in rat motor cortex. *Acta Neurobiol Exp (Warsz)* 56:397–405.

Hikosaka O, Rand MK, Miyachi S, and Miyashita K (1995) Learning of sequential movements in the monkey: Process of learning and retention of memory. *J Neurophysiol* 74:1652–1661.

Honda M, Deiber MP, Ibanez V, Pascual-Leone A, Zhuang P, and Hallett M (1998) Dynamic cortical involvement in implicit and explicit motor sequence learning. A PET study. *Brain* 121:2159–2173.

Hund-Georgiadis M and von Cramon DY (1999) Motor-learning-related changes in piano players and non-musicians revealed by functional magnetic-resonance signals. *Exp Brain Res* 125:417–425.

Huntley GW (1997) Correlation between patterns of horizontal connectivity and the extent of short-term representational plasticity in rat motor cortex. *Cereb Cortex* 7:143–156.

Hyden H and Lange PW (1983) Modification of membrane-bound proteins of the hippocampus and entorhinal cortex by change in behavior in rats. *J Neurosci Res* 9:37–46.

Jackson PL, Forget J, Soucy M-C, Leblanc M, Cantin J-F, and Doyon J (1997) Consolidation of visuomotor skills in humans: A psychophysical study. *Soc Neurosci Abstr* 23:1052.

Jacobs KM and Donoghue JP (1991) Reshaping the cortical motor map by unmasking latent intracortical connections. *Science* 251:944–947.

Jenkins IH, Brooks DJ, Nixon PD, Frackowiak RS, and Passingham RE (1994) Motor sequence learning: A study with positron emission tomography. *J Neurosci* 14:3775–3790.

Jueptner M, Frith CD, Brooks DJ, Frackowiak RS, and Passingham RE (1997a) Anatomy of motor learning. II. Subcortical structures and learning by trial and error. *J Neurophysiol* 77:1325–1337.

Jueptner M, Stephan KM, Frith CD, Brooks DJ, Frackowiak RS, and Passingham RE (1997b) Anatomy of motor learning. I. Frontal cortex and attention to action. *J Neurophysiol* 77:1313–1324.

Karni A (1996) The acquisition of perceptual and motor skills: A memory system in the adult human cortex. *Cogn Brain Res* 5:39–48.

Karni A, Meyer G, Jezzard P, Adams MM, Turner R, and Ungerleider LG (1995) Functional MRI evidence for adult motor cortex plasticity during motor skill learning. *Nature* 377:155–158.

Karni A, Meyer G, Rey-Hipolito C, Jezzard P, Adams MM, Turner R, and Ungerleider LG (1998) The acquisition of skilled motor performance: Fast and slow experience-driven changes in primary motor cortex. *Proc Natl Acad Sci USA* 95:861–868.

Karni A and Sagi D (1993) The time course of learning a visual skill. *Nature* 365:250–252.

Kleim JA, Barbay S, Cooper NR, Hogg TM, Reidel CN, Remple MS, and Nudo RJ (2002) Motor learning-dependent synaptogenesis is localized to functionally reorganized motor cortex. *Neurobiol Learn Mem* 77:63–77.

Kleim JA, Barbay S, and Nudo RJ (1998) Functional reorganization of the rat motor cortex following motor skill learning. *J Neurophysiol* 80:3321–3325.

Kleim JA, Lussnig E, Schwarz ER, Comery TA, and Greenough WT (1996) Synaptogenesis and Fos expression in the motor cortex of the adult rat after motor skill learning. *J Neurosci* 16:4529–4535.

Kolb B, Buhrmann K, McDonald R, and Sutherland RJ (1994) Dissociation of the medial prefrontal, posterior parietal, and posterior temporal cortex for spatial navigation and recognition memory in the rat. *Cereb Cortex* 4:664–680.

Krebs HI, Brashers-Krug T, Rauch SL, Savage CR, Hogan N, Rubin RH, Fischman AJ, and Alpert NM (1998) Robot-aided functional imaging: Application to a motor learning study. *Hum Brain Mapp* 6:59–72.

Li CS, Padoa-Schioppa C, and Bizzi E (2001) Neuronal correlates of motor performance and motor learning in the primary motor cortex of monkeys adapting to an external force field. *Neuron* 30:593–607.

Liepert J, Tegenthoff M, and Malin JP (1995) Changes of cortical motor area size during immobilization. *Electroencephalogr Clin Neurophysiol* 97:382–386.

Lu X, Hikosaka O, and Miyachi S (1998) Role of monkey cerebellar nuclei in skill for sequential movement. *J Neurophysiol* 79:2245–2254.

McDonald R and White NM (1993) A triple dissociation of memory systems: Hippocampus, amygdala, and dorsal striatum. *Behav Neurosci* 107:3–22.

Middleton FA and Strick PL (1997) Cerebellar output channels. *Int Rev Neurobiol* 41:61–82.

Milak MS, Shimansky Y, Bracha V, and Bloedel JR (1997) Effects of inactivating individual cerebellar nuclei on the performance and retention of an operantly conditioned forelimb movement. *J Neurophysiol* 78:939–959.

Muellbacher W, Ziemann U, Boroojerdi B, Cohen L, and Hallett M (2001) Role of the human motor cortex in rapid motor learning. *Exp Brain Res* 136:431–438.

Muellbacher W, Ziemann U, Wissel J, Dang N, Kofler M, Facchini S, Boroojerdi B, Poewe W, and Hallett M (2002) Early consolidation in human primary motor cortex. *Nature* 415:640–644.

Nissen MJ and Bullemer P (1987) Attentional requirements of learning: Evidence from performance measures. *Cogn Psychol* 19:1–32.

Nudo RJ, Jenkins WM, and Merzenich MM (1990) Repetitive microstimulation alters the cortical representation of movements in adult rats. *Somatosens Mot Res* 7:463–483.

Nudo RJ and Milliken GW (1996) Reorganization of movement representations in primary motor cortex following focal ischemic infarcts in adult squirrel monkeys. *J Neurophysiol* 75:2144–2149.

Nudo RJ, Milliken GW, Jenkins WM, and Merzenich MM (1996) Use-dependent alterations of movement representations in primary motor cortex of adult squirrel monkeys. *J Neurosci* 16:785–807.

Nudo RJ, Plautz EJ, and Milliken GW (1997) Adaptive plasticity in primate motor cortex as a consequence of behavioral experience and neuronal injury. *Semin Neuroscience* 9:13–23.

Pascual-Leone A, Grafman J, Clark K, Stewart M, Massaquoi S, Lou JS, and Hallett M (1993) Procedural learning in Parkinson's disease and cerebellar degeneration. *Ann Neurol* 34:594–602.

Pascual-Leone A, Grafman J, and Hallett M (1994) Modulation of cortical motor output maps during development of implicit and explicit knowledge. *Science* 263:1287–1289.

Penhune VB and Doyon J (2002) Dynamic cortical and subcortical networks in learning and delayed recall of timed motor sequences. *J Neurosci* 22:1397–1406.

Picard N and Strick PL (1996) Motor areas of the medial wall: A review of their location and functional activation. *Cereb Cortex* 6:342–353.

Plautz EJ, Milliken GW, and Nudo RJ (2000) Effects of repetitive motor training on movement representations in adult squirrel monkeys: Role of use versus learning. *Neurobiol Learn Mem* 74:27–55.

Randic M, Jiang MC, and Cerne R (1993) Long-term potentiation and long-term depression of primary afferent neurotransmission in the rat spinal cord. *J Neurosci* 13:5228–5241.

Rauch SL, Savage CR, Brown HD, Curran T, Alpert NM, Kendrick A, Fischman AJ, and Kosslyn S (1995) A PET investigation of implicit and explicit sequence learning. *Hum Brain Mapp* 3:271–286.

Rauch SL, Whalen PJ, Savage CR, Curran T, Kendrick A, Brown HD, Bush G, Breiter HC, and Rosen BR (1997) Striatal recruitment during an implicit sequence learning task as measured by functional magnetic resonance imaging. *Hum Brain Mapp* 5:124–132.

Rey-Hipolito C, Adams MM, Ungerleider L, and Karni A (1997) When practice makes perfect: Time dependent evolution of skilled motor performance. *Soc Neurosci Abstr* 23:1052.

Sakai K, Hikosaka O, Miyauchi S, Takino R, Sasaki Y, and Putz B (1998) Transition of brain activation from frontal to parietal areas in visuomotor sequence learning. *J Neurosci* 18:1827–1840.

Sanes JN, Dimitrov B, and Hallett M (1990) Motor learning in patients with cerebellar dysfunction. *Brain* 113:103–120.

Sanes JN and Donoghue JP (2000) Plasticity and primary motor cortex. *Annu Rev Neurosci* 23:393–415.

Sanes JN, Wang J, and Donoghue JP (1992) Immediate and delayed changes of rat motor cortical output representation with new forelimb configurations. *Cereb Cortex* 2:141–152.

Sawaki L, Boroojerdi B, Kaelin-Lang A, Burstein AH, Butefisch CM, Kopylev L, Davis B, and Cohen LG (2002) Cholinergic influences on use-dependent plasticity. *J Neurophysiol* 87:166–171.

Schlaug G, Knorr U, and Seitz R (1994) Intersubject variability of cerebral activations in acquiring a motor skill: A study with positron emission tomography. *Exp Brain Res* 98:523–534.

Seitz RJ, Roland E, Bohm C, Greitz T, and Stone-Elander S (1990) Motor learning in man: A positron emission tomographic study. *Neuroreport* 1:57–60.

Shadmehr R and Brashers-Krug T (1997) Functional stages in the formation of human long-term motor memory. *J Neurosci* 17:409–419.

Shadmehr R and Holcomb HH (1997) Neural correlates of motor memory consolidation. *Science* 277:821–825.

Shadmehr R and Holcomb HH (1999) Inhibitory control of competing motor memories. *Exp Brain Res* 126:235–251.

Squire LR (1992) Declarative and nondeclarative memory: Multiple brain systems supporting learning and memory. *J Cogn Neurosci* 4:232–243.

Tanji J (1996) New concepts of the supplementary motor area. *Curr Opin Neurobiol* 6:782–787.

Thach WT (1997) Context–response linkage. *Int Rev Neurobiol* 41:599–611.

Toni I, Krams M, Turner R, and Passingham RE (1998) The time course of changes during motor sequence learning: A whole-brain fMRI study. *Neuroimage* 8:50–61.

Topka H, Cohen LG, Cole RA, and Hallett M (1991) Reorganization of corticospinal pathways following spinal cord injury. *Neurology* 41:1276–1283.

Ungerleider LG (1995) Functional brain imaging studies of cortical mechanisms for memory. *Science* 270:769–775.

Van Mier H (2000) Human learning. In: Toga AW and Mazziotta JC (eds), *Brain Mapping: The Systems*. San Diego: Academic Press, pp 605–620.

Van Mier H, Tempel LW, Perlmutter JS, Raichle ME, and Petersen SE (1998) Changes in brain activity during motor learning measured with PET: Effects of hand of performance and practice. *J Neurophysiol* 80:2177–2199.

Whishaw IQ and Pellis SM (1990) The structure of skilled forelimb reaching in the rat: A proximally driven movement with a single distal rotatory component. *Behav Brain Res* 41:49–59.

White NM (1997) Mnemonic functions of the basal ganglia. *Curr Opin Neurobiol* 7:164–169.

Willingham DB (1998) A neuropsychological theory of motor skill learning. *Psychol Rev* 105:558–584.

Willingham DB and Koroshetz WJ (1993) Evidence for dissociable motor skills in Huntington's disease patients. *Psychobiology* 21:173–182.

Wise SP, Moody SL, Blomstrom KJ, and Mitz AR (1998) Changes in motor cortical activity during visuomotor adaptation. *Exp Brain Res* 121:285–299.

Withers GS and Greenough WT (1989) Reach training selectively alters dendritic branching in subpopulations of layer II–III pyramids in rat motor-somatosensory forelimb cortex. *Neuropsychologia* 27:61–69.

# 14

# Cortical Reorganization and the Rehabilitation of Movement by CI Therapy After Neurological Injury

VICTOR W. MARK AND EDWARD TAUB

Since the 1980s, considerable advances have been made in two important areas of neuroscience: (1) the description and measurement of injury-related and use-dependent cortical reorganization for specific sensorimotor functions and (2) the application of behavioral neuroscience findings on intensive use-dependent learning to restitution of purposive movement following its disruption. The latter results have also been related to cortical reorganization. In this chapter, we will discuss the behavioral mechanisms of use-dependent cortical reorganization for the enhancement of purposive movement, particularly in regard to rehabilitation after neurological injury.

## Cortical Reorganization in Sensorimotor Cortex and Therapeutical Implications

### Fundamental Investigations of Cortical Sensorimotor Plasticity in Animals

Sherrington and colleagues (Brown and Sherrington, 1912; Leyton and Sherrington, 1917) in the early twentieth century determined that focal cortical stimulation could result in variable motor responses, which suggested that the correspondence between anatomical structure and function was not fixed. Nonetheless, only in the past decade has a plastic model for structural–functional correlation in mature animals become widely accepted (Sanes et al., 1990). Work by Merzenich and colleagues was seminal in inspiring the current interest in cortical remapping. Initial studies associated somatosensory cortical remapping in primates (based on intracortical microelectrode recording) with peripheral deafferentation via either nerve section (Merzenich et al., 1983a, 1983b) or digit amputation (Merzenich et al., 1984). In either case, when somatosensory cortex that was formerly associated primarily with input from a body region was deafferented, the nervous system responded by an extension of cutaneous receptive fields from adjacent representational zones of still-intact somatic regions into the deafferented cortical zone. These findings suggested that cortical reorganization is opportunistic, ensuring that viable neuronal real estate (including associated subcortical structures) is invariably neurophysiologically active after overcoming transient unresponsiveness following acute peripheral injury. This process, in which regions of cortex with an intact afferent supply invade an adjacent deafferented cortical region, may be characterized as injury-related cortical reorganization.

Subsequent findings demonstrated that cortical remapping can also occur when there is an increase of behaviorally relevant somatosensory input produced by increased use of a body part. Merzenich and colleagues (Jenkins et al., 1990; Recanzone et al., 1992a–1992c) showed that when monkeys were trained either to regulate finger pressure on a vibrating surface or to detect differences in tactile vibratory frequencies through their fingertips, the corresponding somatosensory representations of the fingertips were enlarged. Thus, cortical reorganization may be associated with enhanced somatosensory discriminative ability and therefore may have adaptive significance. These findings supported the hypothesis that the functional correlation between cortical areas and somatic regions is *use-dependent* in the adult and can be constantly modified.

In additional research, the surgical fusion of digits in adult monkeys, which tends to synchronize the tactile afferent input from formerly independently functioning structures (thus in effect relaying environmental information from a single syndactylous digital region), resulted in a fusion of the cortical representation zones of those digits (Clark et al., 1988). Compatible observations by Wang et al. (1995) demonstrated that controlling the synchronization of tactile stimulation applied to the physically independent digits dramatically affected the organization of the representations of the digits in somatosensory cortex. Somatosensory cortex thus becomes reorganized according to whether peripheral stimulation arrives simultaneously from two peripheral foci or whether there is a temporal delay between the two inputs. Although cortical plasticity in response to changing environmental stimuli would appear to have adaptive value, this blending of previously discretely represented digits in somatosensory cortex may have functionally disadvantageous effects. Byl et al. (1996a) trained two monkeys to repetitively and rapidly grasp a handle for food rewards using all fingers simultaneously. Over several months performance efficiency declined, even when there was no clear evidence of peripheral tissue injury. Both monkeys used progressively less force to grip the handle, and one reduced its dominant hand use for other tasks. The representational maps of the digits recorded following this prolonged training resembled the changes that had been previously found in monkeys that had undergone surgically induced syndactyly (Clark et al., 1988). Although the contribution of nociceptive inputs to these cortical and motor changes could not be excluded, the findings suggested that syndactyly and prolonged repetitive use of the fingers synchronously may effect similar changes in digit representations in somatosensory cortex. The performance decline in the monkeys that repetitively grabbed the handle resembled changes seen in humans with repetitive strain injuries, or performance dystonia, and suggested therefore that this occupational hazard has, at least in part, a central neurologic basis.

Motor cortex has also been found to be responsive to peripheral somatic changes in adult mammals. Acute motor nerve lesioning in rats may be followed by reorganization of the primary motor cortex regions that are associated with purposive movement of specific body parts, as indicated by intracortical electrical stimulation studies (Sanes et al., 1988; Donoghue et al., 1990). Such changes may occur over a few hours. Since altered feedback from the environment was presumed to mediate these central changes, Sanes, Donoghue, and colleagues suggested that altered kinesthesis secondary to paralysis may have been involved. Findings consistent with the foregoing were reported by Nudo et al. (1996), who recorded expanded representations of the digits in monkeys whose cortical hand area was partially destroyed and who were then trained to extract food from progressively smaller wells. Thus, just as somatosensory reorganization may be importantly associated with improving vibrotactile discrimination, primary motor cortex reorganization may be importantly involved in use-dependent acquisition of motor skills. Important support for this possibility comes from the work of Ungerleider (1995) and Karni and coworkers (1995). Moreover, in research in humans who had practiced stereotyped finger movements repetitively (Muellbacher et al., 2001), motor cortical representations of the involved muscles (as determined from transcranial magnetic stimulation [TMS]) were associated with augmented motor evoked potentials in the muscles only during the training period itself, not when the skill had effectively been learned (as determined from follow-up assessment).

## Cortical Reorganization Adaptations to Injury and Altered Limb Use in Humans

### Adaptations to Injury and Altered Limb Use in Humans

Since the above research and related studies have demonstrated that alterations in peripheral input can influence cerebral functional–anatomic correspondences, it is not unexpected that increased somatosensory input, central neurologic injury, or somatic injuries that secondarily reduce afferent input may also be associated with cortical reorganization in humans. Thus, the treatment of anatomic syndactyly in humans via surgical separation of the digits has been found to be associated with individuation of the somatosensory representations of the involved fingers (Mogilner et al., 1993). This somatosensory reorganization consequent to rendering the sensory input from the digits nonsimultaneous would appear to be adaptive in that it enhances the cutaneous discriminability of independent input from the newly liberated digits. In contrast, the extensive injury-related reorganization of somatosensory cortex after forelimb amputation, as shown by measuring focal cortical magnetic field changes to cutaneous stimulation (Elbert et al., 1994, 1997; Borsook et al., 1998), is highly correlated with the frequently accompanying phantom limb pain (Flor et al., 1995; Birbaumer et al., 1997). This may result from a preferential disinhibition of nociceptive afferents (Rausell et al., 1992) to the surgically affected body part representations in somatosensory cortex.

Similar alterations in function may appear in otherwise healthy subjects who force their limbs to work in extreme manners. Fingertip reading of Braille may be accompanied by expansion of the somatosensory cortical representations of the involved digit (Pascual-Leone and Torres, 1993), and this would seem to be adaptive toward enhancing cutaneous sensitivity, as shown in monkey research cited above. However, Braille readers who use several digits simultaneously (thus becoming functionally syndactylous) often develop a topographically disordered somatosensory representation of the digits. When this occurs, there is also a correlative confusion when attempting to detect individual finger stimulation. However, the fusion of individual finger representations may also be advantageous in enabling the efficient synthesis of these inputs for enhanced comprehension in three-finger Braille readers (Sterr et al., 1998a, 1998b). The somatosensory cortical expansion of digit representations in professional musicians (Elbert et al., 1995) would seem to be adaptive for performance. In some cases, however, the increased somatosensory input associated with musical practice can lead to fused digit representations, which are associated with focal hand dystonia during performance, a nonpainful use-dependent decrease in dexterity (Bara-Jimenez et al., 1998; Elbert et al., 1998). The fused representations are consistent with the above-cited research by Clark et al. (1988) and Byl et al. (1996a) in monkeys. Thus, the digits of musicians engaged in extensive practice may become effectively syndactylous due to ultrarapid fingerings that perhaps overwhelm the ability of somatosensory areas to resolve temporally discrete sensory inputs from the individual digits. Prolonged active application of synchronous force in the digits may also be involved (Byl et al., 1996a).

## *Reorganization Associated with Limb Nonuse Following Cerebral Injury*

In our research and clinical treatment programs, we have routinely found that stroke patients with chronic hemiparesis show considerable retention of movement to command by the more-affected limb, despite its nonuse or minimal use during the real-life situation, although this observation seems to have been reported only once before (Andrews and Stewart, 1979). Even more surprising, such patients do not *maintain* purposive use of the more-affected limb at home, even though they have demonstrated improved activity during standard physical therapy. Standard physical therapy is often insufficient to promote spontaneous limb use during real-life daily living activities, since it commonly actively encourages lack of use by the more-affected extremity (Sabari et al., 2001).

Similar phenomena had previously been described by Taub and colleagues (summarized in Taub, 1980) following deafferentation of one forelimb in monkeys by dorsal rhizotomy. Initially, this procedure results in immediate inability to use the limb under any circumstances. However, if the functioning contralateral limb is restrained several months after surgery, the monkey can resume limb use for daily living activities (e.g., feeding, locomotion). If the constraint is maintained for only a few days, the monkey resumes relying exclusively on the unaffected limb after the constraint is removed. However, if the constraint is maintained for several more days and then removed, the monkey persistently uses that forelimb for self-care, climbing, ambulation, and other activities of daily living in the colony environment. Thus, the chronic failure to use the affected limb is not absolute, but rather is motivational and learning-dependent, after a poorly understood process of recovery of motor capacity has occurred. This chronic failure of limb use has been termed *learned nonuse* (Taub, 1980). Immediately following hemideafferentation, monkeys have been observed to risk self-injury during locomotion when they fail to move the affected limb. These punishing experiences likely inhibit future attempts to use the affected limb.

The similarity of phenomena following unilateral forelimb deafferentation in monkeys and stroke in humans suggested that learned nonuse contributes to chronic hemiparesis following stroke or other structural brain injury in humans (Taub, 1980; Taub et al., 1993). In our laboratory, we identify patients with presumptive learned nonuse by contrasting their relatively preserved movements to command in the more-affected limb with their self-reported failure to use the limb in real-life activities at home, as reflected by a semistructured interview termed the *Motor Activity Log* (MAL) (Taub et al., 1993; Uswatte and Taub, 1999). Patients who meet the clinical criteria for learned nonuse following stroke demonstrate reduced cortical representation of the more-affected hand in the corresponding motor cortices during TMS (Liepert et al., 1998, 2000). These observations are consistent with the findings from experimental studies in primates indicating that the size of the cortical representation of a limb or limb segment is related to the extent of its use (Jenkins et al., 1990; Recanzone et al., 1992a–1992c).

## Reorganization in Response to Therapy for Learned Nonuse

Standard physical therapy for stroke hemiparesis promotes only marginal improvement, at best, compared with nonspecific treatment (Ernst 1990; de Pedro-Cuesta et al., 1992). Furthermore, since standard physical therapy often emphasizes reliance on the less-affected extremity (Sabari et al., 2001), this likely contributes to the learned nonuse and functional hemispheric asymmetry in the motor representations of the limbs that we discussed above. Accordingly, recovery of purposeful use in the more-affected limb is hindered behaviorally as well as physiologically.

The research by Taub and colleagues in hemideafferented monkeys demonstrated that enduring restoration of bilateral limb use could be achieved by restraining the unaffected limb for at least several days. Consequently, following publication of a suggested treatment protocol derived from the primate deafferentation research (Taub, 1980), an initial clinical trial adopted one-half of this protocol, the restraint component (Wolf et al., 1989). This was termed the *forced use* paradigm, and it produced reliable but small treatment effects. Subsequently, the full recommended therapeutic regimen was implemented, resulting in treatment effects that were one-half to a full magnitude larger in terms of effect size. This approach was termed *constraint-induced movement* (*CI*) *therapy*. The standard CI therapy approach requires the patient to wear a mitt on the less-affected limb for up to 90% of waking hours during the 2 or 3 weeks of treatment (Fig. 14-1). The patient undergoes *massed practice* of the more-affected limb, using it to perform various grasping, pushing, lifting, and other manual actions repeatedly over a period of 7 hours a day (with at least 1 hour of rest) under the supervision of a physical or occupational therapist. Finally, activities are graduated to more difficult tasks after the patient accomplishes simpler ones, which is part of the process termed *shaping*. Results from the initial CI therapy trials in humans demonstrated improved spontaneous use of the more-affected limb in real-life activities (as reflected in the MAL). The effect size of such treatment was about 3.3 (Taub et al., 1999) and persisted for at least 2 years. Maximal motor

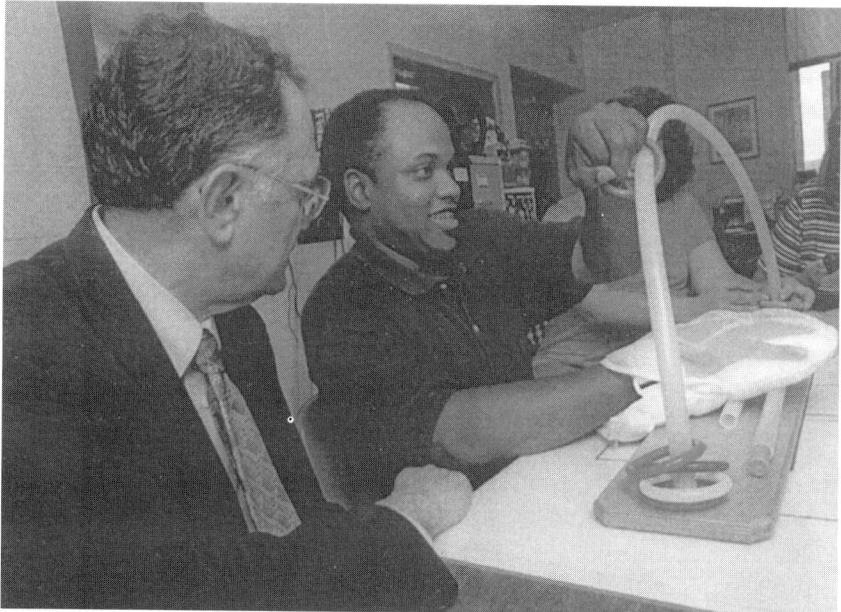

**Figure 14-1.** Demonstration of standard constraint-induced (CI) therapy for upper extremity hemiparesis, which involves restraint of the less-affected upper extremity with a mitt for 90% of waking hours and massed practice with the more-affected upper extremity for up to 7 hours per day with rest periods for 2–3 weeks of treatment.

ability when a patient is requested to carry out test tasks in the laboratory also improved significantly, but to a lesser extent (effect size of about 0.9). Thus, CI therapy has the effect of minimizing the disparity between movement capacity and actual amount of use of the more-affected arm in the real-life situation. The treatment has been validated against placebo-treated stroke patient controls (Taub et al., 1993, 1999). Moreover, repeated MAL assessments before treatment do not significantly change (Miltner et al., 1999; Liepert et al., 2000). Thus, CI therapy appears to be effective due primarily to massed practice of functionally relevant tasks, with a lesser contribution made by restraint of the less-affected arm. Its effectiveness does not result simply from an enhanced desire to move or increased attention from the therapist. One might also note that CI therapy has been found to be effective in patients whose extent of paresis represents that of 50–75% of the population with chronic stroke and significant residual motor deficit (Taub et al., 1999).

Since CI therapy counteracts the behavioral asymmetry of limb activity that existed prior to treatment, it is not surprising that it reverses the interhemispheric asymmetry in functionally excitable motor cortex, as demonstrated by TMS (Liepert et al., 1998, 2000). The expansion of the motor cortex representation of the more-affected upper extremity occurs in parallel with improvement on the MAL (Liepert et al., 2000), thus reinforcing the value of the MAL as an index of functional motor status. In a neuroelectric source localization study of learned nonuse patients (Kopp et al., 1999), the main area of activation associated with purposive finger tapping had shifted from the premotor area to the supplementary motor area immediately following CI therapy. However, upon reexamination 3 months later, the associated electric source dipole was found to have shifted to the opposite hemisphere. Conclusions drawn from this study must be tempered by the recognition that these results were obtained from a sample of only four patients. However, they provisionally suggest not only that CI therapy improves spontaneous use of the more-affected limb, but also that the contralateral cortical reorganization that occurs immediately after the end of treatment may facilitate subsequent recruitment of ipsilateral motor areas to maintain improved purposive limb movement.

## *Reorganization in Response to Treatment for Focal Hand Dystonia*

Focal hand dystonia is a condition involving manual incoordination that occurs in individuals, including musicians, who engage in extensive and forceful use of the digits. To date, no treatment has been found to be effective. Using magnetic source imaging, Elbert et al. (1998) found that musicians with focal hand dystonia exhibit a use-dependent overlap or smearing of the representational zones of the digits of the dystonic hand in somatosensory cortex. Similar results were obtained by Bara-Jimenez et al. (1998), and abnormalities in hand motor maps were observed by Byrnes et al. (1998). Digital overuse had previously been found to produce a similar phenomenon in monkeys by Byl and coworkers (1996a, 1997). The motor dysfunction is accompanied by decrements in somatosensory perceptual ability (Byl et al., 1996b; Bara-Jimenez et al., 2000a, 2000b). However, there is no evidence indicating whether the sensory disorder underlies the motor problem or is simply correlative with it. Since the deficit in focal hand dystonia that is disabling is clearly motor in nature (whatever else it may involve), and since behavioral mechanisms apparently underlie both the cortical disorder and the involuntary incoordination of movement, Candia and coworkers (1999, in press) hypothesized that a behavioral intervention could be of value in reducing or eliminating the motor manifestations of the condition. The procedures employed in this treatment approach to focal hand dystonia were derived in part from CI therapy, involving restraint of a body part, massing of practice, and training by shaping.

Eight professional musicians (six pianists and two guitarists) with long-standing symptoms were studied; they had previously received several different treatments, each without success. The therapy involved immobilization by splint(s) of one or more of the digits other than the focal dystonic finger. The musicians were required to carry out repetitive exercises with the focal dystonic finger in coordination with one or more of the other digits for 1.5–2.5 hours daily (depending on patient fatigue) over a period of 8 consecutive days (14 days in one case) under a therapist's supervision. The practice was thus massed; practice of this intensity and duration was very taxing and was at the limit of patient capability. After the end of the primary period of treatment, the patients continued practicing the exercises with the splint for 1 hour every day or every other day at home in combination with progressively longer periods of repertoire practice without the splint. Patient status was quantified with two measurement instruments: (1) a dexterity/displacement device that continuously recorded digital displacement during metronome-paced movements of two fingers (spectral analysis of the records provided information concerning the smoothness of the movements before, during, and after training) and (2) a dystonia evaluation scale (DES) on which patients, when not wearing the splint, rated how well they were performing movement sequences and passages from their repertoire that had tended to generate dystonic movements in the past.

All patients showed significant and substantial improvements without the splint at the end of treatment on both measures. The improvement persisted for the 24 months of follow-up and in five of the eight cases became greater with further practice of the therapeutic exercises after the end of laboratory treatment. Half of the subjects returned to the normal or almost normal range of digit function during music performance. There was one regression 9 months posttreatment following noncompliance with the home practice requirement for 6 months. Four of the patients were orchestral musicians and had never stopped their professional activities. However, four of the patients were soloists who had been forced to stop performing because of focal dystonia; they have now resumed performing in concert.

Unpublished data by Elbert, Candia, Taub, and coworkers indicate that the therapy breaks apart the fused representations of the digits of the dystonic hand; this is correlative with the improved performance. However, anomalously, the topographic relation of the digit representational zones often does not return to its characteristic order.

The treatment of performance dystonia using this approach is less well established than is CI therapy for hemiparesis. Thus, further studies are required to verify the effectiveness of the intervention and to determine whether such improvement can be generalized to other forms of focal dystonia. Since the publication of the findings of Candia et al. (1999), a different approach has been advocated by Priori et al. (2001), which involves the complete immobilization of the dystonic hand in performing musicians for more than 90% of the entire day for several weeks, followed by gradually lengthening periods of musical performance. Unsurprisingly, removal of the restraint is immediately followed by clumsiness in the affected hand, but by 1 week after removal of the restraint the seven musicians in the study reported lessening of their dystonic symptoms as they began to resume practice. Sustained benefit was found in most patients for at least several months.

These two different studies suggest that some form of immobilization counteracts performance dystonia, but it is unclear whether the results are comparable when individual fingers are exercised versus when the entire hand is forced to relax for several weeks, since different assessments were used. The findings of Priori et al. (2001) suggest that prolonged immobilization—which would be expected to reduce the hand representation in motor cortex (Liepert et al., 2000)—may be sufficient to restore individual representation of the digits in somatosensory cortex. These observations suggest that further studies should be performed to compare these two different interventions for their comparative efficacy and the extent to which they produce plastic changes in the hand representation in both somatosensory and motor cortex.

## *Other Applications of CI Therapy*

CI therapy, not surprisingly, can be used with forms of neurological injury other than stroke, where learned nonuse might be expected to be operative. These include aphasia (Pulvermüller et al., 2001; Taub, in press) and traumatic brain injury (Taub et al., 1999; Shaw et al., in press). Preliminary results (Taub et al., 1999; Weiss et al., in press) also indicate that the massed practice principle derived from CI therapy may be effective in reducing phantom limb pain by increasing the use of the unused residual limb after upper extremity amputation. In addition, the CI therapy approach appears to benefit ambulation in patients with incomplete spinal cord injury (Taub et al., 2000) and nonneurologic hip fractures (Taub et al., 2001). These observations are consistent with the stroke studies in that they suggest that nonuse is modifiable through massed practice and shaping. In turn, this suggests that chronically impaired locomotion following orthopedic injury can be, at least in part, a learned disorder. Chronically impaired locomotion, therefore, is expected to be related, at least partially, to either learned nonuse or, in the case of stroke and hip fracture, learned misuse (Taub et al., 1999). The disorder in each of these conditions involves alterations in the organization and function of the central nervous system (CNS), and their amelioration by CI therapy or its adaptations can be expected to be associated with marked alterations in CNS activity, as has been shown for stroke and focal hand dystonia.

Since massed practice can overcome nonuse following stroke, another possible target for such intervention would be akinesia associated with parkinsonian illnesses. This would be a different application than we have seen thus far, since the nonuse in such illnesses arises apparently from progressive neuronal degeneration, rather than alterations in the contingencies of punishment and reward, although this occurrence is not excluded in a progressive neurologic disorder. In contrast to the comparatively static impairments in stroke, spinal cord injury, and hip fracture, CI therapy for neurodegenerative disorders will be less likely to have a sustained benefit. Nonetheless, due to the possibility that there are functional and neurophysiological similarities between learned nonuse following stroke and Parkinson's disease, a trial of CI therapy for the latter may be warranted, at least in patients who are primarily affected by akinesia rather than tremor.

As we have seen, the discriminative tactile functions of monkeys may improve with massed practice (Jenkins et al., 1990; Recanzone et al., 1992a–1992c). Extended sensory training may improve somatosensory impairment associated with stroke in humans (Carey et al., 1993; Yekutiel and Guttman, 1993). In our outpatient CI therapy clinic at the University of Alabama at Birmingham, stroke patients occasionally ask whether their associated hemihypesthesia may be improved. Trials have not been conducted to formally assess the benefits of intensive motor retraining as used in CI therapy for restitution of somatosensory function. As Recanzone et al. (1992a–1992c) indicate, sensory restoration requires active attention. Thus, any intervention for somatosensory deficit in humans would not succeed simply through prolonged passive exposure to a tactile stimulus. It remains to be determined what would constitute the most effective training tasks for improving somatosensory deficits following CNS injury in humans. However, many of our clinic CI therapy patients indicate that they have had somatosensory improvement following treatment, even though this was not the objective of the intervention. This outcome should not be surprising, since somatosensory function and purposive movement are interdependent. Consequently, reorganization of somatosensory cortex likely attends nonuse following stroke, and it likely attends improved purposive movement following CI therapy as well. Both processes may alter somatosensory perception.

## Concluding Remarks

Use-dependent cortical reorganization is a fundamental property of the CNS. We have considered this only in regard to sensorimotor function, but it undoubtedly involves any cerebral areas that receive potentially modifiable neurophysiological input in relation to purposive activity. As we have indicated, cortical reorganization is opportunistic. When input to the CNS changes, the CNS rapidly adapts. Deficient afferentation from one body region is responded to by augmenting the cortical representation of adjoining regions. Increased utilization of a body region is responded to by expanding its cortical representation. These changes are probably fundamental to adaptation to the diverse demands placed upon the organism by the environment and therefore have substantial survival value.

Injury-related cortical reorganization can be associated with maladaptive outcomes, as seen in the maintenance of learned nonuse, performance hand dystonia, phantom limb pain, and tinnitus (Mühlnickel et al., 1998; see also Chapter 12, this volume). However, by understanding the extent and patterns of reorganization that accompany disability, it may be possible to validate and improve interventions that utilize similar reorganizational mechanisms to counteract disabilities.

## References

Andrews K and Stewart J (1979) Stroke recovery: He can but does he? *Rheumatol Rehabil* 18:43–48.

Bara-Jimenez W, Catalan MJ, Hallett M, and Gerlott C (1998) Abnormal somatosensory homunculus in dystonia of the hand. *Ann Neurol* 44:828–831.

Bara-Jimenez W, Shelton P, and Hallett M (2000b) Spatial discrimination is abnormal in focal hand dystonia. *Neurology* 55:1869–1873.

Bara-Jimenez W, Shelton P, Sanger T, and Hallett M (2000b) Sensory discrimination capabilities in human hand dystonia. *Ann Neurol* 47:377–380.

Birbaumer N, Lutzenberger W, Montoya P, Larbig W, Unerte K, Grodd W, Flor H, and Taub E (1997) Effects of regional anesthesia on phantom limb pain are mirrored in changes in cortical reorganization. *J Neurosci* 17:5503–5508.

Borsook D, Becerra L, Fishman S, Edwards A, Jennings CL, Stojanovic M, Papinicolas L, Ramachandran VS, Gonzalez RG, and Breiter H (1998) Acute plasticity in the human somatosensory cortex following amputation. *Neuroreport* 9:1013–1017.

Brown TG and Sherrington CS (1912) On the instability of a cortical point. *Proc R Soc London Ser B* 85:250–277.

Byl NN, Merzenich MM, Cheung S, Bedenbaugh P, Nagarajan SS, and Jenkins WM (1997) A primate model for studying focal dystonia and repetitive strain injury: Effects on the primary somatosensory cortex. *Phys Ther* 77:269–284.

Byl NN, Merzenich MM, and Jenkins WM (1996a) A primate genesis model of focal dystonia and repetitive strain injury: I. Learning-induced dedifferentiation of the representation of the hand in the primary somatosensory cortex in adult monkeys. *Neurology* 47:508–520.

Byl NN, Nagarajan S, and McKenzie AL (2000) Effect of sensorimotor training on structure and function in three patients with focal hand dystonia. *Soc Neurosci Abstr* 26:680.

Byl N, Wilson F, and Merzenich M (1996b) Sensory dysfunction associated with repetitive strain injuries of tendinitis and focal hand dystonia: A comparative study. *J Orthop Sports Phys Ther* 23:234–244.

Byrnes ML, Thickbroom GW, Wilson SA, Sacco P, Shipman JM, Stell R, and Mastaglia FL (1998) The corticomotor representation of upper limb muscles in writer's cramp and changes following botulinum toxin injection. *Brain* 121:977–988.

Candia V, Elbert T, Altenmüller E, Rau H, Schäfer T, Rockstroh B, and Taub E (in press) A treatment for focal hand dystonia of pianists and guitarists based on behavioral principles. *Arch Phys Med Rehabil.*

Candia V, Elbert T, Altenmüller E, Rau H, Schäfer T, and Taub E (1999) Constraint-induced movement therapy for focal hand dystonia in musicians. *Lancet* 353:42.

Carey LM, Matyas TA, and Oke LE (1993) Sensory loss in stroke patients: Effective training of tactile and proprioceptive discrimination. *Arch Phys Med Rehabil* 74:602–611.

Clark SA, Allard T, Jenkins WM, and Merzenich MM (1988) Receptive fields in the body-surface map in adult cortex defined by temporally correlated inputs. *Nature* 332:444–445.

de Pedro-Cuesta J, Widén-Holmqvist L, and Bach-y-Rita P (1992) Evaluation of stroke rehabilitation by randomized controlled studies: A review. *Acta Neurol Scand* 86:433–439.

Donoghue JP, Suner S, and Sanes JN (1990) Dynamic organization of primary motor cortex output to target muscles in adult rats. II. Rapid reorganization following motor nerve lesions. *Exp Brain Res* 79:492–503.

Elbert T, Candia V, Altenmüller E, Rau H, Sterr A, Rockstroh B, Pantev C, and Taub E (1998) Alteration of digital representations in somatosensory cortex in focal hand dystonia. *Neuroreport* 9:3571–3575.

Elbert T, Flor H, Birbaumer N, Knecht S, Hampson S, Larbig W, and Taub E (1994) Extensive reorganization of the somatosensory cortex in adult humans after nervous system injury. *Neuroreport* 5:2593–2597.

Elbert T, Pantev C, Wienbruch C, Rockstroh B, and Taub E (1995) Increased cortical representation of the fingers of the left hand in string players. *Science* 270:305–307.

Elbert T, Sterr A, Flor H, Rockstroh B, Knecht S, Pantev C, Wienbruch C, and Taub E (1997) Input-increase and input-decrease types of cortical reorganization after upper extremity amputation in humans. *Exp Brain Res* 117:161–164.

Ernst E (1990) A review of stroke rehabilitation and physiotherapy. *Stroke* 21:1081–1085.

Flor H, Elbert T, Knecht S, Wienbruch C, Pantev C, Birbaumer N, Larbig W, and Taub E (1995) Phantom-limb pain as a perceptual correlate of cortical reorganization following arm amputation. *Nature* 375:482–484.

Jenkins WM, Merzenich MM, Ochs MT, Allard T, and Guic-Robles E (1990) Functional reorganization of primary somatosensory cortex in adult owl monkeys after behaviorally controlled tactile stimulation. *J Neurophysiol* 63:82–104.

Karni A, Meyer G, Jezzard P, Adams MM, Turner R, and Ungerleider LG (1995) Functional MRI evidence for adult motor cortex plasticity during motor skill learning. *Nature* 377:155–158.

Kopp B, Kunkel A, Mühlnickel W, Villringer K, Taub E, and Flor H (1999) Plasticity in the motor system correlated with therapy-induced improvement of movement after stroke. *Neuroreport* 10:807–810.

Leyton ASF and Sherrington CS (1917) Observations on the excitable cortex of the chimpanzee, orang-utan and gorilla. *Q J Exp Physiol* 11:135–222.

Liepert J, Miltner W, Bauder H, Sommer M, Dettmers C, Taub E, and Weiller C (1998) Motor cortex plasticity during constraint-induced movement therapy in stroke patients. *Neuroscience Letters* 250:5–8.

Liepert J, Bauder H, Miltner W, Taub E, and Weiller C (2000) Treatment-induced cortical reorganization after stroke in humans. *Stroke* 31:1210–1216.

Merzenich MM, Kaas JH, Wall J, Nelson RJ, Sur M, and Felleman D (1983a) Topographic reorganization of somatosensory cortical areas 3b and 1 in adult monkeys following restricted deafferentation. *Neuroscience* 8:33–55.

Merzenich MM, Kaas JH, Wall JT, Sur M, Nelson RJ, and Felleman DJ (1983b) Progression of change following median nerve section in the cortical representation of the hand in areas 3b and 1 in adult owl and squirrel monkeys. *Neuroscience* 10:639–665.

Merzenich MM, Nelson RJ, Stryker MP, Cynader MS, Schoppmann A, and Zook JM (1984) Somatosensory cortical map changes following digit amputation in adult monkeys. *J Comp Neurol* 224:591–605.

Miltner W, Bauder H, Sommer M, Dettmers C, and Taub E (1999) Effects of constraint-induced movement therapy on patients with chronic motor deficits after stroke. A replication. *Stroke* 30:586–592.

Mogilner A, Grossman JA, Ribary U, Joliot M, Volkmann J, Rapaport D, Beasley RW, and Llinás RR (1993) Somatosensory cortical plasticity in adult humans revealed by magnetoencephalography. *Proc Natl Acad Sci USA* 90:3593–3597.

Muellbacher W, Ziemann U, Boroojerdi B, Cohen L, and Hallett M (2001) Role of the human motor cortex in rapid motor learning. *Exp Brain Res* 136:431–438.

Mühlnickel W, Elbert T, Taub E, and Flor H (1998) Reorganization of auditory cortex in tinnitus. *Proc Natl Acad Sci USA* 95:10340–10343.

Nudo RJ, Milliken GW, Jenkins WM, and Merzenich MM (1996) Use-dependent alterations of movement representations in primary motor cortex of adult squirrel monkeys. *J Neurosci* 16:785–807.

Pascual-Leone A and Torres F (1993) Plasticity of the sensorimotor cortex representation of the reading finger in Braille readers. *Brain* 116:39–52.

Pons TP, Garraghty PE, Ommaya AK, Kaas JH, Taub E, and Mishkin M (1991) Massive cortical reorganization after sensory deafferentation in adult macaques. *Science* 252:1857–1860.

Priori A, Pesenti A, Cappellari A, Scarlato G, and Barbieri S (2001) Limb immobilization for the treatment of focal occupational dystonia. *Neurology* 57:405–409.

Pulvermüller F, Neininger B, Elbert T, Mohr B, Rockstroh B, Koebbel P, and Taub E (2001) Constraint-induced therapy of chronic aphasia after stroke. *Stroke* 32:1621–1626.

Rausell E, Cusick CG, Taub E, and Jones EG (1992) Chronic deafferentation in monkeys differentially affects nociceptive and nonnociceptive pathways distinguished by specific calcium-binding proteins and down-regulates gamma-aminobutyric acid type A receptors at thalamic levels. *Proc Natl Acad Sci* 89:2571–2575.

Recanzone GH, Jenkins WM, Hradek GT, and Merzenich MM (1992a) Progressive improvement in discriminative abilities in adult owl monkeys performing a tactile frequency discrimination task. *J Neurophysiol* 67:1015–1030.

Recanzone GH, Merzenich MM, and Jenkins WM (1992c) Frequency discrimination training engaging a restricted skin surface results in an emergence of a cutaneous response zone in cortical area 3a. *J Neurophysiol* 67:1057–1070.

Recanzone GH, Merzenich MM, Jenkins WM, Grajski KA, and Dinse HR (1992b) Topographic reorganization of the hand representation in cortical area 3b owl monkeys trained in a frequency-discrimination task. *J Neurophysiol* 67:1031–1056.

Sabari JS, Kane L, Flanagan SR, and Steinberg A (2001) Constraint-induced motor relearning after stroke: A naturalistic case report. *Arch Phys Med Rehabil* 82:524–528.

Sanes JN, Suner S, and Donoghue JP (1990) Dynamic organization of primary motor cortex output to target muscles in adult rats. I. Long-term patterns of reorganization following motor or mixed peripheral nerve lesions. *Exp Brain Res* 79:479–491.

Sanes JN, Suner S, Lando JF, and Donoghue JP (1988) Rapid reorganization of adult rat motor cortex somatic representation patterns after motor nerve injury. *Proc Natl Acad Sci USA* 85:2003–2007.

Shaw SE, Morris DM, Uswatte G, McKay S, Abernathy S, Meythaler JM, and Taub E (in press) Constraint-induced movement therapy for recovery of upper extremity function following traumatic brain injury. *Arch Phys Med Rehabil.*

Sterr A, Müller MM, Elbert T, Rockstroh B, Pantev C, and Taub E (1998a) Changed perceptions in Braille readers. *Nature* 391:134–135.

Sterr A, Müller MM, Elbert T, Rockstroh B, Pantev C, and Taub E (1998b) Perceptual correlates of changes in cortical representation of fingers in blind multifinger Braille readers. *J Neurosci* 18:4417–4423.

Taub E (1980) Somatosensory deafferentation research with monkeys: Implications for rehabilitation medicine. In: Ince LP (ed), *Behavioral Psychology in Rehabilitation Medicine: Clinical Applications.* Baltimore: Williams & Wilkins (pp 371–401).

Taub E (in press) CI therapy: A new rehabilitation technique for aphasia and motor disability after neurological injury. *Klinik Forschung.*

Taub E, Miller NE, Novack TA, Cook EW, Fleming WC, Nepomuceno CS, Connell JS, and Crago JE (1993) Technique to improve chronic motor deficit after stroke. *Arch Phys Med Rehabil* 74:347–354.

Taub E, Uswatte G, Mark V, Willcutt C, Pearson S, Jannett T, and King DK (2000) CI therapy extended from stroke to spinal cord injured patients. *Soc Neurosci Abstr* 26:544.

Taub E, Uswatte G, Mark V, Bussey C, Pearson S, Jannett T, Bryson C, and King DK (2001) CI therapy for lower extremities extended from CNS damage to fractured hip. *Soc Neurosci Abstr* 27:2208.

Taub E, Uswatte G, and Pidikiti R (1999) Constraint-induced movement therapy: A new family of techniques with broad application to physical rehabilitation—a clinical review. *J Rehabil Res Dev* 36:237–251.

Ungerleider LG (1995) Functional brain imaging studies of cortical mechanisms for memory. *Science* 270:769–775.

Uswatte G and Taub E (1999) Constraint-induced movement therapy: New approaches to outcome measurement in rehabilitation. In: Stuss DT, Winocur G, and Robertson IH (eds.), *Cognitive Neurorehabilitation.* Cambridge: Cambridge University Press, pp 215–229.

Wang X, Merzenich MM, Sameshima K, and Jenkins WM (1995) Remodelling of hand representation in adult cortex determined by timing of tactile stimulation. *Nature* 378:71–75.

Weiss T, Miltner WHR, Adler T, Brückner L, and Taub E (1999) Decrease in phantom limb pain associated with prosthesis-induced increased use of an amputation stump. *Neurosci Lett* 272:131–134.

Wolf SL, Lecraw DE, Barton LA, and Jann BB (1989) Forced use of hemiplegic upper extremities to reverse the effect of learned nonuse among chronic stroke and head-injured patients. *Exp Neurol* 104:125–132.

Yekutiel M and Guttman E (1993) A controlled trial of the retraining of the sensory function of the hand in stroke patients. *J Neurol Neurosurg Psychiatry* 56:241–244.

# 15

## Conclusion:
## Contributions of Inhibitory Mechanisms to Perceptual Completion and Cortical Reorganization

LIISA A. TREMERE, RAPHAEL PINAUD,
AND PETER DE WEERD

In preceding chapters, a number of physiological processes have been described that suggest ways in which single cells in sensory systems can participate in interpolation. In Chapters 4 and 5, activity increases in single neurons are described, taking place on a time scale of milliseconds or seconds, driven by the surround of their receptive fields (RFs). Expansions of the classical RF, occurring within minutes of deafferentation of sensory cortical neurons (Chapters 10 and 12), provide another example of neural interpolation. Under particular conditions, slow changes in cortical topographical maps of the receptive sheet can take place, over the course of months or even years, in which the representation of one part of the environment becomes invaded by neighboring parts. This chapter investigates the role of these different types of neural interpolation in perceptual completion, skill learning, and recovery from peripheral injury. It focuses on findings in visual and somatosensory modalities, but some findings in auditory and motor domains are discussed as well.

*Neural interpolation* refers to the lateral spread of excitatory activity in cortex, which is limited by competing inhibition. The spatial extent and structure of a neuron's RF reflect a particular balance between excitation and inhibition. These RF properties thus gauge the interplay between inhibition and neural interpolation. The chapter will start, therefore, with a review of the identified contributions of inhibitory mechanisms to normal RF properties.

In the second section, contributions of neural interpolation to normal perception will be discussed. Specifically, a link will be proposed between the short-term effects of disinhibition on neural interpolation and perceptual completion phenomena. Sustained disinhibition following deafferentation is proposed to promote slow patterns of neural interpolation, leading to long-term cortical reorganizations that, once completed, can modify the way in which stimuli are perceptually completed. A similar interplay between inhibitory mechanisms and interpolation may be triggered during skill learning. It will be proposed that attention can trigger a state of disinhibition resulting in the promotion of plastic changes in cortex that can lay down a *memory* for the practiced skill. In sum, while the role of inhibition in RF formation and the enabling of plasticity has been recognized before, we propose that the interplay between inhibition and cortical interpolation, operating at different time scales, provides a common basis for understanding disparate aspects of perception, skill learning, attention, and recovery from injury.

## Inhibition, Filling-In, and Remapping

### Contributions of Inhibition to Sensory Function

The response properties of sensory neurons are to a significant extent shaped by inhibition. Inhibitory modulation is a common aspect of sensory function, and some general features of inhibitory mechanisms will be reviewed. This will provide a framework within which the concept of neural interpolation can be defined.

*Common Aspects of GABAergic Contributions in Different Sensory Systems*
Sensory cortical neurons receive a mixture of excitatory and inhibitory inputs. Inhibitory effects are mediated through the neurotransmitter GABA (gamma-aminobutyric acid). The most prevalent GABA receptor belongs to the $GABA_A$ subtype. The action of GABA on the $GABA_A$ receptor permits the influx of chloride, which causes hyperpolarization and, consequently, neuronal inhibition (Connors et al., 1988). Activation of the $GABA_A$ receptor can block action potentials or reduce excitability by shunt inhibition, and can shorten or shape an ongoing excitatory response. The $GABA_A$ receptor is the principal source of fast-acting cortical inhibition and can significantly influence cell signaling. In the neocortex approximately 25% of the neuronal population is GABAergic, making it the dominant inhibitory system (Krnjevic, 1984; Hendry et al., 1990; Jones, 1993). Furthermore, the primary visual area (V1) and primary somatosensory area (SI) show a similar distribution of GABAergic neurons in different cortical layers. Hendry et al. (1987) and Jones (1993) showed that in both sensory systems, the greatest proportions of GABAergic neurons exist in cortical layers 2, 3, and 4. Similar immunocytochemical profiles were reported in the somatosensory systems of other species including the rat, cat, and raccoon (Akhtar and Land, 1991; Doetsch et al., 1993; Li et al., 1994). These data indicate a special role for inhibitory mechanisms in superficial layers of sensory cortex.

Pyramidal neurons project either to different structures or cortical areas (feedforward and feedback projections) or within the same cortical area through axon collaterals (vertical or horizontal projections). The effects of each of these types of projections are modulated by local inhibitory neurons, which show a variety of morphologies (Jones, 1993). Primary sensory cortex receives thalamic afferents in layer 4, after which information is sent to superficial layers (2 and 3) and subsequently to deep layers (5 and 6). Inhibitory interneurons play an important role in the progressive increase in size and complexity of RF characteristics along this processing pathway (Bolz et al., 1989; Douglas et al., 1989; Armstrong-James et al., 1992). Primary sensory cortex forwards its outputs to layer 4 of the next cortical processing stage, from where it also receives feedback, which originates predominantly in deep cortical layers. Within cortical areas, there is substantial horizontal connectivity, predominantly in superficial layers (Schwark and Jones, 1989; McGuire et al., 1991; Tanifuji et al., 1994). Sensory RFs are a product of the balance between excitatory and inhibitory inputs provided by all their anatomical connections. Therefore, GABA contributes significantly to the definition of RFs and the response properties of sensory cortical neurons (Sillito, 1975a, 1975b, 1979; Laskin and Spencer, 1979; Hicks and Dykes, 1983; Bolz et al., 1989; Freund and Meskenaite, 1992; Jones, 1993; Gupta et al., 2000).

*GABAergic Contributions to Response Properties of the Classical RF*
The *classical RF* refers to the region in sensory space from which a neuron can be stimulated with a single isolated stimulus (e.g., an oriented luminance bar for a visual neuron). The acronym RF will be used to refer to the classical RF. The idea that local GABAergic circuitry helps to shape RF properties of sensory neurons (e.g., Benevento et al., 1972; Blakemore and Tobin, 1972; Creutzfeldt et al., 1974) was proposed shortly after the discovery that neurons in the visual cortex are tuned to the direction of movement and orientation of luminance-defined bars and edges (Hubel and Wiesel, 1959, 1962). Many studies showed that microiontophoretic application of bicuculline methiodide (BMI, a $GABA_A$ antagonist) resulted in expansions of the classical RF and in the loss of direction sensitivity and orientation tuning and, on occasion, reversed or reorganized the ON and OFF subregions of the classical RF, implying a role for GABA in the definition of these RF properties. Such studies have been done in the visual system (Sillito, 1977; Eysel et al., 1998; Pernberg et al., 1998) and in the somatosensory system (Mountcastle and Powell 1959; Laskin and Spencer 1979; Gardner and Costanzos, 1980a, 1980b; Alloway et al., 1989; Park and Pollak, 1994). In both the visual system (Eysel et al., 1998) and the somatosensory system (Kyriazi et al., 1998; Tremere et al., 2001a), most cells whose properties were affected by BMI application were found in superficial cortical layers. These observations concur with immunocytochemical studies showing a dominance of GABAergic cells in layers 2 and 4 (see previous section).

*GABAergic Contributions to Modulatory Responses Elicited*
*by Stimulation of the RF Surround*
The classical RF of cortical sensory neurons is surrounded by a region that, when stimulated alone by a small stimulus, elicits little or no response, but that can

modulate responses to stimuli presented in the classical RF. Stimuli in the surround generally suppress responses to stimuli inside the RF. This holds true in the visual (Maffei and Fiorentini, 1976; Nelson and Frost, 1978; Allman et al., 1985; Desimone and Schein, 1987; Schein and Desimone, 1990; Knierim and Van Essen, 1992; Levitt and Lund, 1997; Hupe et al., 2001) as well as in the somatosensory systems (Laskin and Spencer, 1979; Goldreich et al., 1998). From a modeling perspective, a classical RF and its surround can be considered as a *single* entity that can be approximated with a *Difference of Gaussians* (DOG) model. In this model, a broad Gaussian distribution of inhibition is subtracted from a narrower Gaussian distribution of excitation, with a higher maximum, to yield an excitatory classical RF enveloped in a suppressive surround (Laskin and Spencer, 1979; Sceniak et al., 2001). A DOG approach was used originally by Enroth-Cugell and Robson (1966) to model the antagonistic properties of the classical RFs of retinal ganglion cells, and was used later to model the classical RF of simple cells (Marcelja, 1980; Stork and Wilson, 1990). From an anatomical perspective, it is reasonable to consider the classical RF and the suppressive surround as *separate* entities. The classical RF of sensory neurons is derived to a significant extent from thalamic input, or inputs from a lower-order cortical region, while lateral cortico-cortical connections have been proposed as the anatomical substrate for the suppressive surround. Axon collaterals of pyramidal cells can extend laterally for 5 mm or more in visual (Gilbert and Wiesel, 1989; McGuire et al., 1991; Levitt et al., 1994) and somatosensory cortex (DeFelipe et al., 1986; Huntley and Jones, 1991), as well as in other neocortical regions (Lund et al., 1993). They make direct excitatory connections on other pyramidal cells, but they can also make connections on local GABAergic neurons (Winfield et al., 1981; McGuire et al., 1991) that may inhibit nearby pyramidal cells. The existence of local GABAergic circuitry thus limits the effects of remote excitatory inputs. Hence, the inhibitory surround can be interpreted as providing containment for the horizontal spread of excitatory signals across cortex. The horizontal spread of excitatory signals from active cortical regions into inactive regions along lateral cortical connections is an example of neural interpolation.

## *GABAergic Modulation of Limits on Neural Interpolation: Short-Term Effects of Disinhibition*

A restricted cortical region blocked from its normal afferent input will show disinhibition, which has two sources. First, a lack of afferent drive will necessarily reduce the drive for local inhibitory circuits. Second, the level of intracellular GABA itself is activity-dependent. A lack of neural activity interferes directly with the availability (or structural integrity) of glutamic acid decarboxylase (GAD), an enzyme that turns glutamate into GABA. Activity-dependent effects on GAD, and ensuing disinhibition, may occur fast enough (Jones, 1993; see also Li et al., 2001) to explain the rapid changes in RF structure observed in cortical regions deprived of their normal input. These ideas, and their relevance for perceptual completion, will be discussed separately for the visual and somatosensory systems.

## GABAergic Modulation of the Spatial Limits
## of Neural Interpolation in the Visual System

The role of GABA will be discussed in three physiological effects that can influence the size or structure of RFs of visual cortical neurons. The possibility that these physiological effects influence or enable neural interpolation processes relevant for particular types of perceptual completion will be considered.

Dynamic RF expansions have been reported in neurons with RFs at the edge of a scotoma induced by restricted homonymous retinal lesions (Chapter 10). Gilbert and Wiesel (1992) showed that RFs expanded in area by a factor of 5, on average, within minutes of lesioning. Even more remarkable, similar expansions of the classical RF were shown after the insertion of an *artificial scotoma* within a dynamic visual texture (Pettet and Gilbert, 1992). An artificial scotoma typically consists of a large, homogeneous stimulus that exceeds the size of the RF and does not drive the neuron, thereby acting as an occluder of the textured background. The data, combined with the finding that BMI application can expand V1 RFs (Eysel et al., 1998), indicate that RF expansion results from disinhibition, allowing previously ineffective excitatory inputs to become effective in driving the cell. Both the absence of visual contrast within the artificial scotoma and the stabilization of its edges may contribute to the disinhibition.

Expanded classical RFs in V1 indicate an expanded spatial reach of a neural interpolation process, which may provide a physiological basis for perceptual completion across artificial scotomas. Specifically, the expansion of a neuron's classical RF inside the artificial scotoma may bring the textured background inside the RF, causing the neuron to signal the texture. This idea, however, is not supported by the data. In Pettet and Gilbert's study (1992), RF expansions did not exceed the size of the artificial scotoma. Additionally, bringing the textured background inside the expanded RF shrank the RF back to its normal size. This may be related to an increased excitatory drive and an associated reinstatement of normal lateral inhibition. Nevertheless, RF expansions in permanently deafferented V1 neurons (due to a retinal lesion) may be more stable and may initiate a process of cortical remapping of the visual field.

De Weerd et al. (1995) reported another physiological phenomenon indicative of neural interpolation. They trained monkeys to fixate away from a gray square (artificial scotoma) on a dynamic texture, and found that neurons in V2 and V3 (but not V1) with RFs inside the square increased their response after 5–10 seconds of fixation, without any physical change to the stimulus (Chapter 5). This effect did not reflect a change in the classical RF, but it may have resulted from an adaptation of inhibitory inputs from the surround, allowing previously ineffective excitatory inputs to become effective. De Weerd, Gattass, Desimone, and Ungerleider (unpublished data; see Fig. 15-1) found explicit support for a link between disinhibition and neural interpolation. They showed that large surround stimuli produced measurable inhibition, and that the strength of this inhibition predicted the magnitude of response increases during eccentric fixation of the artificial scotoma. These fast response increases, driven by texture in the RF surround, suggest a temporary remapping of the visual environment onto cor-

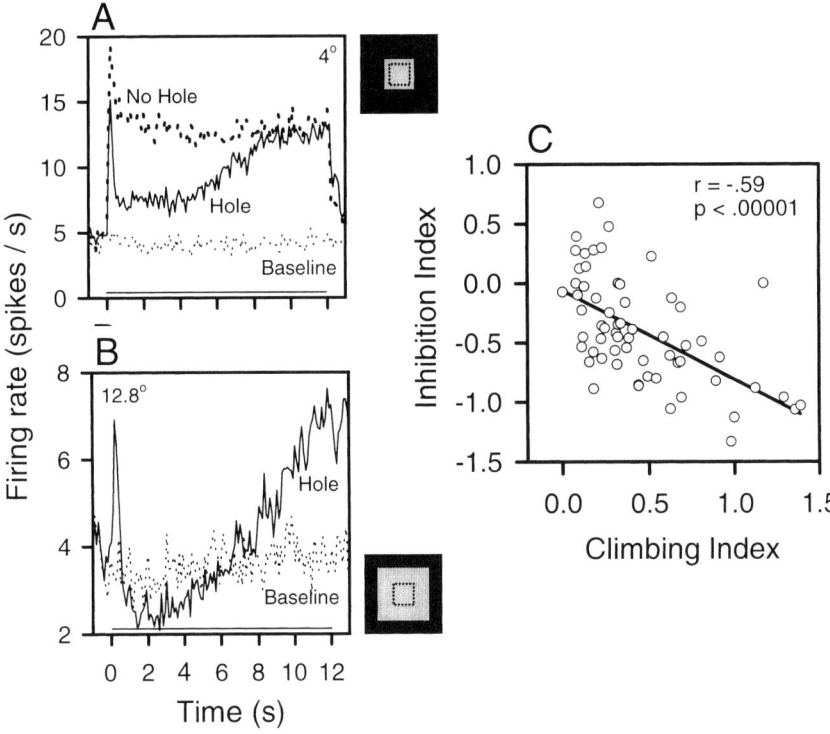

**Figure 15-1.** Contribution of inhibition to perceptual filling-in. (A) Average responses of V2 and V3 neurons in the No Hole condition (texture physically filled in over the receptive field [RF]), in the Hole condition (artificial scotoma over the RF), and in the Baseline condition (spontaneous activity). The duration of stimulation is indicated by the horizontal line above the abscissa. Insets illustrate the presentation of a 4 degree artificial scotoma over the RF (gray) surrounded by a dynamic line texture (symbolized by the black region; see Fig 5-1 in Chapter 5). The stippled line indicates the boundaries of the classical RF. Neurons included in the histograms ($N = 48$) showed a significant increase in activity in the Hole condition ($p < .05$ on the two-tailed paired $t$-test) in a total population of 93. Activity increases were quantified by a *climbing index* in which activity in a 9.5–12 second time window was subtracted from activity in a 1.5–4 second time window and divided by the sum. The time required for the average activity to reach a firing plateau correlates with the perception of perceptual completion. (B) Effects of inhibition revealed by remote stimulation. Stimulation with a dynamic texture far outside the RF results in inhibition for several seconds, starting just after a brief onset transient. Presentation of this stimulus is not accompanied by perceptual completion. Same 48 neurons as shown in (A). (C) Correlation between inhibition and activity increases (climbing indices). The inhibition index (see B) is calculated by subtracting the activity in the Hole condition in a 1.5–4 second time window from activity in the baseline condition and dividing it by the sum of those activities. Inhibition and climbing indices were calculated individually in 62 neurons (out of a population of 93) with positive climbing indices, and a negative correlation between both indices was obtained (the more negative the inhibition index, the stronger the inhibition). The data indicate that higher climbing indices are associated with stronger inhibition. Hence, activity increases associated with perceptual completion result from the adaptation of an inhibitory mechanism.

tex induced by a temporary source of disinhibition. It is possible that when the source of disinhibition is more permanent, such as after infliction of a retinal scotoma, fast response increases in deafferented V2 and V3 neurons might be present as well, which could help initiate the slow structural changes associated with cortical remapping.

At first, the discussed striate and extrastriate RF effects seem unrelated, as classical RF expansions in V1 were observed in anesthetized preparations, while response increases in V2 and V3 during exposure to an artificial scotoma could not be replicated in anesthetized monkeys (De Weerd, Gattass, Desimone and Ungerleider, unpublished). Nevertheless, in conscious animals with a *real* (permanent) scotoma, the possibility remains that long-term changes in the RF structure of V1 neurons, and cortical remapping, are partly driven by feedback from extrastriate cortex, where neural interpolation effects may occur within seconds after lesioning.

The fast neural interpolation effects in V2 and V3 show a time course that is compatible with perceptual filling-in (Chapters 4 and 5). Both take place within seconds of the presentation of the stimulus with the artificial scotoma. The relatively fast time course of perceptual filling-in reduces the plausibility of classical RF expansions in V1 as a basis for texture filling-in, because classical RF expansions take place on a time scale of minutes. Fast (extrastriate) mechanisms of neural interpolation may help explain the fact that newly inflicted *real* scotomas are rarely noticed (Safran et al., 1999).

Bolz et al. (1989) discovered yet another type of disinhibition that could play a role in initiating neural interpolation during exposure to artificial scotomas. They found that inactivation of a layer 6 neuron through localized diffusion of GABA eliminated the end-inhibition of a simple cell in layer 4 removed by several millimeters. This effect was not caused by widespread diffusion of GABA. Instead, it reflected how localized inhibition in one part of cortex caused disinhibition in a remote part of cortex, where it functionally removed the contribution of end-stopping to visual processing.

End-stopped cells may play a crucial role in the coding of boundaries (von der Heydt et al., 1984; Heitger et al., 1998). It has been proposed that active boundary representations produce an inhibitory signal that prevents surface features from spreading beyond physical boundaries (Gerrits and Vendrik, 1970; see also Chapters 2 and 8). Hence, any factor that reduces the strength of the boundary between an artificial scotoma and its background will promote filling-in. One such factor is the adaptation of neural responses activated by the border during prolonged retinal stabilization of the image (Chapters 2, 4, 5, and 8). A further factor can be the lack of visual contrast within artificial scotomas, which can lead to the silencing of layer 6 neurons with RFs inside the artificial scotoma. As discussed above, this effect may contribute to the functional loss of end-stopped mechanisms of boundary representation, thereby promoting filling-in (see also Komatsu et al., 2000).

Some authors have suggested that disinhibition can lead to prolonged (reverberating) signaling and spread of activity in neural networks. Billock (1997) proposed that a thalamo-cortical loop, formed by projections from the lateral geniculate nucleus (LGN) to V1 that are returned by projections from layer 6 of V1 to the LGN, may serve as a substrate for reverberating activity that could contribute to perceptual filling-in. This theory may be relevant for the filling-in of brightness, which involves areas as early as V1 (Chapter 4) but not for the filling-in of more complex visual surface features, such as texture, which has been observed in extrastriate cortex only (De Weerd et al., 1995). Reverberating activity within extrastriate horizontal cortical networks (Iijima et al., 1996) may contribute to the latter type of filling-in.

*GABAergic Modulation of the Spatial Limits of Neural Interpolation in the Somatosensory System*
Analogous to studies in the visual system, pronounced RF expansion of SI neurons has been demonstrated within minutes of amputation, ligation, or anesthesia of digits and other body parts (e.g., Merzenich et al., 1984; Calford and Tweedale, 1991; Rasmusson et al., 1993). As in the visual studies, this effect may reflect the expression of previously ineffective excitatory inputs after disinhibition due to loss of the dominant afferent drive. In line with this idea, application of $GABA_A$ antagonists to the somatosensory cortex yielded significant RF expansions. These expansions, expressed as a percentage over the original RF area, were approximately the same for the primate (231%; Alloway and Burton, 1991), the raccoon (224%; Tremere et al., 2001b), and the cat (approximately 225%; recalculated from Alloway et al., 1989). The work conducted in the primate and cat suggests that RF expansions in the deafferented cortical area were driven by neurons in neighboring digit representations. Hence, as in the visual system, RF expansions can be seen as indicators of an expanded reach of a neural interpolation process, and the evidence supports the idea that this effect is mediated by disinhibition.

In humans, deafferentation in the somatosensory system due to amputation is often followed by the experience of phantom limbs (Wartan et al., 1997). These vivid sensations of a body part that is no longer present are triggered instantaneously by touching cutaneous zones close to the amputated body part. Phantom limbs have been reported within 24 hours of amputation (Doetsch, 1997). They are the equivalent of visual filling-in across retinal scotomas. Expansions of the RFs of deafferented neurons in SI reported in animal studies could provide a basis for phantom sensations. Alternatively, more subtle changes in the balance of excitatory and inhibitory inputs from the surround might correlate with the perception of phantom limbs. By analogy with the visual system, such surround effects might take place in somatosensory cortical neurons outside SI. To test these ideas, a study of neural correlates of perceptual completion through an artificial scotoma in the somatosensory system would be informative. A somatosensory artificial scotoma would consist of a nonstimulated region of the receptive sheet surrounded by a stimulated region. Possibly, response increases of somatosensory neurons with RFs inside the artificial scotoma might be correlated with a sensation of perceptual filling-in of the artificial scotoma, as observed in the visual system. To our knowledge, these studies have not been done. However, fast perceptual completion of artificial scotomas has been described in the auditory system. Dannenbring (1976) demonstrated that tonal glides interrupted by a burst of white noise (artificial scotoma) are perceived as continuous. For example, a 500 ms burst inserted in the middle of a tonal glide lasting for 2000 ms was perceptually filled in, resulting in the illusory perception of a continuously gliding tone. Sugita (1997) showed that some neurons in A1 that did not respond well to the artificial scotoma responded well when it was inserted in the tonal glide, suggesting that these neurons contributed to this form of auditory filling-in.

*Balancing of Excitation and Inhibition in*
*Neocortical Circuits and Perceptual Completion*
The changes in RF size or structure described above are unlikely to be due to plastic changes in connectivity. Rather, these changes in RF size reflect increased effects of distant excitatory inputs, reflecting properties of existing cortical circuitry. This hypothesis was confirmed elegantly by Das and Gilbert (1995), who showed that the point spread function of optical imaging signals predicted the extent of RF expansion. Optical imaging is sensitive to subthreshold events and therefore can reveal spread of neural signal that cannot be revealed by standard extracellular recordings. The spread of the excitatory signal revealed in this way was consistent with the presence of long-range lateral connections spanning distances on the order of 5 mm (McGuire et al., 1991). Computational studies show that a physiologically plausible model of the lateral connectivity in sensory cortex (Xing and Gerstein, 1994, 1996) indeed predicts realistic RF expansions for various degrees of disinhibition.

Perceptual filling-in across artificial scotomas is delayed by a few seconds, and this argues for a role of disinhibition in this type of perceptual completion. On the other hand, perceptual filling-in of brightness (and other features) across visual surfaces or long-term visual scotomas can be observed within milliseconds of presenting a visual image (Chapter 4). These types of filling-in reflect a default, stable balance between neural interpolation and inhibition in the visual system.

## *GABAergic Modulation of Limits on Neural Interpolation: Long-Term Effects Enabled by Disinhibition*

RF expansions are a functional consequence of deafferentation, but under conditions of permanent deafferentation they can herald the beginning of a slow structural reorganization of the cortex. In the somatosensory cortex, remapping takes place during which cortical representations of deafferented parts of the receptor sheet become invaded by representations of neighboring, intact parts (e.g., Rasmusson, 1982; Merzenich et al., 1984; Calford and Tweedale, 1988; reviewed by Buonomano and Merzenich, 1998). The most spectacular remapping has been described in the monkey by Pons et al. (1991), who discovered that years after a deafferentation of the cortical regions in somatosensory cortex (SI) normally devoted to the arm and hand, these regions could be activated by stimulating the face (Fig 15-2). The distance over which cortex had reorganized in different monkeys was 10–14 mm. The data suggest that deafferentation triggers a slow neural interpolation process, proceeding over months or even years, during which deafferented cortical territory becomes driven by increasingly far-removed cortical sites. This view is supported by progressive changes in the trigger zones for phantom limbs following amputation (Doetsch, 1997; see also Ramachandran and Blakeslee, 1998) and by slow cortical remapping demonstrated in experiments using somatosensory evoked magnetic fields (Weiss et al., 2000). A related slow reorganization of motor maps has been described after peripheral nerve injury (Donoghue and Sanes, 1987) or amputation (Pascual-Leone, 1996; Karl et al., 2001), as well as in studies using transcranial magnetic stimulation (Pascual-Leone et al., 1996; Karl et al., 2001). Furthermore, long-term modifications of tonotopic maps in A1 have been shown after partial cochlear damage (Robertson and Irvine, 1989), and analogous changes of retinotopic maps have been observed in visual cortex (Chino et al., 1995; Darian-Smith and Gilbert, 1995; Kaas, 1995). There is compelling evidence that long-term remapping is associated with sprouting of horizontal axon collaterals. For example, this finding was reported in area 17 of the cat 8 months after deafferentation (Darian-Smith and Gilbert, 1994). Divergence of thalamocortical projections could contribute to remapping as well. There is convincing evidence for that idea in the somatosensory system (Jones, 2000) but not in the visual system (Darian-Smith and Gilbert, 1995).

Because a disinhibited cortical region has a reduced threshold for activation, remote excitatory inputs that under normal conditions would be ineffective could become effective. Hence, deafferented cortex is a prime candidate for the development of new functional connections with neurons outside the disinhibited region, provided that the disinhibition lasts long enough. The following sections review evidence suggesting that a reduction of GABAergic function is maintained for several months following deafferentation, creating a time window that promotes cortical plasticity. In addition, some evidence will be reviewed compatible with the idea that the deafferented cortex is gradually filled-in with neural activity. The link between disinhibition and plasticity is an important feature of early development as well. During early development, the maturation of inhibitory circuits lags behind the maturation of excitatory circuits. This creates a time window (the critical period) during which neuronal connections are more easily molded by a mixture of activity-dependent and activity-independent mechanisms (Yuste and Sur, 1999).

*GABA and Remapping in the Visual System*
To test the idea that deafferentation leads to maintained disinhibition, Rosier et al. (1995) used immunocytochemistry and showed reduced GABAergic activity in a cortical region in cat area 17 that had become deafferented by a binocular homonymous retinal lesion 2 weeks earlier. In support of this finding, other studies found that prolonged deafferentation leads to reductions in mRNA for $GABA_A$ receptors and GAD, an enzyme involved in the synthesis of GABA (Jones, 1993;

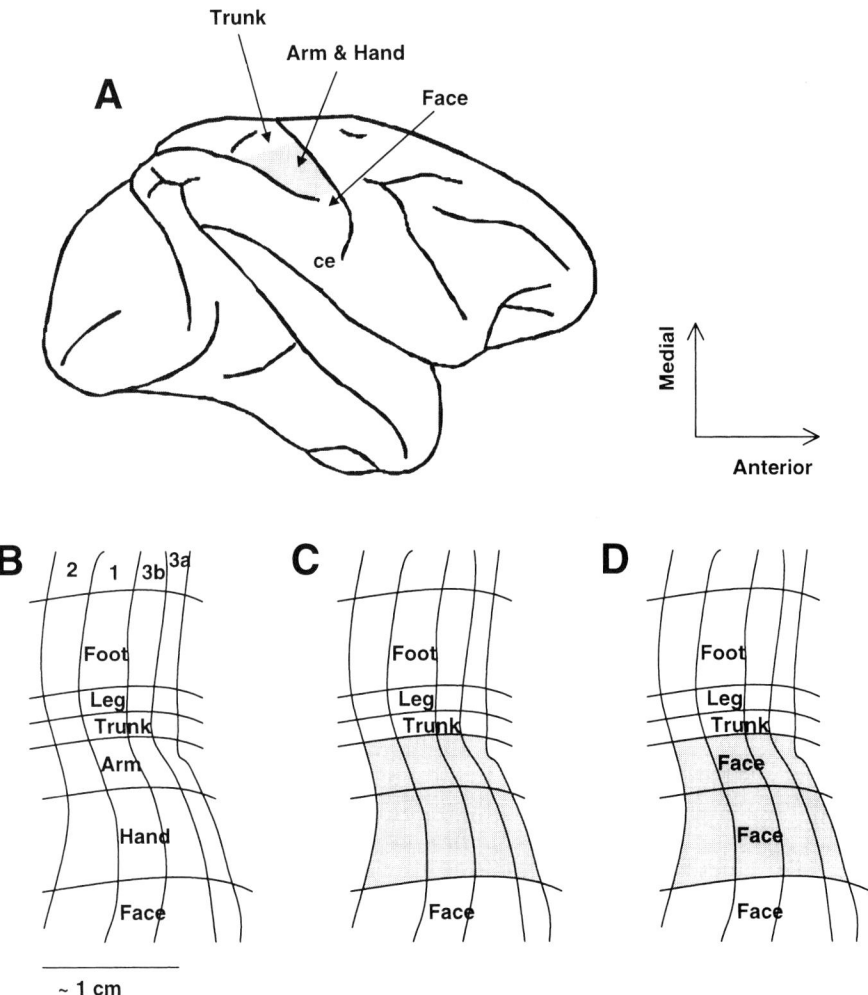

**Figure 15-2.** Effects of deafferentation on topography in somatosensory cortex (after Pons et al., 1991). (A) Lateral view of the monkey brain, with indications of the approximate location of representation of the trunk, arm and hand (in gray), and face. Mapping experiments to determine topography were done by recording from neurons in SI while determining tactile receptive fields (RFs) on the cutaneous surface. (B) Standard somatotopic map in SI after unfolding of the central sulcus (ce in A). Areas 1 and 2 are visible on the dorsal surface posterior to the central sulcus, whereas areas 3a and 3b are buried in the posterior wall and fundus of the central sulcus. (C) Deafferentation by dorsal rhizotomy. The deafferented area is shown in gray. (D) Results of a mapping experiment 12 years after deafferentation. The cortical region representing the hand had invaded deafferented cortex. The fact that it is the face rather than the trunk representation that expanded into deafferented cortex may reflect the fact that the face is innervated more densely and is likely to be stimulated more than the representation of the trunk. The strengthening of lateral connections through Hebbian mechanisms between deafferented cortex and adjacent normal cortex is more likely to occur for adjacent cortex that is strongly activated.

Benson et al., 1994). Furthermore, Arckens et al. (2000) showed that after 3 months, GABAergic immunocytochemistry in the deafferented region returned to normal. Arckens et al. (2000) also tracked changes in glutamate immunoreactivity at several time points after placement of the lesion, indicating that while glutamate levels were down after deafferentation, the region characterized by decreased glutamate levels grew smaller with time, until after 3 months the deafferented cortex was similar to surrounding cortex. Since glutamate levels are positively correlated with neural activity, this finding suggested that the deafferented zone became gradually interpolated with neural activity over a period of about 3 months. The gradual nature of this slow neural filling-in process suggests that the larger the deafferented zone is, the longer the time required for completion of the process. This may explain why extensive peripheral damage can cause reorganization over years in the somatosensory cortex and motor cortex. It is also possible that the 3-month time window for disinhibition acts as an initiator for cortical remodeling that might continue after inhibition has returned to normal (Darian-Smith and Gilbert, 1994). Immuncytochemical changes in GABA and glutamate have also been demonstrated in extrastriate cortex after deafferentation (Arckens et al., 1998; see also Chapter 10).

*GABA and Remapping in the Somatosensory System*
RFs of neurons in deafferented cortex commonly appear to be abnormally large and poorly defined, an effect that results from disinhibition (see sections on GABAergic modulation of spatial limits of neural interpolation). Disinhibition exposes latent excitatory connectivity and sometimes reveals developmentally outmoded excitatory circuitry. For example, Korodi and Toldi (1998) found that disinhibition caused neurons normally responsive to the whiskers alone to become driven by the forepaw digits and vice versa. This suggested a preexisting overlap in the anatomical connectivity for the whiskers and digits that became masked by inhibition during normal early development.

The contributions of GABAergic systems to early development invites the question of tracking the contribution of GABA to reorganization after deafferentation in the adult. This experiment was carried out in the raccoon by applying BMI at various time intervals after deafferentation (Rasmusson et al., 1993; Tremere et al., 2001a, 2001b). In this species, digit amputation leads to a silencing of deafferented neurons for about 2 weeks. BMI application during that period did not modify responsiveness. After that time, abnormally large and poorly defined excitatory RFs appeared on distal pads, which were further enlarged (or revealed) by BMI application. After roughly 3 months, many RFs on the distal digits were normal in size, and BMI application revealed RF expansions similar in size to those observed in normal neurons. Thus, as the new excitatory drive became stronger and better defined, there was a gradual normalization of inhibitory mechanisms. Thus, as in the visual system, there is a period of disinhibition following deafferentation, which promotes plasticity and remapping. The recruitment of new excitatory drive eventually leads to a reinstatement of normal inhibition.

*Balancing of Excitation and Inhibition in*
*Neocortical Circuits, Remapping, and Perceptual Completion*
There are two interesting links between perceptual completion and the outcome of slow neural interpolation (remapping). First, in the visual system, the underestimation of the dimensions of objects that cross old retinal scotomas suggests that the remapped cortex ultimately starts to contribute directly to perceptual completion (Safran et al., 1999). Second, we speculate that changes in the balance of inhibition and excitation correlated with perceptual completion of real scotomas could play a role in initiating the more permanent disinhibition in deafferented cortex that permits plasticity and remapping. In the visual system, it is possible that RF expansions and ensuing remapping in V1 may be driven in part by fast changes in excitation and inhibition in extrastriate cortex correlated with perceptual completion. Thus, perceptual completion would instigate cortical plasticity, the outcome of which, in turn, would influence properties of perceptual completion.

We have considered RF surrounds as homogeneously suppressive and have assumed that disinhibition enhances an isotropic neural interpolation process that may underlie the perceptual completion of surfaces. Slow isotropic (omnidirectional) neural interpolation may also be a reasonable model for slow cortical reorganization following infliction of permanent receptor damage. However, inhibitory RF surrounds can also be inhomogeneous (Jones et al., 2001), and they could facilitate the interpolation between local measures of discontinuities related to contours in the image while suppressing local information that is unlikely to be related to those contours (Field et al., 2000). Because the distribution of inhibition in the surround shapes this anisotropic interpolation process, disinhibition would also destroy mechanisms of contour perception. Hence, the reorganization of deafferented cortex may include the redevelopment of specific circuits involved not only in surface completion across the scotoma, but also in contour completion. Since, in the normal visual system, perceptual completion of contours and surfaces may be carried out by separate neural interpolation mechanisms (Chapters 2 and 8), it indeed is reasonable to expect that recovery after infliction of a scotoma will lead to a reinstatement of both interpolation mechanisms. That idea is supported further by studies of perceptual completion across the blind spot (Chapter 9), suggesting the existence of both anisotropic mechanisms of neural interpolation contributing to contour completion (Fiorani et al., 1992) and isotropic mechanisms of neural interpolation relevant for surface completion (Komatsu et al., 2000).

*Mechanisms of Hebbian Learning Enabled by Disinhibition*
This section focuses on activity-driven mechanisms of cortical plasticity that are enhanced in disinhibited regions of the adult cortex. A disinhibitory state of cortex promotes associative mechanisms of plasticity that strengthen initially weak connections between neurons inside and outside the deafferented cortical region. This idea goes back to Hebb (1949), who suggested that neurons that fire together will increase the strength of their connections. Cellular evidence for this

type of plasticity has been obtained by pairing presynaptic input with postsynaptic depolarization during a stimulation phase and by showing a lasting enhancement of excitatory postsynaptic potentials during a later test phase (Bliss and Lomo, 1973). There is direct evidence that these mechanisms can change RF properties in sensory neurons (e.g., Fregnac and Shulz, 1999).

For associative mechanisms of plasticity to work, there must be a mechanism to detect the coincidence of pre- and postsynaptic activity. This mechanism is provided by the *N*-methyl-D-aspartate (NMDA) glutamatergic receptors; glutamate from the presynaptic neuron paired with postsynaptic depolarization (and spiking) allows calcium influx, which triggers a number of biochemical cascades that lead to long-term potentiation (LTP). Multiple spaced periods of paired stimulation are often required to produce sustained LTP. Sustained LTP requires *de novo* protein synthesis, indicating that genomic intervention is required for synaptic enhancement. The synaptic enhancement may be carried by an increase in the probability of neurotransmitter release from individual release sites on the presynaptic neuron, by an increase in the number of presynaptic release sites, and by an increase in the number of postsynaptic receptors. Some of the genes expressed during sustained LTP have been shown to be involved in the formation and rearrangement of cortical circuits (Wisden et al., 1990), and there is direct evidence for a role of immediate early gene expression in the regulation of cortical plasticity (e.g., Pinaud et al., 2001, 2002). Ultimately, these genomic interventions can lead to the sprouting of new axon collaterals (Darian-Smith and Gilbert, 1994; Donoghue, 1995).

Associative plasticity is typically investigated in pairs of excitatory neurons, but it has been reported between inhibitory and excitatory cells as well. Hebbian plasticity is necessarily competitive, because among multiple sources of input, the strongest modifications in synaptic strength are expected for inputs that are best correlated with postsynaptic depolarization. The cellular mechanisms underlying LTP and other types of Hebbian learning have been reviewed by several authors, including Bear and Abraham (1996), Buonomano and Merzenich (1998), Kandel (2000), and Katz and Shatz (1996).

The facilitation of plasticity by disinhibition is supported by the finding that LTP is enhanced in disinhibited cortex (Hess et al., 1996). A reduction in GABAergic inputs will increase the time period during which (subthreshold) afferent drive caused by an excitatory input is maintained. This increases the time period in which temporal summation can occur, and it enhances the probability of coincident spiking and LTP. The probability of plastic changes can be enhanced further between neurons that fire in synchrony. Synchronous firing has been reported during early development of sensory systems (Kandel et al., 2000), as well as in reorganizing deafferented cortex in the adult (Diamond et al., 1993; Armstrong-James et al., 1994).

The effect of disinhibition is that neighboring neuronal populations with separate response properties start to influence each other. Ensuing plasticity can result in the transfer of response properties from one population to another (after deafferentation), resulting in *desegregation* of the two populations. Desegregation can also be initiated by desegregating the inputs to (or uses of) cell populations, which then can result in the development of common properties. For instance, two surgically attached digits will produce highly correlated inputs to somatosensory cortex. Under these conditions, it has been reported that the separation between digit representations in SI disappears, and that cortical neurons in reorganizing cortex develop RFs spanning the cutaneous surface of both digits (Allard et al., 1991; Merzenich and Jenkins, 1993). Similarly, in the visual system, when boundaries between separate regions in an image are eliminated, activity in the two cortical regions representing the previously segregated regions may become correlated. This may lead to plasticity if the source of desegregation is maintained. The link between desegregation and disinhibition suggests that the mechanism by which attention reduces the time required for filling-in of an artificial scotoma (i.e., desegregation) may rely on a form of disinhibition (Chapter 5).

In summary, cortical deafferentation induces a longer-lasting state of disinhibition that promotes structural remodeling through LTP-like mechanisms. This results in a slow interpolation of neural activity into deafferented cortex. Cortical reorganization can also be triggered by sensory experiences that correspond to biologically meaningful events. How the meaningfulness of stimuli or actions, together with their repetition, might lead to cortical plasticity is the topic of the next section.

## *Disinhibition, Attention, and Skill Learning*

Studies in the somatosensory and motor systems have revealed that the sensory input that coincides with the repeated performance of a particular skill produces cortical reorganization. For example, violinists show an enlarged representation in somatosensory cortex of the hand used to manipulate the strings (Elbert et al., 1995). Hence, a correlate of use (during skill learning) is an expansion of representations, while the correlate of underuse (after deafferentation) is a shrinking (due to invasion by other representations). This suggests that skill learning and deafferentation may invoke similar mechanisms of cortical plasticity, and it raises the question of whether there is a factor during skill learning that promotes plasticity. We suggest that attention, which facilitates skill learning, might help to induce cortical disinhibition, and that the basal forebrain may be instrumental in producing the disinhibition.

The cholinergic basal forebrain is one of several systems implied in arousal and attention (Parasumaran, 2000). Gritti and colleagues (1993) showed that cholinergic projection neurons that form the cholinergic basal forebrain system are intermingled with GABAergic projection neurons. Freund and Meskenaite (1992) showed that at least 25% of the cells targeted by GABAergic projection neurons are cortical GABAergic interneurons. Thus, basal forebrain neurons provide a plausible means of producing disinhibition. In addition, elevated levels of cortical acetylcholine enhance population responses to sensory input in a manner that suggests LTP-like mechanisms (Webster et al., 1991). Therefore, cholinergic projections from the basal forebrain could further enhance cortical plasticity enabled by GABAergic projections onto GABAergic interneurons. The resulting malleability of cortical connections might be exploited by other structures involved in learning and attention such that these connections start to reflect the acquired skill. The hypothesized links between attention, skill learning, the cholinergic basal forebrain, disinhibition, and LTP are discussed further below (see also Chapters 12–14).

Studies that control attention show that repeated stimulation during skill learning will lead to enhanced discrimination of those stimuli only if they are relevant in the context of the task (attended) (Karni and Sagi, 1991, 1993; Ahissar et al., 1992; Ahissar and Hochstein, 1993). Several other studies indicate that attention to a repeated stimulus is required for that stimulation to be effective in causing changes in sensory maps (Recanzone et al., 1992, 1993).

A potential role of the forebrain in the consolidation of a visual discrimination skill has been shown by Karni et al. (1994). They showed that interrupting rapid eye movement (REM) sleep, a sleep stage associated with cholinergic forebrain activity, interferes with the overnight consolidation of the skill (measured as a reduction of improvement from one daily training session to the next). Furthermore, activation of the forebrain has been demonstrated to stimulate remapping induced by electrical stimulation, which supports the possibility that cortical reorganization during skill learning is facilitated by the basal forebrain as well (Kilgard and Merzenich, 1998; see also Mercado et al., 2001).

A link between skill learning, LTP, and disinhibition was shown by Butefisch et al. (2000). They showed that in humans the administration of a drug that enhances $GABA_A$ receptor function, and of another drug that blocks NMDA receptors (that are required for LTP), prevents the electromyographical changes that can normally be triggered by transcranial stimulation directed at the primary motor area (M1) after the learning of a simple motor skill (Chapter 13). It has also been shown that disinhibition facilitates LTP after tetanic stimulation in slice preparations of motor cortex (Hess et al., 1996). Furthermore, the asymptotic daily performance enhancements that characterize skill learning bear a striking resemblance to the asymptotic enhancements of cortical population responses in rat cortex following daily sessions of exposure to repeated weak electrical stimulation, which are hypothesized to induce LTP (Trepel and Racine, 1998). Direct evidence for a link between LTP and motor learning was provided by Rioult-Pedotti et al. (1998, 2000). They found that in the rat, less LTP could be induced in motor cortex representing the forelimb when the forelimb had been used during behavioral skill training. These findings, taken together, support the idea that skill learning depends on LTP-like plasticity in cortex enabled by disinhibition.

A link between skill learning, LTP-like plasticity, and structural reorganization of horizontal connections in M1 has been shown as well. As has been demonstrated for reorganization in visual cortex after deafferentation, several studies suggest that skill learning in rats strengthens horizontal connections in cortical layers 2 and 3 of M1 (Hess and Donoghue 1994, 1996; Donoghue, 1995; Rioult-

Pedotti et al., 1998) and that this change in connective efficacy is at least partly due to LTP-like mechanisms (see also Xerri et al., 1998; Jones et al., 1999).

Recent studies show that attention to relevant stimuli (which is an essential aspect of skill learning) can lead to synchronous activity in populations of neurons involved in the processing of the stimulus (Fries et al., 2001). Synchronous activity may be yet another way to make a population of neurons more sensitive to new excitatory inputs, and it may be instrumental in selective recruitment of neuronal ensembles contributing to the trained skill, such that connections relevant for the trained skill are selectively strengthened. Fronto-parietal mechanisms of selective attention, and associated neuromodulator systems, might play a role in the selection of relevant neuronal ensembles during early phases of learning (Willingham, 1998; Kastner and Ungerleider, 2000; Parasumaran, 2000). Enhanced connectivity in relevant ensembles may lead to enhanced correlated activity or synchrony, strengthening selective plasticity. A study by Laubach et al. (2000) in monkeys demonstrated increases in correlated firing in an ensemble of M1 motor neurons associated with increases in skilled motor performance.

Thus, the hypothesized link between attention, disinhibition, LTP-like mechanisms, activity-dependent changes in the strength of horizontal connections, and skill learning starts to find empirical support. It is important to keep in mind, however, that the details of the plasticity mechanisms may be different in different systems and may depend on the way in which plasticity is induced (e.g., Castro-Alamancos et al., 1995). Nevertheless, the main features of plasticity induced by skill learning and deafferentation are similar, and both may interact. If this idea holds true, then the stimulation of cortex deafferented due to a scotoma or amputation should reverse or prevent the passive invasion of that cortex by surrounding representations. This is exactly what a recent study has demonstrated (Lotze et al., 1999). In this study, some patients started using a myoelectrical prosthesis soon after limb amputation. These patients maintained a normal mapping of body parts on the motor cortex, and they did not show phantom pain, in contrast to patients who did not have a prosthesis. The latter patients did show substantial reorganization and suffered phantom pain. Several studies have demonstrated a correlation between the extent of the phantom limb, or the intensity of pain sensations, and cortical reorganization in motor and somatosensory cortex (Kew et al., 1994; Knecht et al., 1995; Flor et al., 1998). Furthermore, a recent study found that specific movement therapy in stroke patients improved motor function of the paretic arm and resulted in an expansion of the representation of that arm (Nudo et al., 1996; Liepert et al., 1998). Jones et al. (1999) showed a structural basis in rat cortex for the therapeutic effects of movement therapy. The data, taken together, support the idea that top-down, attentive skill learning and bottom-up, passive reorganization trigger a similar type of cortical plasticity. The finding that the development of phantom limbs can be prevented by using a prosthesis suggests the modulation of somatosensory remapping by permissive factors, which may be somatosensory or visual in nature (see Ramachandran and Blakeslee, 1998).

## A Cascade of Plastic Events at Different Time Scales?

We have discussed neural interpolation phenomena taking place on time scales varying from milliseconds to minutes, to weeks and months. The more rapid effects may underlie perceptual completion of surfaces and contours and can be demonstrated in various illusions. Fast perceptual completion effects are thought to reflect lateral interaction effects that make use of existing circuitry that is essential for normal perception. This circuitry has been formed in part through experience during early development. Although this circuitry is relatively stable during adulthood, it is subject to adaptive, plastic changes. Significant changes can occur after peripheral damage to the receptor sheet in sensory systems or during attentive learning of new skills.

In our account of these plastic events, we have stressed the interplay between thalamic afferents and lateral connections within sensory areas. Neurons in sensory cortex also receive prominent feedback from higher-order cortical regions, which partly determines the RF properties of sensory neurons. It is possible, therefore, that at least parts of the changes in RF structure that ultimately can lead to remapping of sensory space upon cortex are driven by feedback. According to a *reverse hierarchy* model proposed to explain skill learning in visual cortex (Ahissar and Hochstein, 1997), the fastest plasticity phenomena would be expected in higher-order areas, with slower—and more permanent—plasticity phenomena gradually trickling down to lower-order areas. Some of the evidence in visual cortex seems to be in agreement with this notion. Dynamic changes in RF size at a time scale of seconds were reported in V2 and V3 but not in V1 (De Weerd et al., 1995). Furthermore, motor learning studies suggest temporary activation of a number of motor structures outside M1 during initial phases of learning, which may facilitate and regulate more permanent plastic changes in M1 and related motor structures (Chapter 13). A study by Pons et al. (1988) showed much stronger plasticity phenomena in SII than in SI, but the time courses and the flexibility of the plastic changes in SI and SII remain to be tested.

While we have stressed the influences of the basal forebrain as a permissive factor for plasticity, fronto-parietal networks of attention are another potential source of feedback during skill learning and associated cortical reorganization. These and other structures may play a role in synchronizing activity in targeted populations of neurons, selected by task demands, such that learning-induced plasticity is specific (Karni and Bertini, 1997) for the learned skill.

## Conclusions

Inhibition plays an important role in normal sensory function. Disinhibition of a cortical region leads to the loss of normal RF properties and to RF expansion. Disinhibition can alter perception, as during the perceptual filling-in of an artificial scotoma. The adaptation of inhibitory inputs, due to retinal stabilization of the image over several seconds, permits previously ineffective excitatory inputs to drive neurons whose RFs are contained within the artificial scotoma, leading to perceptual filling-in. We have argued that dynamic sensory processing and filling-in reflect short-term, functional neuronal interpolation in sensory cortex, whereas long-term changes in sensory input (or motor use) trigger long-term neural interpolation (resulting in reorganization). One common feature of both processes is local disinhibition, and it has therefore been proposed that the maintenance of conditions that normally induce short-term neural interpolation can result in long-term neural interpolation processes and remodeling of cortical organiza-

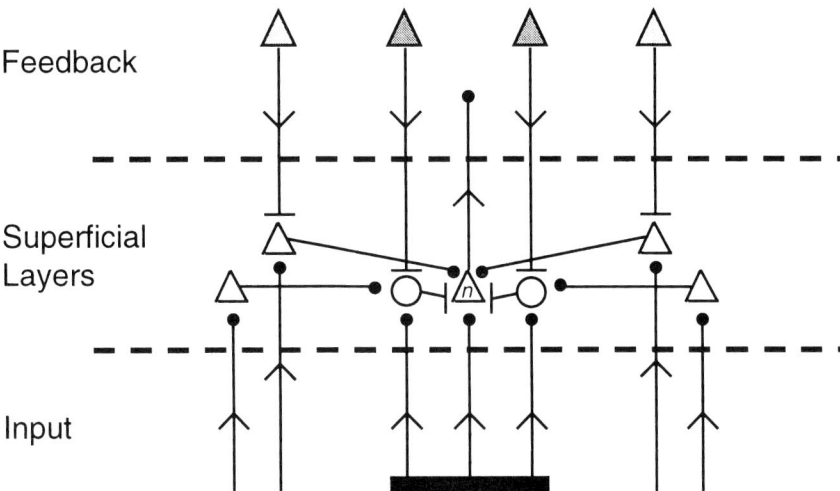

**Figure 15-3.** Hypothetical schematic diagram of cortical circuits involved in reorganization through disinhibition. Triangles represent pyramidal projection neurons. Large open circles represent inhibitory interneurons. Neurons whose axon ends in a small dot make an excitatory connection, and neurons whose axon ends in a small bar make an inhibitory connection. Open triangles are pyramidal neurons in superficial cortical layers, receiving (thalamic) feedforward input, lateral inputs through horizontal connections and interneurons, and feedback. Modulations of inhibition induced by deafferentation, perceptual completion, and skill learning are illustrated for the pyramidal neuron labeled $n$. Blocking afferent input (black horizontal bar) leads to a reduction of activity and of inhibition, such that remote excitatory inputs can start to drive neuron $n$. Because long-range lateral excitatory connections often occur between neurons with similar tuning properties (McGuire et al., 1991), unmasking of excitatory connections can lead to a transfer of these tuning properties and related aspects of cortical organization into the deafferented region. Inhibitory neurons do not always receive direct thalamic input, but for simplicity, this has not been taken into account in this diagram. During perceptual completion, inhibitory input or feedback from neural networks involved in representing the boundary between the artificial scotoma and the background prevents lateral spread of activity (light gray pyramidal neurons on the left and right). Adaptation of boundary representations reduces these inhibitory influences, causing remote excitatory inputs to drive neuron $n$. Attention may cause an enhancement of inhibitory feedback inputs (dark gray triangles) onto inhibitory circuitry, leading to disinhibition and promotion of cortical plasticity.

tion. After termination of remodeling, rewired cortex in primary and other sensory areas may become a substrate for fast neural interpolation through deafferented regions. Cortical reorganization induced by skill learning may be facilitated by a state of disinhibition promoted by mechanisms of attention. Thus, the finding that a balance between excitation and inhibition in neural circuits can be manipulated just as well by bottom-up factors such blocking of afferent input, and by cognitive factors such as attention, reveals the interweaving of mechanisms that support seemingly unrelated aspects of behavior, such as perceptual completion, recovery of function after injury, and skill learning (Fig 15-3).

The literature on perceptual filling-in, on deafferentation, RF expansions, and cortical reorganizations, and on skill learning and attention has developed into strong but separate traditions of research, further divided among the different sensory modalities and the motor system. By contrast, the approach of this book was to investigate the relationships between mechanisms involved in perceptual completion, cortical remodeling or remapping, attention, and skill learning. Apart from a conceptual enhancement of our understanding of each of those phenomena, this approach may help prescribe interventions after accidental injury designed to strengthen desirable aspects of cortical reorganization and to prevent undesirable side effects (Ziemann et al., 1998; Jones et al., 1999). Ultimately, such interventions may become applicable to enhance skill learning in a variety of circumstances relevant to our daily lives.

## References

Ahissar E, Vaadia E, Ahissar M, Bergman H, Arieli A, and Abeles M (1992) Dependence of cortical plasticity on correlated activity of single neurons and on behavioral context. *Science* 257:1412–1415.

Ahissar M and Hochstein S (1993) Attentional control of early perceptual learning. *Proc Natl Acad Sci USA* 90:5718–5722.

Ahissar M and Hochstein S (1997) Task difficulty and the specificity of perceptual learning. *Nature* 387:401–406.

Akhtar ND and Land PW (1991) Activity-dependent regulation of glutamic acid decarboxylase in the rat barrel cortex: Effects of neonatal versus adult sensory deprivation. *J Comp Neurol* 307:200–213.

Allard T, Clark SA, Jenkins WM, and Merzenich MM (1991) Reorganization of somatosensory area 3b representations in adult owl monkeys after digital syndactyly. *J Neurophysiol* 66:1048–1058.

Allman J, Miezin F, and McGuinness E (1985) Direction- and velocity-specific responses from beyond the classical receptive field in the middle temporal visual area (MT). *Perception* 14:105–126.

Alloway KD and Burton H (1991) Differential effects of GABA and bicuculline on rapidly- and slowly-adapting neurons in primary somatosensory cortex of primates. *Exp Brain Res* 85:598–610.

Alloway KD, Rosenthal P, and Burton H (1989) Quantitative measurements of receptive field changes during antagonism of GABAergic transmission in primary somatosensory cortex of cats. *Exp Brain Res* 78:514–532.

Arckens L, Eysel UT, Vanderhaeghen JJ, Orban GA, and Vandesande F (1998) Effect of sensory deprivation on the GABAergic circuitry of the adult cat visual system. *Neuroscience* 83:381–391.

Arckens L, Schweigart G, Qu Ying, Wouters G, Pow DV, Vandesande F, Eysel UT, and Orban GA (2000) Cooperative changes in GABA, glutamate and activity levels: The missing link in cortical plasticity. *Eur J Neurosci* 12:4222–4232.

Armstrong-James M, Diamond ME, and Ebner FF (1994) An innocuous bias in whisker use in adult rats modifies receptive fields of barrel cortex neurons. *J Neurosci* 14:6978–6991.

Armstrong-James M, Fox K, and Das-Gupta A (1992) Flow of excitation within rat barrel cortex on striking single vibrissae. *J Neurophysiol* 68:1356–1358.

Bear MF and Abraham WC (1996) Long-term depression in the hippocampus. *Annu Rev Neurosci* 19:437–462.

Benevento LA, Creutzfeldt OD, and Kuhnt U (1972) Significance of intracortical inhibition in the visual cortex. *Nature* 238:124–126.

Benson DL, Huntsman MM, and Jones EG (1994) Activity-dependent changes in GAD and preprotachykinin mRNAs in visual cortex of adult monkeys. *Cereb Cortex* 4:40–51.

Billock VA (1997) Very short-term visual memory via reverberation: A role for the cortico-thalamic excitatory circuit in temporal filling-in during blinks and saccades? *Vision Res* 37:949–953.

Blakemore C and Tobin EA (1972) Lateral inhibition between orientation detectors in the cat's visual cortex. *Exp Brain Res* 15:439–440.

Bliss TV and Lomo T (1973) Long-lasting potentiation of synaptic transmission in the dentate area of the anaesthetized rabbit following stimulation of the perforant path. *J Physiol* 232:331–356.

Bolz J, Gilbert CD, and Wiesel TN (1989) Pharmacological analysis of cortical circuitry. *Trends Neurosci* 12:292–296.

Buonomano DV and Merzenich MM (1998) Cortical plasticity: From synapses to maps. *Annu Rev Neurosci* 21:149–186.

Butefisch CM, Davis BC, Wise SP, Sawaki L, Kopylev L, Classen J, and Cohen LG (2000) Mechanisms of use-dependent plasticity in the human motor cortex. *Proc Natl Acad Sci USA* 97:3661–3665.

Calford MB and Tweedale R (1988) Immediate and chronic changes in responses of somatosensory cortex in adult flying fox after digit amputation. *Nature* 332:446–448.

Calford MB and Tweedale R (1991) C-fibres provide a source of masking inhibition to primary somatosensory cortex. *Proc R Soc Lond B Biol Sci* 243:269–275.

Castro-Alamancos MA, Donoghue JP, and Connors BW (1995) Different forms of plasticity in somatosensory and motor areas of the neocortex. *J Neurosci* 15:5324–5333.

Chino YM, Smith EL 3rd, Kaas JH, Sasaki Y, and Cheng H (1995) Receptive-field properties of deafferentated visual cortical neurons after topographic map reorganization in adult cats. *J Neurosci* 15:2417–2433.

Connors BW, Malenka RC, and Silva LR (1988) Two inhibitory postsynaptic potentials, and $GABA_A$ and $GABA_B$ receptor-mediated responses in neocortex of rat and cat. *J Physiol* 406:443–468.

Creutzfeldt OD, Kuhnt U, and Benevento LA (1974) An intracellular analysis of visual cortical neurones to moving stimuli: Responses in a co-operative neuronal network. *Exp Brain Res* 21:251–274.

Dannenbring GL (1976) Perceived auditory continuity with alternately rising and falling frequency transitions. *Can J Psychol* 30:99–114.

Darian-Smith C and Gilbert CD (1994) Axonal sprouting accompanies functional reorganization in adult cat striate cortex. *Nature* 368:737–740.

Darian-Smith C, and Gilbert CD (1995) Topographic reorganizartion in the striate cortex of the adult cat and monkey is cortically mediated. *J Neurosci* 15:1631–1647.

Das A and Gilbert CD (1995) Long-range horizontal connections and their role in cortical reorganization revealed by optical recording of cat primary cortex. *Nature* 375:780–784.

DeFelipe J, Conley M, and Jones EG (1986) Long-range focal collateralization of axons arising from cortico-cortical cells in monkey sensory-motor cortex. *J Neurosci* 6:3749–3766.

Desimone R and Schein SJ (1987) Visual properties of neurons in area V4 of the macaque: Sensitivity to stimulus form. *J Neurophysiol* 57:835–868.

De Weerd P, Gattass R, Desimone R, and Ungerleider LG (1995) Responses of cells in monkey visual cortex during perceptual filling-in of an artificial scotoma. *Nature* 377:731–734.

Diamond ME, Armstrong-James M, and Ebner FF (1993) Experience-dependent plasticity in adult rat barrel cortex. *Proc Natl Acad Sci USA* 90:2082–2086.

Doetsch GS (1997) Progressive changes in cutaneous trigger zones for sensation referred to a phantom hand: A case report and review with implication for cortical reorganization. *Somatosens Mot Res* 14:6–16.

Doetsch GS, Norelle A, Mark EK, Standage GP, Lu SM, and Lin RC (1993) Immunoreactivity for GAD and three peptides in somatosensory cortex and thalamus of the raccoon. *Brain Res Bull* 31:553–563.

Donoghue JP (1995) Plasticity of adult sensorimotor representations. *Curr Opin Neurobiol* 5:749–754.

Donoghue JP and Sanes JN (1987) Peripheral nerve injury in developing rats reorganizes representation pattern in motor cortex. *Proc Natl Acad Sci USA* 84:1123–1126.

Douglas RJ, Martin KAC, and Whitteridge D (1989) A canonical microcircuit for neocortex. *Neural Comput* 1:480–488.

Elbert T, Pantev C, Wienbruch C, Rockstroh B, and Taub E (1995) Increased cortical representation of the fingers of the left hand in string players. *Science* 270:305–307.

Enroth-Cugell C and Robson JG (1966) The contrast sensitivity of retinal ganglion cells of the cat. *J Physiol* 187:517–552.

Eysel UT, Shevelev IA, Lazareva NA, and Sharaev GA (1998) Orientation tuning and receptive field structure in cat striate neurons during local blockade of intracortical inhibition. *Neuroscience* 84:25–36.

Field DJ, Hayes A, and Hess RF (2000) The roles of polarity and symmetry in the perceptual grouping of contour fragments. *Spat Vis* 13:51–66.

Fiorani M Jr, Rosa MG, Gattass R, and Rocha-Miranda CE (1992) Dynamic surrounds of receptive fields in primate striate cortex: A physiological basis for perceptual completion? *Proc Natl Acad Sci USA* 89:8547–8551.

Flor H, Elbert T, Muhlnickel W, Pantev C, Wienbruch C, and Taub E (1998) Cortical reorganization and phantom limb phenomena in congenital and traumatic upper-extremity amputees. *Exp Brain Res* 119:205–212.

Fregnac Y and Shulz DE (1999) Activity-dependent regulation of receptive field properties of cat area 17 by supervised Hebbian learning. *J Neurobiol* 41:69–82.

Freund TF and Meskenaite V (1992) Gamma-aminobutyric acid–containing basal forebrain neurons innervate inhibitory interneurons in the neocortex. *Proc Natl Acad Sci USA* 89:738–742.

Fries P, Reynolds JH, Rorie AE, and Desimone R (2001) Modulation of oscillatory neuronal synchronization by selective visual attention. *Science* 291:1560–1563.

Gardner EP and Costanzos RM (1980a) Spatial integration of multipoint stimuli in primary somatosensory cortical receptive fields of alert monkeys. *J Neurophysiol* 43:420–443.

Gardner EP and Costanzos RM (1980b) Temporal integration of multipoint stimuli in primary somatosensory cortical receptive fields of alert monkeys. *J Neurophysiol* 43:444–468.

Gerrits HJM and Vendrik AJH (1970) Simultaneous contrast, filling-in process and information processing in man's visual system. *Exp Brain Res* 11:411–440.

Gilbert CD and Wiesel TN (1989) Columnar specificity of intrinsic cortico-cortical connections in cat visual cortex. *J Neurosci* 9:2432–2442.

Gilbert CD and Wiesel TN (1992) Receptive field dynamics in adult primary visual cortex. *Nature* 356:150–152.

Gritti I, Mainville L, and Jones BE (1993) Codistribution of GABA- with acetylcholine-synthesizing neurons in the basal forebrain of the rat. *J Comp Neurol* 329:438–457.

Gupta A, Wang Y, and Markram H (2000) Organizing principles for a diversity of GABAergic interneurons and synapses in the neocortex. *Science* 287:273–278.

Hebb D (1949) *The Organization of Behavior: A Neuropsychological Theory.* New York: John Wiley & Sons.

Heitger F, von der Heydt R, Peterhans E, Rosenthaler L, and Kübler O (1998) Simulation of neural contour mechanisms: Representing anomalous contours. *Image Vis Comput* 16:407–421.

Hendry SH, Fuchs J, de Blas AL, and Jones EG (1990) Distribution and plasticity of immunocytochemically localized GABA receptors in adult monkey visual cortex. *J Neurosci* 10:2438–2450.

Hendry SH, Schwark HD, Jones EG, and Yan J (1987) Numbers and proportions of GABA-immunoreactive neurons in different areas of monkey cerebral cortex. *J Neurosci* 7:1503–1519.

Hess G, Aizenman CD, and Donoghue JP (1996) Conditions for the induction of long-term potentiation in layer II/III horizontal connections of the rat motor cortex. *J Neurophysiol* 75:1765–1778.

Hess G and Donoghue JP (1994) Long-term potentiation of horizontal connections provides a mechanism to reorganize cortical motor maps. *J Neurophysiol* 71:2543–2547.

Hess G and Donoghue JP (1996) Long-term depression of horizontal connections in rat motor cortex. *Eur J Neurosci* 8:658–665.

Hicks TP and Dykes RW (1983) Receptive field size for certain neurons in primary somatosensory cortex is determined by GABA-mediated intracortical inhibition. *Brain Res* 274:160–164.

Hubel DH and Wiesel TN (1959) Receptive fields of single neurons in the cat's striate cortex. *J Physiol* 148:574–619.

Hubel DH and Wiesel TN (1962) Receptive fields, binocular interaction, and functional architecture in the cat's visual cortex. *J Physiol* 160:106–154.

Huntley GW and Jones EG (1991) The emergence of architectonic field structure and areal borders in developing monkey sensorimotor cortex. *Neuroscience* 44:287–310.

Hupe JN, James AC, Girard P, and Bullier J (2001) Response modulations by static texture surround in area V1 of the macaque monkey do not depend on feedback connections from V2. *J Neurophysiol* 85:146–163.

Iijima T, Witter MP, Ichikawa M, Tominaga T, Kajiwara R, and Matsumoto G (1996)

Entorhinal–hippocampal interactions revealed by real-time imaging. *Science* 272:1176–1179.

Jones EG (1993) GABAergic neurons and their role in cortical plasticity in primates. *Cereb Cortex* 3:361–372.

Jones EG (2000) Cortical and subcortical contributions to activity-dependent plasticity in primate somatosensory cortex. *Annu Rev Neurosci* 23:1–37.

Jones HE, Grieve KL, Wang W, and Sillito AM (2001) Surround suppression in primate V1. *J Neurophysiol* 86:2011–2028.

Jones TA, Chu CJ, Grande, LA, and Gregory A (1999) Motor skills training enhances lesion-induced structural plasticity in the motor cortex of adults rats. *J Neurosci* 19:10153–10163.

Kaas J (1995) How cortex reorganizes. *Nature* 375:735–736.

Kandel ER (2000) Cellular mechanisms of learning and the biological basis of individuality. In: Kandel ER, Schwartz JH, Jessell TM (eds), *Principles of Neural Science.* New York: McGraw-Hill Book Companies, pp 1247–1277.

Kandel ER, Jessel TM, and Sanes JR (2000) Sensory experience and the fine-tuning of synaptic connections. In: Kandel ER, Schwartz JH, and Jessell TM (eds), *Principles of Neural Science.* New York: McGraw-Hill Book Companies, pp 1115–1130.

Karl A, Birbaumer N, Lutzenberger W, Cohen LG, and Flor H (2001) Reorganization of motor and somatosensory cortex in upper extremity amputees with phantom limb pain. *J Neurosci* 21:3609–3618.

Karni A and Bertini G (1997) Learning perceptual skills: Behavioral probes into adult cortical plasticity. *Curr Opin Neurobiol* 7:530–535.

Karni A and Sagi D (1991) Where practice makes perfect in texture discrimination: Evidence for primary visual cortex plasticity. *Proc Natl Acad Sci USA* 88:4966–4970.

Karni A and Sagi D (1993) The time course of learning a visual skill. *Nature* 365:250–252.

Karni A, Tanne D, Rubenstein BS, Askenasy JJ, and Sagi S (1994) Dependence on REM sleep of overnight improvement of a perceptual skill. *Science* 265:679–682.

Kastner S and Ungerleider LG (2000) Mechanisms of visual attention in the human cortex. *Annu Rev Neurosci* 23:315–341.

Katz LC and Shatz CJ (1996) Synaptic activity and the construction of cortical circuits. *Science* 274:1133–1138.

Kew JJM, Ridding MC, Rothwell JC, Passingham RE, Leigh PN, Sooriakumaran S, Frackowiak RSJ, and Brooks DJ (1994) Reorganization of cortical blood flow and transcranial magnetic stimulation maps in human subjects after upper limb amputation. *J Neurophysiol* 72:2517–2524.

Kilgard MP and Merzenich MM (1998) Cortical map reorganization enabled by nucleus basalis activity. *Science* 279:1714–1717.

Knecht S, Henningsen H, Elbert T, Flor H, Hohling C, Pantev C, Birbaumer N, and Taub E (1995) Cortical reorganization in human amputees and mislocalization of painful stimuli to the phantom limb. *Neurosci Lett* 201:262–264.

Knierim JJ and Van Essen DC (1992) Neuronal responses to static texture patterns in area V1 of the alert macaque monkey. *J Neurophysiol* 67:961–980.

Komatsu H, Kinoshita M, and Murakami I (2000) Neural responses in the retinotopic representation of the blind spot in the macaque V1 to stimuli for perceptual filling-in. *J Neurosci* 20:9310–9319.

Korodi K and Toldi J (1998) Does the cortical representation of body parts follow both injury to the related sensory peripheral nerve and its regeneration? *Neuroreport* 9:771–774.

Krnjevic K (1984) Some functional consequences of GABA uptake by brain cells. *Neurosci Lett* 47:283–287.
Kyriazi H, Carvell GE, Brumberg JC, and Simons DJ (1998) Laminar differences in bicuculline methiodide's effects on cortical neurons in the rat whisker/barrel system. *Somatosens Mot Res* 15:146–156.
Laskin SE and Spencer WA (1979) Cutaneous masking. II. Geometry of excitatory and inhibitory receptive fields of single units in somatosensory cortex of the cat. *J Neurophysiol* 42:1061–1082.
Laubach M, Wessberg J, and Nicolelis MA (2000) Cortical ensemble activity increasingly predicts behaviour outcomes during learning of a motor task. *Nature* 405:567–571.
Levitt JB and Lund JS (1997) Contrast dependence of contextual effects in primate visual cortex. *Nature* 387:73–76.
Levitt JB, Yoshioka T, and Lund JS (1994) Intrinsic cortical connections in macaque visual area V2: Evidence for interaction between different visual streams. *J Comp Neurol* 342:551–570.
Li CX, Waters RS, Oladehin A, Johnson EF, McCandlish CA, and Dykes RW (1994) Large unresponsive zones appear in cat somatosensory cortex immediately after ulnar nerve cut. *Can J Neurol Sci* 21:233–247.
Li YM, Qu Y, Vandenbussche E, Arckens L, and Vandesande F (2001) Analysis of extracellular γ-aminobutyric acid, glutamate and aspartate in cat visual cortex by in vivo microdialysis and capillary electrophoresis-laser induced fluorescence detection. *J Neurosci Methods* 105:211–215.
Liepert J, Bauder H, Sommer M, Miltner WHR, Dettmers C, and Weiller C (1998) Effects of constraint induced movement therapy on motor cortex organization in chronic stroke patients. *Neuroimage* 7:S24 (4th International Conference on Functional Mapping of the Human Brain).
Lotze M, Grodd W, Birbaumer N, Erb M, Huse E, and Flor H (1999) Does use of a myoelectric prosthesis prevent cortical reorganization and phantom limb pain? *Nat Neurosci* 2:501–502.
Lund JS, Yoshioka T, and Levitt JB (1993) Comparison of intrinsic connectivity in different areas of macaque monkey cerebral cortex. *Cereb Cortex* 3:148–162.
Maffei L and Fiorentini A (1976) The unresponsive regions of visual cortical receptive fields. *Vision Res* 16:1131–1139.
McGuire BA, Gilbert CD, Rivlin PK, and Wiesel TN (1991) Targets of horizontal connections in macaque primary visual cortex. *J Comp Neurol* 305:370–392.
Mercado E, Bao S, Orduna I, Gluck MA, and Merzenich MM (2001) Basal forebrain stimulation changes cortical sensitivities in complex sound. *Neuroreport* 12:2283–2287.
Merzenich MM and Jenkins WM (1993) Reorganization of cortical representations of the hand following alterations of skin inputs induced by nerve injury, skin island transfers, and experience. *J Hand Ther* 6:89–104.
Merzenich MM, Nelson RJ, Stryker MP, Cynader MS, Schoppmann A, and Zook JM (1984) Somatosensory cortical map changes following digit amputation in adult monkeys. *J Comp Neurol* 224:591–605.
Mountcastle VB and Powell TP (1959) Neural mechanisms subserving cutaneous sensibility with special reference to the role of afferent inhibition in sensory perception and discrimination. *Bull Johns Hopkins Hosp* 105:201–232.
Nelson JI and Frost B (1978) Orientation selective inhibition from beyond the classical receptive field. *Brain Res* 139:359–365.
Nudo RJ, Wise BM, SiFuentes F, and Milliken GW (1996) Neural substrates for the ef-

fects of rehabilitative training on motor recovery after ischemic infarct. *Science* 272:1791–1794.

Parasumaran R (Ed) (2000) *The Attentive Brain.* Cambridge, MA: MIT Press.

Park TJ and Pollak GD (1994) Azimuthal receptive fields are shaped by GABAergic inhibition in the inferior colliculus of the mustache bat. *J Neurophysiol* 72:1080–1102.

Pascual-Leone A, Peris M, Tormos JM, Pasucal-Leone AP, and Catala MD (1996) Reorganization of human cortical motor output maps following traumatic forearm amputation. *Neuroreport* 7:2068–2070.

Pernberg J, Jirmann KU, and Eysel UT (1998) Structure and dynamics of receptive fields in the visual cortex of the cat (area 18) and the influence of GABAergic inhibition. *Eur J Neurosci* 10:3596–3606.

Pettet MW and Gilbert CD (1992) Dynamic changes in receptive-field size in cat primary visual cortex. *Proc Natl Acad Sci USA* 89:8366–8370.

Pinaud R, Penner MR, Robertson HA, and Currie RW (2001) Upregulation of the immediate early gene arc in the brains of rats exposed to environmental enrichment: Implications for molecular plasticity. *Mol Brain Res* 91:50–56.

Pinaud R, Tremere LA, Penner MR, Hess FF, Robertson HA, and Currie RW (2002) Complexity of sensory environment drives the expression of candidate-plasticity gene, nerve growth factor induced-A. *Neuroscience* 112:573–582.

Pons TP, Garraghty PE, and Mishkin M (1988) Lesion-induced plasticity in the second somatosensory cortex of adult macaques. *Proc Natl Acad Sci USA* 85:5279–5281.

Pons TP, Garraghty PE, Ommaya AK, Kaas JH, Taub E, and Mishkin, M (1991) Massive cortical reorganization after sensory deafferentation in adult macaques. *Science* 252:1857–1860.

Ramachandran VS and Blakeslee S (1998) *Phantoms in the Brain.* New York: William Morrow and Company.

Rasmusson DD (1982) Reorganization of raccoon somatosensory cortex following removal of the fifth digit. *J Comp Neurol* 205:313–326.

Rasmusson DD, Louw DF, and Northgrave SA (1993) The immediate effects of peripheral denervation on inhibitory mechanisms in the somatosensory thalamus. *Somatosens Mot Res* 10:69–80.

Recanzone GH, Merzenich MM, Jenkins WM, Grajski KA, and Dinse HR (1992) Topographical reorganization of the hand representation in cortical area 3b of owl monkeys trained in a frequency discrimination task. *J Neurophysiol* 67:1031–1056.

Recanzone GH, Schreiner GE, and Merzenich MM (1993) Plasticity in the frequency representation of primary auditory cortex following discrimination training in adult owl monkeys. *J Neurosci* 13:87–103.

Rioult-Pedotti MS, Friedman D, and Donoghue JP (2000) Learning-induced LTP in neocortex. *Science* 290:533–536.

Rioult-Pedotti MS, Friedman D, Hess G, and Donoghue JP (1998) Strengthening of horizontal connections following skill learning. *Nat Neurosci* 1:230–234.

Robertson D and Irvine DRF (1989) Plasticity of frequency organization in auditory cortex of guinea pigs with partial unilateral deafness. *J Comp Neurol* 282:456–471.

Rosier AM, Arckens L, Demeulemeester H, Orban GA, Eysel UT, Wu YL, and Vandesande F (1995) Effect of sensory deafferentation on immunoreactivity of GABAergic cells and on GABA receptors in the adult cat visual cortex. *J Comp Neurol* 359:476–489.

Safran AB, Achmard O, Duret F, and Landis T (1999) The "thin man" phenomenon: A sign of cortical plasticity following inferior homonymous paracentral scotomas. *Br J Ophthalmol* 83:137–142.

Sceniak MP, Hawken MJ, and Shapley R (2001) Visual spatial characterization of macaque V1 neurons. *J Neurophysiol* 85:1873–1887.
Schein JJ and Desimone R (1990) Spectral properties of V4 neurons in the macaque. *J Neurosci* 10:3369–3389.
Schwark HD and Jones EG (1989) The distribution of intrinsic corical axons in area 3b of cat primary somatosensory cortex. *Exp Brain Res* 78:501–513.
Sillito AM (1975a) The effectiveness of bicuculline as an antagonist of GABA and visually evoked inhibition in the cat's striate cortex. *J Physiol* 250:287–304.
Sillito AM (1975b) The contribution of inhibitory mechanisms to the receptive field properties of neurones in the striate cortex of the cat. *J Physiol* 250:305–329.
Sillito AM (1977) Inhibitory processes underlying the directional specificity of simple, complex and hypercomplex cells in the cat's visual cortex. *J Physiol* 271:699–720.
Sillito AM (1979) Inhibitory mechanisms influencing complex cell orientation selectivity and their modification at high resting discharge levels. *J Physiol* 289:33–53.
Sugita Y (1997) Neuronal correlates of auditory induction in the cat cortex. *Neuroreport* 8:1155–1159.
Tanifuji M, Sugiyama T, and Murase K (1994) Horizontal propagation of excitation in rat visual cortical slices revealed by optical imaging. *Science* 266:1057–1059.
Tremere L, Hicks TP, and Rasmusson DD (2001a) Role of inhibition in cortical reorganization of the adult raccoon revealed by microiontophoretic blockade of GABA(A) receptors. *J Neurophysiol* 86:94–103.
Tremere L, Hicks TP, and Rasmusson DD (2001b) Expansion of receptive fields in raccoon somatosensory cortex in vivo by GABA(A) receptor antagonism: Implications for cortical reorganization. *Exp Brain Res* 136:447–455.
Trepel C and Racine RJ (1998) Long-term potentiation in the neocortex of the adult freely moving rat. *Cereb Cortex* 8:719–729.
von der Heydt R, Peterhans E, and Baumgartner G (1984) Illusory contours and cortical neuron responses. *Science* 224:1260–1262.
Wartan SW, Hamann W, Wedley JR, and McColl I (1997) Phantom pain and sensation among British veteran amputees. *Br J Anaesth* 78: 652–659.
Webster HH, Rasmusson DD, Dykes RW, Schliebs R, Schober W, Bruckner G, and Biesold D (1991) Long-term enhancement of evoked potentials in raccoon somatosensory cortex following co-activation of the nucleus basalis of Meynert complex and cutaneous receptors. *Brain Res* 545:292–296.
Weiss T, Miltner WH, Huonker R, Friedel R, Schmidt I, and Taub E (2000) Rapid functional plasticity of the somatosensory cortex after finger amputation. *Exp Brain Res* 134:199–203.
Willingham DB (1998) A neurophysiological theory of motor skill learning. *Psychol Rev* 105:558–584.
Winfield DA, Brooke RNL, Sloper JJ, and Powell TPS (1981) A combined Golgi electron microscope study of the synapses made by the proximal axon and recurrent collaterals of a pyramidal cell in the somatic sensory cortex of the monkey. *Neuroscience* 6:1217–1230.
Wisden W, Errington ML, Williams S, Dunnett SB, Waters C, Hitchcock D, Evan G, Bliss TV, and Hunt SP (1990) Differential expression of immediate early genes in the hippocampus and spinal cord. *Neuron* 4:603–614.
Xerri C, Merzenich MM, Peterson BE, and Jenkins W (1998) Plasticity of primary somatosensory cortex paralleling sensorimotor skill recovery from stroke in adult monkeys. *J Neurophysiol* 79:2119–2148.

Xing J and Gerstein GL (1994) Simulation of dynamic receptive fields in primary visual cortex. *Vision Res* 34:1901–1911.

Xing J and Gerstein GL (1996) Networks with lateral connectivity. I. Dynamic properties mediated by the balance of intrinsic excitation and inhibition. *J Neurophysiol* 75:184–199.

Yuste R and Sur M (1999) Development and plasticity of the cerebral cortex: From molecules to maps. *J Neurobiol* 41:1–6.

Ziemann U, Corwell B, and Cohen LG (1998) Modulation of plasticity in human motor cortex after forearm ischemic nerve block. *J Neurosci* 18:1115–1123.

# Index

Abraham, W.C., 308
Abrams, P.L., 163
Achard, O., 217
Adams, M.M., 267, 268f, 283
Adaptation, delayed, 83, 84, 85
Albright, T.D., 201
Allard, T., 284
Alpert, N.M., 261
Altenmüller, E., 287, 289
Ambler, J.S., 196
Amodal completion, 39, 41
   attention spreading, modal and, 144–48, 145f
   binocular and monocular filled-in surfaces and, 33
   blind spot filling-in v., xv–xvii
   decision of, xvi
   definition of, 33, 39
   depth and, 146–47
   FACADE and, 18, 33, 34
   functional roles similar to modal and, 132–34, 133f
   illusory color/brightness and, 145f, 146–47
   isolating filling-in and modal v., 130–31
   Kanizsa square and, 130f
   Metelli Rule and, 142–43, 142f, 144
   occluded regions and, 132, 135
   ON- and OFF-filling-in, 168
   parallel vision and, 134, 135, 136f, 137, 139, 140, 141, 144
   pop-out stimulus and, 135, 136f, 137
   preattentive, 135, 136f, 137, 138f, 139
   shape completion process and, 134
   visual attention and, 134
   visual-search tasks, modal and, 135, 136f, 137–39, 138f, 140f, 141–44, 142f, 148
Amsler grid, 98, 98f
Anchoring, 25
Anderson, J.R., 261

Anisotropic diffusion, 20, 22
Anosognosia, xx
ANOVA (analysis of variance) method, 261
Anson, R., 183
Anstis, S., 82
Anton's syndrome, 207
Aphasia, 289
Apperceptive completion of gestalt, 208
Arckens, L., 304, 306
Arnold, J.B., 261
Arrington, K.F., 22, 163
Artificial scotoma, xi, 198, 303
   attention and, 51
   creation of, xii
   filling in of, xv, 99, 217–18
   neural interpolation and, 300f, 301–2
   neurophysical mechanism of, xii–xiii, 82, 82f, 84
   retinal lesions and, 198
   RF and, 300f, 301, 302, 303, 312–13
   stablized images and, 59
   as temporary remapping, xiii
   texture filling-in and, 82, 82f, 84, 96–97
   (delayed) texture filling-in of, 92, 93f, 94, 95
Askenasy, J.J., 310
Association fields, 154–55
Association processing, 202
Asymmetry between near and far, 26, 28, 32, 33
Attention
   depth and, 146–47
   feature binding (color), 110
   for figure-ground segregation and texture filling-in, 90–92
   modal and amodal completion and, 134, 135
   modal and amodal completion and spreading of, 144–48, 145f

Attention (*Continued*)
  pathological visual completion and biased spatial, 218–19, 220*f*
  between physically present fragments, 146
  qualia and, xvii
  between regions, 144, 145*f*, 146
  skill learning, disinhibition and, 309–11
  visual cortex and, 50–51
Auditory cortical, human. *See* Plasticity, human auditory cortical
Auditory evoked magnetic fields (AEF), 231, 242.244
Auditory illusion, 242
Azzi, J.C.B., 180–81

Backward masking, 60–61, 62*f*
Ballard, D.H., 155
Bara-Jimenez, W., 287
Barbay, S., 265, 272
Barbieri, S., 289
Baseler, H., 46
Battersby, W.S., 212*f*
Baumann, R., 181
Baumgartner, G., 41
BCS. *See* Boundary Contour System (BCS)
Bear, M.F., 308
Benda, B.J., 256
Bender, M.B., 212*f*, 213
Benson, R.R., 44
Bernardes, R.F., 181
Bicuculline methiodide (BMI), 297, 306
Billock, V.A., 301–2
Binocular cortical neurons, 191–92, 192*f*
Binocular fusion, 26, 29*f*
Bipole cells, 30, 31*f*, 181
Bizzi, E., 256
Blair, N., 189, 191
Blind spot, 202, 210, 307
  amodal completion v. filling-in, xv–xvii
  brightness/luminance and, 65
  color and, 106, 108, 109, 110, 111
  filling-in, xiv–xv, xv, 4, 22, 59, 177–80, 178*f*, 179*f*, 184
  interpolation, 38
  irrevocable, qualia quality of, xviii
  irrevocable sensory representation and, xix
  large RF over, 42
  modal completion and, 128–29, 130*f*
  monocular vision and, 1, 128–29
  natural, xi–xii, xiii, xiv, xix, 38, 94–95, 97, 177
  neural machinery for, xv
  peripheral visual field and, 129
  photoreceptors devoid in, 1
  in retina, 16, 21, 177
  sewn up and, 129, 202
  shrinkage of, 97
  surface interpolation and, xvi
Blindsight, 207, 216–17
Blomstrom, KJ., 255
Bolz, J., 301
Border ownership, 41, 51, 124
  coding principles, surface processing and, 152, 153*f*, 154
  figure-ground and, 154, 164–65, 170
  visual completion, spatial occlusion and, 164–67, 166*f*, 170
Border signals
  color filling-in, and surface signals, 116–20, 117*f*, 118*f*, 119*f*, 121, 122*f*, 123–24
Born, R.T., 163
Boroojerdi, B., 262, 273
Bosking, W.H., 183
Bottom-up processing, xviii, 4, 110, 156*f*, 314
Boundary Contour System (BCS), 22, 24
  boundary-gating, 31
  definition of, 19
  depth-selective, 30–32
  FCS interaction with, 28–29, 29*f*, 30–34
Boundary grouping, 152
  anisotropic diffusion, filling-in and, 20, 22
  asymmetry between near and far in, 26, 28, 32, 33
  binocular fusion, da Vinci Stereopsis and, 26, 29*f*
  bipole cells, hypercomplex cells and, 29–30, 31*f*
  boundary enrichment and, 34
  boundary invisibility and, 16, 17*f*, 18–19, 20, 33, 41, 108
  from boundary-surface complementarity to consistency, 28, 32, 34
  brightness constancy, contrast and assimilation and, 22–25, 23*f*
  FACADE, surface filling-in and, 16–28, 34
  insensitivity to contrast polarity and, 17*f*, 18
  luminance discontinuities with, 23*f*, 24
  monocular, 28–30, 29*f*
  multiple scales into multiple boundary depths and, 26–27
  object recognition v. seeing unoccluded parts and, 27–28, 27*f*
  proximity-luminance covariation and, 31
  relative depths of, 30
  size-disparity correlation and, 29–30, 29*f*, 32

three-dimensional vision, figure-ground
    separation and, 25–28, 27f, 32
  T-junctions and, 28, 30–32, 31f
Boundary processing
  boundary finding, completion and, 154–55
  coding principle, visual neural mechanism
    for surface processing and, 152, 153f,
    154
  feedback for, 151–52
Boundary pruning
  figure-ground separation influenced by,
    32–33
Boundary representations, 167, 313f
  for texture filling-in, 81–85
  texture filling-in and background penetrating failing, 91
Brady, T.J., 44
Braille, 284
Brain
  completing boundary/surface information
    in, 16
Brain imaging, functional, 223–24
Brain, processing streams of
  boundary formation with, 17f, 18–19
  complementary properties, computation
    and, 15–16, 21–22, 23, 28, 32, 34
  complex cells, 14f, 16, 18
  hierarchical resolution of uncertainty of,
    14t, 15–16, 20, 21–22
  interactions between, 15
  interblob cortical, 14f, 16, 18
  multiple stages of, 14t, 15
  specialized v. non-independent, 13, 15
  symmetry-breaking and parallel, 22
Brashers-Krug, T., 261
Bregman-Kanizsa display, 27f, 33, 34
Brewster, David, xi–xii, 129
Brightness. *See also* Discounting the illuminant; Luminance
  anchoring, 162–63
  assimilation, 23f, 24–25
  backward masking, disruption of surface
    completion and, 60–61, 62f
  cells, 79
  color, darkness and, 108
  color, illusions and, 113, 124, 125, 128
  constancy, 23f, 24, 73–74, 75f, 76
  contrast, 23f, 24, 69
  contrast v. homogenous, 87
  critical flicker fusion rate of, 66
  (perceived) depth and, 13, 20
  dichoptic and monoptic presentation for,
    61, 62f
  dwell time and spreading of, 65

  end gaps and, 30
  fast v. slow filling-in and, 66, 68
  flank modulation and, 72
  grey v. black stimulus center and, 72
  high cutoff frequency and, 68
  illumination conditions of, 74, 75f, 76
  illusory, 131, 134, 144f, 146–47
  "in phase and out phase" modulation of,
    74
  induction, 66, 67f, 68–70, 71f, 72–73, 76
  isomorphic representation not correlated to,
    59
  Kanizsa square and, 17f, 18, 32
  lateral interactions in visual cortex and,
    73–74, 75f, 76
  low (temporal) cutoff frequency and, 66,
    68, 77
  luminance modulation and, 68, 70, 72–73
  luminance sweeps, filling-in precepts and,
    63, 64f, 65
  luminance-constrast borders, start/stop filling-in and, 60
  modulation rates v. induction of, 66, 67f,
    68
  Mondrian stimuli and, 60, 74, 75f, 76
  neural responses correlated, in induction
    paradigm, 69–70, 71f, 72–73
  neurophysical investigations, filling-in and,
    69–70, 71f, 72–74, 75f, 76–77, 78f, 79
  perception, 22–25, 23f, 73–74, 75f, 76
  proximity-luminance covariation and, 31
  psychophysical investigations, filling-in
    and, 60–61, 62f, 63, 64f, 65–66, 67f,
    68–69
  scale-dependent, 66, 68
  slower/lower modulation, spatial frequency
    and larger, 66, 71f, 72–73, 77
  spatiotemporal dynamics and (dynamic) induction of, 66, 67f, 68–69, 73
  spreading activation in primary visual cortex and, 76–77, 78f, 79
  squarewave grating and, 66, 67f
  striate cortex and, 60, 69
  surface formation and, 20, 21, 69, 160
  visible, 33
  visible effect of invisible cause and, 23f,
    24–25, 108
  in (primary) visual cortex, 69–70, 71f,
    72–74, 75f, 76–77, 78f, 79
Bringuier, V., 77
Brown, T.G., 281
Buffer, short-term, xvii
Bullemer, P., 258
Bullier, J., 55

Buomomano, D.V., 308
Burstein, A.H., 273
Bütefisch, C.M., 273, 310
Byl, N.N., 282, 284

Calford, M.B., 196
Candia, V., 287–89
Cappellari, A., 289
Cartesian theater, xv
Catalan, M.J., 287
Caudal forelimb area (CFA), 265
Cerebral blood flow (rCBF), 259, 272f
Chavene, F., 77
Chino, Y.M., 189, 191
Cholinergic basal forebrain, 309–10, 312
Chong, C.D.R., 52
Churchland, P., xix
CI therapy. *See* Constraint-induced movement therapy (CI)
Clark, S.A., 284
Classen, J., 256, 257f, 258, 275
Climbing activity, 92, 93f, 94, 217, 300f
Cognitive interpretation
 of 2D displays, 4
Cohen, L.G., 256, 257f, 258, 275
Cohen, M.A., 22, 159
Color, xiv, 4–5, 17f, 76, 90, 91, 210
 constancy, 39, 120, 121
 different, of annulus, 59
 end gaps and, 30
 impairment of perception of, 5
 motion and, 13
 neon, spreading, 17f, 20, 34
 proximity-luminance covariation and, 31
 surface formation and, 19–20, 21
 without seeing, 33
Color filling-in
 afterimage, adapting color and, 125
 artificial image stabilization and, 106
 blind spot in, 106, 108, 109, 110, 111
 blurred edge v. sharp edge for, 112–13, 112f, 113f, 116, 117f, 118f, 120
 border ownership and, 124
 brightness and, 124, 125
 color selectivity, color-selective cells and, 112, 112f, 115–16, 117–18, 118f, 119f, 120–21, 123
 cortical coding of figures in, 114–16
 decay of border signals and, 123–24
 delayed, 108, 111–14, 112f, 113f
 edge cells/signals and, 115, 119f, 120, 122f, 124
 fading and, 108
 fixation and, 106, 112–13, 123, 125
 illusory (change of color and), 113, 125, 128, 131, 134, 145f, 146–47
 immediate, 111–12
 isomorphic filling-in theory for, 107, 109–10, 111, 116, 121, 123
 lateral (horizontal) connections and, 110, 111
 literature rcview for, 111–12
 neural representation v. perception and, 107–8, 108f–109f
 neural signals, behavioral responses and, 120–23, 123–125122f
 object file (bottom-up processing) and, 110
 optimal color, complementary color and, 116–17, 117f, 118f, 119–20
 with scotoma, 106, 108, 110
 surface and border signals and, 116–20, 117f, 118f, 119f, 121, 122f, 123–25
 surface filling-in and, 107
 symbolic color representation theory for, 108f, 109f, 110, 121
 texture filling-in and, 125
 theory, 108f, 109f, 110
 Troxler's effect and, 106
Commissurotomy, xiii
Complementarity, 15–16, 21–22, 23, 28, 32, 34
Completion, perceptual, 1, 5, 7, 18, 38, 39, 307
Conjunctive junction groupings, 167
Connell, J.S., 285
Consolidation, 262–63
Constraint-induced movement therapy (CI)
 for focal hand dystonia, 288–89
 for learned nonuse, 286–87, 286f
Contextual shape processing, 39–40
 attention and, 50–51
 functional neuroimaging of visual cortex and, 43–51, 44f, 45f, 47f, 49f
 Gestalt grouping, symmetry and, 39, 39f, 44, 45–47, 47f
 illusory contour shape v. stereo-defined shape and, 48, 49f
 interpolation of, 52
 isomorphic and symbolic process and, 50, 53
 object recognition and, 50, 51
 single-neuron properties in macaque cortex and, 40–43, 51–53
 surface, shape and, 47–50, 49f
Contour(s)
 cells, 156f, 157–58, 167
 cessation of, activity, 111
 completion of, 5

detection of, 181
feature, 19
fragmented circular, 158, 158f
illusory, 4, 17f, 18, 41, 44, 48, 49f, 50, 84, 158
integration, 157, 158f, 180–81
interpolation, xvi, 3, 4, 5, 41, 184
real, 39
Contrast, 89, 153f, 163
detection, 156f, 157
lateral spreading of, 168
ON- and OFF-, 160f, 161, 162, 163, 165, 166f, 168
signals, 165–66, 170
suppression, 167
Contrast polarity, 153f, 162f, 166f, 168
insensitivity to, 17f, 18
ON and OFF and, 162, 166f, 168
sensitivity to, 17f, 21
Cook, E.W., 285
Cooper, N.R., 265, 272
Cornsweet's luminance pattern
Cortical neurons, 240–41
binocular, 191–92, 192f, 198
reactivated, 197–98, 199
RF and, 198, 297–98
Cortical point-spread function, 76
Cortical system, 2–3
Cortico-cerebellar circuits, 254–55, 274
Cortico-striatal circuits, 254–55, 274
Cortico-subcortical circuits, 254
Crabbe, G., 131–32
Crago, J.E., 285
Craik-O'Brien-Cornsweet effect, 25, 161, 161f
Cytochrome oxidase (CO), 178f, 180, 196f, 201f

Da Vinci Stereopsis, 26, 34
Dale, A.M., 48, 52
Dang, N., 262
Dannenbring, G.L., 303
Darian-Smith, C., 195
Das, A., 303
Davis, B.C., 273
Davis, G., 137, 138, 138f, 139, 140f, 143f, 145f, 146
De Haan, B., 107, 110, 114
De Valois, K.K., 66
De Valois, R.L., 66
De Weerd, P., xii, 42, 46, 84, 89, 90, 91, 92, 94, 299
De Weert, C.M., 141
Deafferentation, 2, 5, 7, 295

disinhibition, attention, skill learning and, 309–11
disinhibition, remapping and, 304, 305f, 306
functional, 239–42
interpolation and, 304
movement and, 281–82, 285–86, 302
permanent, 6, 303–4
phantom limbs, amputation and, 302
reorganization, auditory cortex and, 232–33, 232f, 237, 239–42, 247
retinal injury and, 81
DeHaan, B., 83
Demeulemeester, H., 304
Dennett, D.C., xiii, xv, xix, 4, 22, 85
DePriest, D.D., 200
Depth, 30
attention, modal/amodal completion and, 146–47
BCS, 30–32
brightness and, 13, 20
FCS, 30–31
figure-ground separation and relative, 30
multiple, boundary, 26–27
Desimone, R., 84, 89, 91, 92, 94, 97, 299
Dextromethorphan (DM), 273
Difference of Gaussians (DOG), 298
Diffusion
as computational metaphor, 160–61, 160f
Digit (finger) training task, 265, 266f
Dinse, H.R., 290
Dipole moment/location, 234, 237, 240, 241f, 243f, 245, 246f, 247n1
Direction-sensitive cells, 164
Discounting the illuminant, 29f
constraints of neural filling-in mechanisms, surface and, 161–63, 162f
in surface filling-in, 19–20, 21–22, 23f, 24, 31
Disinhibition
attention, skill learning and, 309–11, 312–14
desegregation and, 308–9
GABAergic modulations on neural interpolation and long-term effects on, 303–4, 305f, 306–9
GABAergic modulations on neural interpolation and short-term effects on, 298–99, 300f, 301–3
Hebbian learning enabled by, 307–309
reorganization through, 312–14, 313f
Disk-ring stimulation, 112–13, 112f, 117f, 133f
Distractor interference, 146–47

Donoghue, J.P., 272, 283, 310
Dorsolateral prefrontal cortex (DLPFC), 264f
Doyon, J., 259, 260f, 270, 271, 271f
Driver, J., 137, 138, 138f, 139, 140f, 143f, 145f, 146
Duret, F., 217
Durgin, F.H., xvi
Dynamic induction, 66, 67f, 68–69
Dystonia, 287–89

Early development, 304, 308
Edge cells, 115, 119f, 120, 123, 124
EEG (electroencephalographic), 51
Egusa, H., 31
Ehrenstein figure, 84
Elbert, T., 232, 287–89
Elston, G.N., 200
End gaps, 20, 30
End-stopped cells, 301
Engel, S.A., 48
Enns, J.T., 136f, 137, 139
Equivalent current dipole (ECD) model, 237, 247n1
Evans, A.C., 259, 260f
Extra-RF effects, 180
  fast-acting disinhibition of, 7
  modulation of, 5–6
  perceptual filing-in, cortical plasticity and, 7–8
Eye
  lesioned v. normal, 191
Eysel, U.T., 218, 304, 306

FACADE
  binocular fusion, grouping, da Vinci Stereopsis and, 26
  boundary enrichment and, 34
  boundary grouping, surface filling-in and, 16–28, 34
  boundary invisibility for, 16, 17f, 18–19, 20, 33
  from boundary-surface complementarity to consistency, 28, 32, 34
  brightness constancy, contrast and assimilation and, 22–25, 23f
  macrocircuit of BCS and FCS, 28–30, 29f
  meaning of, 34
  multiple scales into multiple boundary depths and, 26–27
  object recognition v. seeing unoccluded parts and, 27–28, 27f
  principles and mechanisms, 28–34, 29f, 31f
  surfaces, seeing and, 19–22
  three-dimensional surface capture, filling-in and, 25
  three-dimensional vision, figure-ground separation and, 25–28, 27f
Facchini, S., 262
FCS. See Feature Contour System (FCS)
Feature Contour System (FCS), 24
  BCS interaction with, 28–29, 29f, 30–34
  definition of, 21–22
  depth-selective, 30–31
  monocular, 29f, 31
Feature-integration theory, 135
Feedback, 2, 167
  bipole/hypercomplex cell, 30
  boundary processing, coding, visual completion and, 154–59
  cellular, retina, LGN, 19
  color, 111
  complementarity/consistency, 28
  contrast signals and inhibitory, 165
  cortical, 73, 155
  EEG, 51
  FCS-to-BCS, 32–33, 34
  inhibitory, 165, 313f, 314
  of lateral connectivity, 41, 52–53
  MT Cells and modulatory, 164
  neuron properties in Macaque cortex and, 40–43, 51, 52, 53
  reorganization and, 236
  in retinotopic areas, 50
  reverse hierarchy by, 97, 312
  RF, 183, 218
Feedforward, 3, 34, 40, 51, 52, 156, 159, 236, 313f
  convergent, integration, 154
  RF and, 218
Feineigle, P.A., 45
Felleman, D., 281
Field, D.J., 30
Figure-ground (segregation), 5, 81
  (directed) attention, texture filling-in and, 90–92
  border ownership and, 154, 164–67, 170
  boundary pruning influence on, 32–33
  delayed, 43
  FACADE and, 21, 22, 25–28, 30
  relative depths and, 30
  scotomas and, 99
  single-neuron properties in Macaque cortex and, 41–43
  stabilized, border, 42
  textural filling-in, degradation and, 92, 99
  textural filling-in, perceptual salience and, 89–90, 90f
  texture filling-in, horizontal connections, lateral spread of neutaral activity, 95–96
  3D vision and, 22, 25–28, 27f, 32

Filling-in domains (FIDO), 24, 26, 29, 29f, 32
  binocular, 29f, 33–34
  brightness and, 32
  illuminant-discounted, 29f, 31
  monocular, 29f, 31, 32–33
Filling-in, perceptual
  cognitive, 177
  finding out v., xix
  meaning of, xv, 59, 81, 128
  neural v.., x, 128
  qualia laden, xvii–xix
  sewn up and, 129, 202
  two types of, 177
Findlay, J.M., 219
Finger training task, 265, 266f, 267, 268f
Fiorani, M., xvi, 41, 95, 180–81
Fischl, B., 48
Fischman, A.J., 261
Fitzpatrick, D., 183
Fixation
  color filling-in and, 106, 112–13, 123, 125
  hemianopic, 215, 220f
  texture filling-in and, 83, 86, 92, 96, 99
Fleming, W.C., 285
Flickering stimuli, 82
fMRI. *See* Functional magnetic resonance imaging
Focal hand dystonia, 287–89
Forebrain, 309–10, 312
Frackowiak, R.S., 258
Fregnac, Y., 77
Freund, T.F., 309
Friedman, D., 310
Friedman, H.S., 112
Friston, K.J., 51, 258
Frost, B.J., 181
Frutiger, S.A., 261
Fuchs, W., 210, 212t
Functional magnetic resonance imaging (fMRI)
  motor skills, reorganization and, 252, 258–59, 260f
  neural field large in, 43
  as neuroimaging, 43–44, 44f, 49, 49f, 51–52
  temporal/spatial resolution poor for, 43

GABA, 198
GABAergic circuitry
  classical RF and, 297
  in different sensory systems, 296–97
  disihibition, attention and, 309–10
  disinhibition's long-term effects, neural interpolation and, 303–4, 305f, 306–9
  disinhibition's short-term effects, neural interpolation and, 298–99, 300f, 301–3
  Hebbian learning and, 308
  motor learning and, 272, 273
  remapping in visual system and, 304, 306
  RF surround and, 297–98
  somatosensory system, spatial limits of neural interpolation and, 302–3
  visual system, spatial limits of neural interpolation and, 299, 300f, 301–2
GAD. *See* Glutamic acid decarboxylase (GAD)
Gain control mechanism, (Neural), 157, 169
Gama-aminobutyric acid (GABA). *See* GABA
Gamma band response, 243f, 244
Gandolfo, F., 256
Garraghty, PE, 6, 303
Gassel, M.M., 211, 212f, 214
Gattass, R., xvi, 41, 92, 94, 95, 180–81, 299
Gawryszenski. L.G., 181
Gedanken experiment, 63
Gelade, G., 135
Gene expression, 308
Geometry, 15, 19
Gerlott, C., 287
Gerrits, H.J.M., 83, 107, 110, 114, 168
Gestalt grouping, 39, 39f, 44, 45–47, 47f, 131, 164, 210, 244
  apperceptive completion of, 208
  texture segregation for, 46
Gilbert, C.D., xii, 96, 97, 182, 183, 189, 190, 195, 232, 299, 301, 303
Girard, P., 55
Girard-Madoux, P., 212f
Glaeser, L., 77
Glaucoma, 98–99
Glutamic acid decarboxylase (GAD), 298, 304, 306
Goodale, M.A., 180–81
Gordon, J., 167
Gore, J.C., 45
Grabowecky, M., 137, 138f, 139
Grafman, J., 258
Grafton, S.T., 258, 261
Grajski, K.A., 290
Gregory, Richard, xii
Gregory, R.L., 183
Gritti, I., 309
Gross, C.G., 201
Grossberg, S., 22, 23, 25, 30, 31, 159, 181

Halgren, E., 52
Hallett, M., 256, 257f, 258, 262, 287
Halligan, P.W., 213f

Hansen, T., 160
Harden, C., 97
Harris, J.M., 91
Hayes, A., 30
Hazeltine, E., 261
He, Z.J., 135, 136f, 139
Hebb, D., 307
Hebbian learning, 307–9
Heilman, K.M., 218
Heim, S., 232
Heinen, S.J., 189, 190
Heisenberg Uncertainity Principle, 15
Hemianopia, xiii, 97, 207, 208, 210, 214, 221
  fixation gaze with, 215
  pseudo, 218
  weakness of attention of, 219
Hendry, S.H., 296
Hermann grid, 25
Hess, G., 30, 310
Hindlimb area (HKA), 265
Hirsch, J.A., 183
Hocking, D., 195
Hogan, N., 261
Hogg, T.M., 265, 272
Hole/No Hole condition, 300f
Homunculus, xiii
Horizontal connections, 30, 53, 73–76, 169, 218, 311–12, 313f
  boundary processing and, 152, 154, 168
  color filling-in and, 108f, 110, 111
  containment of, 298
  cortical plasticity and, 272
  RF and, 183, 198
  single-neuron properties in Macaque cortex and, 40–43, 52
  surface processing and, 159
  texture filling-in, lateral spread of neural activity, figure-ground segregation and, 95–96
  visual cortex and weak, 195
Horizontal connections. *See also* Lateral connectivity
Hornak, J., 213f, 219
Horton, J., 195
Hradek, G.T., 290
Hubel, D.H., 40
Human rabbit, xix–xx
Huntley, G.W., 272
Hupe, J.M., 55
Hypercomplex cells, 29–30, 31f

Illuminant. *See* Discounting the illuminant
Illusory color
  color filling-in and, 113, 125, 128, 131, 134, 145f, 146
Illusory contour, 4, 16, 17t, 18, 44, 113, 125, 128, 129, 130f, 148. *See also* Kanizsa square
  boundary processing, visual completion and, 153f, 154, 155, 158
  inward, oriented forming, 17f, 18
  isomorphic and symbolic process and, 50, 53
  single-neuron, contextual shape processing and, 41
  stereo-defined shape v. shape of, 48, 49f
  texture filling-in and, 84
Illusory square. *See* Illusory contour
Image reflectance, distortions, 23f, 24
Independent component analysis, 244
Inferotemporal cortex, 5, 13, 14t
Inhibition, 312. *See also* Disinhibition
  deafferentation and modulation of, 313f
  excitation balancing, neocortical circuits and, 307
  excitation balancing, perceptual completion and, 303
  formation of RF, 296
  GABAergic circuitry and, 272, 273, 296–98
  Gaussian distribution of, 298
  perceptual filling-in and contribution by, 299, 300f
  remapping, filling-in and, 296–312
  sensory function and, 296–98
Injury. *See* Peripheral injury
Injury, neurological, 290–91
  reorganization, altered limb and, 283–84
  reorganization, CI therapy's other applications and, 289–90
  reorganization, focal hand dystonia treatment and, 287–89
  reorganization, limb nonuse and, 284–85
  reorganization, therapy for learned nonuse and, 285–87, 286f
Interblob cortical processing stream, 14f, 16, 18
Interpolation
  anisotropic, 307
  blind spot/scotoma, 38, 95, 178, 179f, 180–84
  contextual, 52, 53
  for continuity (of normal perception), 8
  contour, xvi, 3, 4, 5, 41, 184
  disinhibition's long-term effects and GAGAergic modulation of limits on neural, 303–4, 305f, 306–9
  disinhibition's short-term effects and GAGAergic modulation of limits on neural, 298–99, 300f, 301–3

figure-ground segregation for, 91
higher-order, 50
neural, 295–96, 298–99, 300f, 301–4, 305f, 306–9, 312, 313–14
occlusion and, 3, 4
remapping and, 81
RF, 178, 179f, 180–82, 182f, 184, 295
of spatially collinear stimulus, 179, 181
surface, xvi, xx, 3, 4, 5
symbolic, 49–50
texture filling-in and fast, 85–89, 87f, 88f, 99
texture filling-in and slow, 85, 99
texture filling-in, boundary representation and, 81–84, 96, 99
varying time scales for, 7
of visual information, 2
Interstimulus interval (ISI), 270, 271f
Invisibility
boundary, 16, 17f, 18–19, 20, 33, 41, 108
Ipsilateral stimulation, 42
Isochronous baseline condition (ISO), 270, 271f
Isomorphic representation, 81, 154
filling-in theory, 107, 109–10, 111, 116, 121, 123
symbolic process v., 50, 53
visual cortex, 3–4, 5, 49–50, 53, 59, 92
Ito, M., 182, 183
Ivry, R., 261

Jackson, S.R., 213f, 216
Jacobs, K.M., 272
James, A.C., 55
James-Galton, M., 211
Jeannerod, M., 212f
Jenkins, W.M., 262, 266f, 269, 282, 283, 284, 290
Jezzard, P., 267, 268f, 283
Jiang, H., 44
Jones, B.E., 309
Jones, E.G., 296

Kaas, J.H., 6, 189, 191, 200, 281, 303
Kaelin-Lang, A., 273
Kamitani, Y., 217
Kandel, E.R., 308
Kanizsa, G., 141
Kanizsa square, 16, 17f, 18, 21, 27–28, 32, 34, 38, 39f, 46, 47f, 48, 49, 49f, 137, 138f130f, 142f, 143, 152, 153f, 154
Kanizsa-Minguzzi, 25
Kanizsa-Varin, 34
Kapadia, M.K., 97, 182
Karni, A., 267, 268f, 283, 310

Kasamatsu, T., 183
Kastner, S., 46, 96
Katz, L.C., 308
Kaufman, L., 247n1
Kawabata, N., 183
Kellman, P.J., 30, 129, 131, 139–40, 148, 167, 168
Kelly, F., 30
Kennedy, W.A., 44
Kinsbourne, M., xiii
Kleim, J.A., 265, 272
Knierim. J.J., 96
Koch, C., 51
Koffka-Benussi ringeffect, 25
Kofler, M., 262
Kooistra, C.A., 218
Kopylev, L., 273
Korodi, K., 306
Krebs, H.I., 261
Krubitzer, L.A., 189, 191, 200
Kwong, K.K., 44

Lamme, V.A., 42, 51, 96
Lamotrigine (LG), 273
Land Modrian, 25
Landis, T., 97, 217
Lando, J.F., 283
Langston, A.L., 189, 191
Lashley, K., 83
Lateral connectivity, 41, 52–53
Lateral geniculate nucleus (LGN), 13, 14t, 15, 16, 69, 70, 73, 107, 161–162115, 187, 199–200, 302
dLGN, 178f, 180, 182f
restricted retinal lesions on neurons in, 195, 196f, 197
Lateral occipital complex (LOC), 50, 56
gestalt grouping and, 47f
neuroimaging and, 44–45, 45f
recognition and, 50
symbolic process in, 49
3D structure, global perception and, 48–49
Lateral spreading. See Horizontal connections
Learned condition (LRN), 270, 271f
Learned nonuse, 285–87, 286
Ledden, P.J., 44
Lesions
edge frequencies, 233–34, 239, 247
functional, 239–42
motor, 283
Lesions, retinal, 5–6. See also Reorganization
artificial scotoma and, 198
bilateral, 189
binocular v. monocular, 199
functional consequences of, 199

Lesions, retinal (*Continued*)
  LGN neurons and restricted, 195, 196*f*, 197
  localization, 212*f*–213*f*, 215–16, 216*f*
  monocular, 188–89, 190–95, 233
  MT (middle temporal) cells and, 200–202, 201*f*
  occipital, 216–17, 216*f*, 221–22, 223
  parietal, 216–17, 216*f*, 219, 221–22, 223–24
  restricted monocular, 190–92, 193*f*–194*f*, 195, 195*f*
  RF and borders of, 218
Levi, D.H., 97
Levi, D.M., xvi, 97
Leyton, A.S.F., 281
LGN. *See* Lateral geniculate nucleus (LGN)
Li, C., 256
Liepert, J., 256, 257*f*, 258
Lightness scission, 25
Lincoln, N.B., 219
Lingelbach, B., 66
LOC. *See* Lateral occipital complex (LOC)
Lombert, S.G., 55
Long-term depression, 242, 272
Long-term potentiation, 242, 272–73, 308
  attention, disinhibition and, 309–11
Lou, L., 90, 91
Lu, A.K., 48
Luminance. *See also* Brightness
  constraint of modal completion and, 141–44
Luminance sweeps, 63, 64*f*, 65

M1. *See* Motor cortex (M1)
Magnetic resonance imaging (MRI), 243*f*, 247, 267, 271*f*
Magnetoencephalographic (MEG) technique, 50, 52, 231, 235*f*, 239–41, 242, 244, 245, 247*n*1
Mainville, L., 309
Malach, R., 44
Marcel, A.J., 213*f*, 216, 222
Marois, R., 45
Marques, R.F., 181
Marshall, J.C., 213*f*
Massed practice (therapy), 286, 289–90
Mattingley, J.B., 146
Maunsell, J.H.R., 200
Mazziotta, J.C., 258
McCarthy, R.A., 211, 213*f*
McCollough effect, 22, 134
McLoughlin, N., 22
MEG. *See* Magnetoencephalographic (MEG) technique

Memory
  cells, 256
  short-term, xvii, xviii, xix
Mendola, J.D., 48, 52
Merzenich, M.M., 232, 262, 266*f*, 269, 281, 282, 283, 284, 290, 308
Meskenaite, V., 309
Metelli Rule
  amodal completion and, 142–43, 142*f*, 144
  inconsistent with, 142*f*, 143–44
  modal completion and, 141–44, 142*f*
Meyer, G., 267, 268*f*, 283
Michotte, A., 131–32
Middle temporal (MT) cells/neurons, 163–64, 200–202, 201*f*
Miller, N.E., 285
Milliken, G.W., 262, 266*f*, 269, 283
Milner, A.D., 180–81
Mingolla, E., 22, 181
Mishkin, M., 6, 303
Mitz, A.R., 255
Mizobe, K., 183
Modal completion, 38
  attention spreading, amodal and, 144–48, 145*f*
  blind spot and, 128–29, 130*f*
  definition of, 33
  depth and, 146–47
  filled-in with illusory brightness and color for, 131
  in front of surrounding inducers, 132
  functional roles similar to amodal and, 132–34, 133*f*
  illusory color/brightness and, 145*f*, 146–47
  isolating filling-in and amodal v., 130–31
  Kanizsa square and, 130*f*
  literature and, 135–48
  luminance and constraint of, 141–44
  Metelli Rule and, 141–44, 142*f*
  parallel vision and, 134, 135, 138–39, 140*f*, 141, 144
  shape and, 131, 132
  shape completion process and, 134
  visual attention and, 134
  visual-search tasks, amodal and, 135, 136*f*, 137–39, 138*f*, 140*f*, 141–44, 142*f*, 148
Mondrian stimulus, 60, 74, 75*f*, 76
Monocular lesions, 188–89, 190–92, 193*f*–194*f*, 195, 195*f*, 233
Monocular processing, 28–29
Moody, S.L., 255
Moore, C., 48

Motion
    color and, 13
    visual, 163–64
Motor Activity Log (MAL), 285–87
Motor area, supplementary (SMA), 254, 255, 270
Motor cortex (M1)
    functional reorganization, physiological/neurobiological correlates of, 271–73
    functional reorganization, retention of motor skill learning and, 270–71, 271f, 274
    functional reorganization after extensive practice, animal data and, 263, 264f, 265, 266f
    functional reorganization after extensive practice, human data and, 267, 268f–269f, 269–70
    peripheral somatic changes and, 283
    rapid functional reorganization, animal data and, 255–56
    rapid functional reorganization, human data and, 256–62, 257f, 260f
    skilled motor behaviors' consolidation and, 262–63
    therapy and, 287
Motor skill learning. *See also* Plasticity, motor skill learning, adult M1 cortex and
    attention, disinhibition and, 309–11
    definition of, 252–53
    functional anatomy of, 254–55
Motoyoshi, I., 86
Movement, interpolation of, 8. *See also* Somatotopy
MRI. *See* Magnetic resonance imaging (MRI)
MT. *See* Middle temporal (MT) cells/neurons
Muellbacher, W., 262
Munker-White, Benary cross, 43
Murakami, I., 183
Musicians, 232, 245, 246f, 247, 288–89

Nakayama, K., 86, 135, 136f, 139, 169
Navon figure, 45
Nealey, T.A., 200
Neglect, 212f–213f, 218–19, 220f
Neglect dyslexia, 219
Nelson, J.I., 181
Nelson, R.J., 281
Neon color spreading, 17f, 20, 34
Nepomuceno, C.S., 285
Neumann, H., 86, 158, 160
Neuroimaging
    flat map of, 44–45, 44f, 45f

fMRI, 43–44, 44f, 49, 49f, 51–52, 252, 258–59, 273
    lack of consistency, motor skills and, 258–61, 260f
    PET, 43, 45, 236, 252, 258–61, 260f, 270, 271f, 273
    of visual cortex and, 43–51, 44f, 45f, 47f, 49f
Neurons. *See* Cortical neurons; Pyramidal neurons; Visual neurons
Nguyen, T.T., 97
Nissen, M.J., 258
NMDA. *See* N-methyl-D-asparte (NMDA)
N-methyl-D-asparte (NMDA), 239, 272, 273, 308, 310
Noë, A., xix, 22
Noise-field campimentry, 98
Nonretinotopic brain regions, 5, 49
Norcia, A.M., 183
Nothdurft, H.C., 96
Novack, T.A., 285
Nudo, R.J., 262, 265, 266f, 269, 272, 283

Object file, 110
Object recognition, 39–40
    seeing unoccluded parts v., 27–28, 27f
Object representations, 154
Occipital lesions, 216–17, 216f, 221–22, 223
Occipital lobe, 44, 44f
Occipitotemporal pathway, 3, 50
Occlusion, 3, 4
Ogmen, H., 97
Oliveira, L., 181
Ommaya, A.K., 6, 303
ON- and OFF- contrast, 160f, 161, 162, 163, 165, 166f, 168
On-center-off-surround network of cells, 23–24, 23f, 157
Orban, G.A., 304, 306
Orientation contrast, 89
Owen, A.M., 259, 260f

Pack, C., 163
Pacmen, 21, 137, 139, 140f
Pantev, C., 287
Pantoja, J.H., 181
Paradiso, M.A., 42, 86, 169
Parallel vision, 134, 135, 136f, 137, 138–39, 140f, 141, 143–44
Parietal cortex, 14t, 271
Pascual-Leone, A., 258
Pathological visual completion
    antiextinction and, 222
    biased spatial attention and, 218–19, 220f

Pathological visual completion (*Continued*)
  definition of, 207
  eccentric fixation and, 215, 223
  eye movement toward affected hemifield and, 214, 223
  functional brain imaging techniques for, 223–24
  interhemispheric interactions for, 221–22
  lesion localization and, 212f–213f, 215–16, 216f
  mental disorientation and, 211
  neglect or extinction for, 212f–213f
  neuroanatomical considerations for, 216f, 215218
  partial and whole shapes in, 209f, 211, 212f–213f, 215–216208–210, 216f, 221, 223
  residual vision in affected hemifield and, 212, 214
  Sprague effect and, 221
  veridical perception of whole shapes and, 211, 212f–213f, 215–16, 216f
Pathological visual completion. *See also* Lesions, retinal
Payne, B.R., 55
Penhume, V.B., 270, 271f
Pentera, L.J., 181
Pereira, A., 181
Perenin, M.T., 212f
Perimetric visual field map, 208, 209f
Peripheral injury, 2. *See also* Deafferentation
  long-term cortical remapping induced by, 6–7
  RF structure and, 5
Peripheral sensory nerves, 232–33
Pesenti, A., 289
Pessoa, L., xix, 22, 86, 160, 166
PET. *See* Positron emission tomography (PET)
Peterhans, E., 41, 181
Petrides, M., 259, 260f
Pettet, M.W., 96, 97, 183, 299
Phantom limb, 6
  reorganization, auditory cortex and, 233, 236–37, 239
  reorganization, movement and, 284–85
  RF and, 302–3
  therapy and, 289, 291, 403
Phelps, M.E., 258
Pigarev, I.N., 96
Pitch, 242, 245
Plant, G.T., 211, 213f
Plasticity. *See also* Reorganization; Remapping
  associative, 308
  by disinhibition, 308–9
Plasticity, cortical, 210, 309–11
  extra-RF effects, perceptual filling-in and, 7–8
  reorganization and, 190–91
Plasticity, cortical sensorimotor, 290–91
  in animals, 281–83
  CI therapy's other applications and, 289–90
  focal hand dystonia treatment and, 287–89
  forced-use, shaping and, 286
  injury adaptations, limb use and, 283–84
  limb nonuse, cerebral injury and, 284–85
  reorganization adaptations to injury in humans and, 283–84
  therapy for learned nonuse, cerebral injury and, 285–87, 286f
Plasticity, human auditory cortical
  following deafferentation, 232–33, 232f, 237, 247
  functional deafferentation and, 239–42
  functional organization of, 231
  learning in discrimination of virtual auditory objects and, 242, 243f, 244
  long-term, 245–47, 274
  in musicians, 232, 245, 246f, 247
  principles of cortical reorganization and, 232–33, 232f
  reorganization in tinnitus and, 235f, 236–39, 238f
  short-term, 239–42, 241f
Plasticity, motor skill learning, adult M1 cortex and
  definition of, 252–53
  functional anatomy of, 254–55
  functional reorganization and retention of, 270–71, 271f, 274
  functional reorganization, physiological/neurobiological correlates of, 271–73
  functional reorganization after extensive practice, animal data and, 263, 264f, 265, 266f
  functional reorganization after extensive practice, human data and, 267, 268f–269f, 269–70
  horizontal connections and, 272
  M1's contribution to consolidation of, 262–63
  rapid functional reorganization, animal data and, 255–56
  rapid functional reorganization, human data and, 256–62, 257f, 260f

single-cell plasticity and, 256
    TMS, TES and, 256–59, 257f, 262, 263, 264f, 273
Plasticity, neuronal, xx
Poewe, W., 262
Polat, U., 183
Pollack, M., 212f
Polley, E.H., 189, 191
Pons, T.P., 6, 303
Pop-out stimulus, 143
    amodal completion and, 135, 136f, 137
    texture filing-in and, 86, 87f, 96
Poppelreuter, Walther, 208–10, 212t, 213, 217, 219
Positron emission tomography (PET), 43, 45, 236
    motor skills, reorganization and, 252, 258–61, 260f, 270, 271f
Postsynaptic potentials, 77
Pow, D.V., 306
Presty, S., 258
Priori, A., 289
Pyramidal neurons, 296–97, 298

Qu Ying, 306
Qualia
    fill-in with, xvii–xix, xx
    as irrevocable, xvii–xix
    (four) laws of, xvii
    linked with attention, xvii
    sensory, xviii
    short-term memory and, xvii, xviii, xix

Raizada, R.D.S., 30
Ramachandran, V.S., 91, 213f
Random-dot stereogram, 132, 133f
Rao, R.P.N., 155
Rapid eye movement (REM), 310
Rau, H., 287, 289
Rauch, S.L., 261
Reaction time (RT), 147
Recanzone, G.H., 232, 290
Receptive field (RF), 187, 295, 297, 308. *See also* Extra-RF effects
    amputation/anesthesia and expansion of, 6
    artificial scotomas and, 300f, 301, 302, 312–13
    attention and, 91
    borders of lesions and, 218
    classical, xii–xiii, 1, 4, 5, 40–41, 181–82, 182f, 198, 297, 299
    collinear, 181, 183
    color filling-in and, 108f, 110, 111, 115, 123
    cutaneous, 282
    as deceptive field, xiii
    dynamic, xx, 218, 299
    edge-selective, 108f, 110
    expansion, 6, 97, 99, 183, 189, 239, 299, 302, 303, 306, 307, 312, 314
    feedback, 183, 218
    fixation and, 92
    GABAergic contributions and, 297–98, 306
    horizontal connections and, 183, 198
    inhibition and, 296, 299, 300f, 307
    interpolated, 178, 179f, 180–82, 182f, 184
    luminance of patches of, 74, 75f, 76
    maps, 194f–195f
    masked, 82, 182f
    of MT, 201f, 202
    neuron and, 69–70, 71f, 72, 74, 75f, 76
    nonclassical, 181–82
    nonlinear, 181
    peripheral injury and, 5
    phantom limb and, 302–3
    primary visual cortex (V1) and, 3
    retinal lesions and changes of, 5–6
    retinotopy and, 3
    sensory, 297
    striate/extrastriate, 301
    surround (extra), 1–2, 5–6, 7–8, 40–41, 297–98
    surround stimulus for, 77, 78f
    surround suppression of, 74, 96, 298
    tactile, 305f
    (dynamic) texture impinging on, 92, 93f, 99
Recognition, 50, 51
Rees, G., 51
Regression techniques, 261–62
Regularity contrast, 89
Regularization theory, 86
Reich, L.N., 97
Reid, R.C., 25
Reidel, C.N., 265, 272
Remapping, 2, 5
    excitation/inhibition in neocortical circuits, completion and, 307
    fast interpolation and, 7–8
    inhibition, filling-in and, 296–312
    interpolation and, 81
    peripheral injury and skill learning inducing, 6–7
    sensorimotor, 282–83
    slow interpolation and, 7–8
    somatosensory system, 303–4, 305f, 306
    of visual space in cortex, scotoma, texture filling-in, 96–97, 307
    visual system, 299–301, 304, 306, 307

Remple, M.S., 265, 272
Rensink, R.A.., 136*f*, 137, 139
Reorganization, 2, 97, 99
  in adult cortex, 233, 242, 255–62, 270–73
  after cortical lesions, 199–202, 201*f*
  bilateral lesions and, 189
  CI therapy's other applications and, 289–90
  cortical, 309–11, 314
  focal hand dystonia treatment and, 287–89
  following deafferentation, 233–34, 235*f*, 236, 237, 247
  forced-use, 286
  functional consequences of retinal lesions with, 199
  functional deafferentation and, 239–42
  functional organization of auditory cortex and, 231
  as healing, 197
  horizontal connections and, 272
  injury adaptations, limb use and, 283–84
  lateral inhibition and, 236
  learning in discrimination of virtual auditory objects and, 242, 243*f*, 244
  lesioned v. normal (nonlesioned) eye and, 191–92, 193*f*–194*f*, 195, 195*f*
  limb nonuse, cerebral injury and, 284–85
  long-term, 245–47, 274
  long-term potentiation and, 242
  M1 after extensive practice, animal data and functional, 263, 264*f*, 265, 266*f*
  M1 after extensive practice, human data and functional, 267, 268*f*–269*f*, 269–70
  M1, animal data and rapid functional, 255–56
  M1, human data and rapid functional, 256–62, 257*f*, 260*f*
  M1, and physiological/neurobiological correlates of functional, 271–73
  monocular lesions and, 188–89, 190–92, 193*f*–194*f*, 195
  MT (middle temporal) cells and, 200–202, 201*f*
  in musicians, 232, 245, 246*f*, 247
  principles of, 232–33, 232*t*
  reactivated cortical neurons with, 197
  recovery mechanisms for, 198
  recovery of responsiveness and, 189–90
  recovery times for, 192, 194*f*, 195, 195*f*, 197
  restricted monocular lesions and, 190–92, 193*f*–194*f*, 195, 195*f*
  restricted retinal lesions on LGN neurons and, 195, 196*f*, 197
  retention of motor skill learning, M1 and functional, 270–71, 271*f*, 274
  in retinotopic representations, 187–88
  sequence of reactivation and, 189–90
  shaping for, 286
  short-term, 239–42, 241*f*
  slow, 303
  somatosensory cortex, 187–88
  striate/extrastriate cortex, filling-in scotoma and, 202
  therapy for learned nonuse, cerebral injury and, 285–87, 286*f*, 289–90
  through disinhibition, 312–14, 313*f*
  in tinnitus, 235*f*, 236–39, 238*f*
  TMS, TES and, 256–59, 257*f*, 262, 273, 285, 287
  use-dependent, 282, 290–91
  of visual cortex following damage, 188–89
Reppas, J.B., 44
Retina. *See also* Lesions, retinal; Visual cortex
  blind spot in, 16, 21, 177
  contralateral, 41
  light impinging on, 13, 14*t*
  stabilization, 110
Retinal ganglion cells, 70
Retinex algorithm, 162–63
Retinex theory, 25
Retinopathy, diabetic, 97
Retinotopy, 3–4, 195
Rey-Hipolito, C., 267, 268*f*
RF. *See* Receptive field (RF)
Rioult-Pedotti, M.S., 310
Rittenhouse, C.D., 42
RMS (root mean squared) field value, 240, 241*f*, 244
Rocha-Miranda, C.E., xvi, 41, 95, 181
Rock, I., 183
Rockstroh, B., 287
Rodman, H.R., 201
Rodriguez-Rodriguez, V., 42
Roelfsema, P.R., 51
Rogers-Ramachandran, D., xiii
Rosa, M.G.P., xvi, 41, 95, 196, 200
Rosen, B.R., 44
Rosier, A.M., 304
Ross, W.D., xvi, 41, 95
Rossi, A.F., 42
Rostral forelimb area (RFA), 265
Rottenberg, D.A., 261
Rubenstein, B.S., 310
Rubin, R.H., 261

Safran, A.B., 97, 217
Sagi, S., 310

Salience, perceptual, 89–90, 90*f*
Sameshine, K., 282
Sanes, J.N., 283
Savage, C.R., 261
Sawaki, L., 273
Scarlato, G., 289
Schäfer, T., 289
Schiller, P.H., 96
Schioppa, C.P., 256
Schmid, L.M., 191
Schofield, B., 183
Schwark, H.D., 296
Schweigart, G., 218, 306
Scopolamine, 273
Scotoma, completion through, 177–80, 178*f*, 179*f*, 303
   half-bars v. full bars and, *179*, 180–81, 182*fi*
   interpolated RF for, 178, 179*f*, 180–82, 182*f*, 184
Scotomas. *See also* Artificial scotomas
   Amsler grid for, 98, 98*f*
   artificial scotomas v., 99
   color filling-in with, 106, 108, 110
   cortical, xiii–xiv, 217–18
   fast texture filling-in for, 94–95
   filling in by surrounding colors/patterns for, xi–xii, 83
   illusionary strip v. horizontal lines and, xiv
   large v. small objects/lines and, xiii–xiv, xvi
   lesions and, 192, 195*f*
   monocular v. binocular, 199
   neural interpolation and, 301, 302
   noise-field campimetry for, 98
   occipital, 217–18
   paracentral homonymous, 217
   permanent, 7
   red color and, xiv
   remapping of visual space in cortex, texture filling-in and, 96–97, 307
   reorganization, striate/extrastriate cortex and filling-in, 202
   retinal imperfections for, 18, 83
   ring, 98–99
   texture filling-in and, 82–84, 82*f*, 87, 94–95, 96–97, 97–99, 98*f*
   TMS inducing, 217
Seach slopes, 135, 139, 143
Selective enhancement, 91
Sensory activation
   top-down v. bottom-up, xviii, 4, 156*f*
Sensory cortex, 1
Sepp, W., 158

Sergent, J., xiii, 211, 213*f*, 215
Serial reaction time (SRT), 258
Shape
   completion process, 131, 132, 134
   illusory contour v. stereo-defined, 48, 49*f*, 50
   outlines of, 151
   whole, 208–10, 212*f*–213*f*
Shaping, 286
Shapley, R., 25, 167
Sharp contrast, 89, 153*f*
Shatz, C.J., 308
Sherrington, C.S., 281
Shimojo, S., 217
Shipley, T.F., 30, 129, 131, 139–40, 148, 167, 168
Shunting, 157
Sidtis, J.J., 261
Signal theory, 162
Silberpfennig, J., 218
Skavenski, A.A., 189, 190
Skill learning, 2
   attention, disinhibition and, 309–11
   long-term cortical remapping induced by, 6–7
Smith, E.., 90, 91
Somatosensory cortex (SMA/SI), 187–88, 232, 259, 282, 309
Somatosensory system
   GABAergic circuitry and, 296–97, 302–3
   remappping and, 303–4, 305*f*, 306
Somatotopy, 3, 6
Souza, A.O., 181
Spatial neglect, 218–19, 220*f*
Spekreijse, H., 42, 51
Spillmann, L., 89
Sprague effect, 221
Sprague, J.M., 221
Squarewave grating, 66, 67*f*
Stabilized images, 59
   color filling-in and, 106
   figure-ground and, 42–43
Sterr, A., 287
Stimulus offset asynchrony (SOA), 60–61
Straight lines, 177
Striate neurons/cortex, 60, 69, 70, 71*f*, 72, 73, 74, 76, 77, 79, 88, 107, 179, 184, 201–2, 222
Stroke hemiparesis, 285
Strother, S.C., 261
Stürzel, F., 89
Sugita, T., 303
Suner, S., 283
Superior temporal sulcus (STS), 201*f*, 231

Sur, M., 281
Surface capture, 20, 25–26, 31
Surface cells, 115, 116, 117*f*, 118–19, 118*f*
Surface completion. *See* Surface filling-in
Surface filling-in. *See also* Texture filling-in
  binocular fusion, grouping, da Vinci Stereopsis and, 26
  boundary bias of, 59
  from boundary-surface complementarity to consistency, 28, 32, 34
  brightness, and fast v. slow, 66, 68
  brightness, backward masking, and disruption of, 60–61, 62*f*, 63, 64*f*, 65
  brightness constancy, contrast and assimilation and, 22–25, 23*f*, 38
  brightness, surface formation and, 20, 21, 69, 160
  brightness/luminance sweeps and precepts of, 63, 64*f*, 65
  discounting illuminant in, 19–20, 21–22, 23*f*, 24, 31, 161–63, 162*f*
  end gaps and, 20, 30
  FACADE, boundary grouping and, 16–28, 34
  Feature Contour System (FCS) for, 21–22, 24
  filling-in domains (FIDO) for, 24, 26, 29*f*, 31–34
  multiple scales into multiple boundary depths and, 26–27
  neural synchronization and, 43
  object recognition v. seeing unoccluded parts and, 27–28, 27*f*
  on-center-off-surround network of cells and, 23–24, 23*f*, 157
  outward, unoriented, 17*f*, 20–21
  seeing from surfaces and, 19–22
  sensitivity to contrast polarity and, 17*f*, 21
  simplest network of, 23*f*, 24
  single-neuron properties and, 42–43
  stabilized figure-ground border and, 42–43
  surface pruning signals for, 33
  surface stimuli for, 42
  3-D surface capture and, 25–26, 34
Surface processing
  coding principle, visual neural mechanism for boundary processing and, 152, 153*f*, 154
  diffusion as computational metaphor for, 160–61, 160*f*, 161*f*
  early active processes of regional completion for, 159–60
  vision complētion for, 159–61, 160*f*

Surface signals
  color filling-in, and border signals, 116–20, 117*f*, 118*f*, 119*f*, 121, 122*f*, 123–25
Surround suppression, 74
Sylvian fissure, 231
Symbolic representation, 49–50, 53
Synaspses, 198, 308
Synchrony, 52, 91, 308, 311
Sziklas, V., 259, 260*f*

Tachistoscopic measures, 209*f*, 210, 215, 219, 220*f*
Tagging, 166–67, 170
  symbolically, 4, 85
Talairach and Tournoux, 272*f*
Tanne, D., 310
Taub, E., 6, 285, 287–89, 303
TES. *See* Transcranial electrical stimulation
Teuber, H.L., 212*f*, 213
Texture filling-in
  anatomical/physiological basis for, 92, 93*f*, 94–99, 98*f*
  artificial scotoma and delayed, 92, 93*f*, 94, 95
  artificial scotoma and, 82, 82*f*, 84, 96–97
  (directed) attention for figure-ground segregation and, 90–92
  background penetrating failing boundary representations and, 91
  boundary representations for, 84–85
  boundary representations, interpolation processes and, 81–84, 82*f*
  cancellation, substitution and, 85
  climbing activity, control activity and, 92, 93*f*, 94, 217, 300*f*
  clinical relevance of, 97–99, 98*f*
  color, surface signals and, 125
  contrast, 89–90, 90*f*
  delayed, adaptation, 83, 84, 85, 91
  fading of, segmentation, 88, 88*f*, 90*f*, 91, 96, 98
  fast, 94–95
  fast interpolation and, 85–89, 87*f*, 88*f*
  figure-ground segregation and, 89–90, 90*f*, 95–96
  horizontal connections, lateral spread of neutaral activity, figure-ground segregation and, 95–96
  interpolation processes and, 81–84, 82*f*, 85–89, 87*f*, 88*f*, 96, 99
  perceptual salience, figure-ground segregation and, 89–90, 90*f*
  pop-out stimulus, 86, 87*f*, 96
  prolonged fixation and, 83, 86, 92, 96, 99

regularization theory and, 86
scotoma and, 82–84, 82f, 87, 97–99, 98f
scotoma and fast, 94–95
scotoma, remapping of visual space in cortex and, 96–97
slow interpolation and, 85
suppression of, 86–88, 87f
as symbolic operation, 87
tagging area and, 85
Troxler's effect and, 82
two-stage process of, 85
Texture perception, 22
Texture segregation, 46
Thalamic sources, 199–200, 297
Thalamocortical network, 236
Therapy. *See also* Constraint-induced movement therapy (CI)
for learned nonuse, 285–87, 286f, 288–89, 311
massed practice, 286, 289–90
Thin man phenomenon, 217
Thines, G., 131–32
Thompson, E., xix, 22
3-D (vision), 21–22, 48
bias for, 39
figure-ground separation and, 25–28, 27f, 32
filling-in and surface capture of, 25–26
LOC, global perception and, 48–49
2D into, 39, 53
Tinnitus
in reorganization, 235f, 236–39, 238f
T-junctions
FACADE principles, boundary, and, 28, 30–32, 31f
groupings of, 166–67
suppression of, 165–67, 166f, 170
TMS. *See* Transcranial magnetic stimulation (TMS)
Todorovic, D., 22, 23, 159
Toldi, J., 306
Tonotopic organization (map), 231, 237–39, 238f, 304
Tootell, R.B., 44, 48
Top-down processing, xviii, 4, 156f, 164
Torjussen, T., 212f, 221
Transcranial electrical stimulation (TES), 256, 258
Transcranial magnetic stimulation (TMS), 252, 304
motor skills, rapid functional reorganization and, 256–59, 257f, 262, 273
pathological visual completion and, 217, 223, 224

repeated, 263, 264f
scotomas induced by, 217
sensorimotor plasticity and, 283, 285, 287
Transparency, 141–44, 145f, 146
Traumatic brain injury, 289
Treisman, A., 135, 137, 138f, 139
Tripathy, S.P., xvi, 97
Troxler, D., 81–82
Troxler's effect, xii, 82, 106, 123
Turner, R., 267, 268f, 283
Tweedale, R., 200
2D, 4, 27–28, 146, 163
interpreted into 3D, 39, 53
Tyler, C.W., 46

Uncertainty
hierarchical resolution of, 14t, 15–16, 20, 21–22
Ungerleider, L.G., 42, 46, 84, 89, 91, 92, 94, 98, 267, 268f, 271, 283, 316
Uswatte, G., 285

Van der Zwan, R., 181
Van Essen, D.C., 96
Vandesande, F., 304, 306
VanTuijl, H.F., 141
Vendrik, A.J.H., 83, 107, 110, 114, 168
Virtual melody, 242, 243f
Vision, completion phenomena in
amodal completion for, 166f, 167–70
aperture problem for, 163–64
border ownership, spatial occlusion and, 164–67, 166f
boundary finding, completion and, 154–55
coding principle, neural mechanism for boundary and surface processing and, 152, 153f, 154, 157, 159
computation of image flow of, 163–64
contour integration for, 157, 158f
diffusion as computational metaphor for, 160–61, 160f, 161f
discounting the illuminant and constraints of neural, 161–63, 162f
early active processes of regional completion for, 159–60
extrastriate, 199–202
integrating perceptual items and, 163–70, 166f
neural gain control mechanism for, 157, 169
object properties and, 151
outlines of shape, invariant surface attributes and, 151
a priori visual knowledge for, 155, 159

Vision, completion phenomena in (*Continued*)
  shunting mechanism for, 157
  spreading mechanism/filling-in for, 151–52
  of surface properties, 151, 159–61, 160f
  templates for, 155, 157
  unified computational framework for, 155, 156f, 157–59, 158f
Visual cortex, 181, 184. *See also* Brain, processing streams of; Cortical neurons
  attention and, 50–51
  brightness induction, and neural responses of, 69–70, 71f, 72–74, 75f, 76–77, 78f, 79
  brightness, spreading activation and, 76–77, 78f, 79
  brightness/lightness perception and constancy, lateral interactions and, 73, 75f, 76
  cortical magnification curves and, 85
  edge cells, surface cells and, 115
  flattened visualization of, 43–45, 44f, 45f, 46, 47f
  fMRI's functionability for, 43–44, 44f, 49, 49f, 51–52
  Gestalt grouping and, 39, 39f, 44, 45–47, 47f
  isomorphic, 3–4, 5, 49–50, 53, 59
  lateral occipital complex (LOC) of, 44–45, 45f, 47f, 48, 50, 56
  natural blind spot and, 38
  (functional) neuroimaging of, 43–51, 44f, 45f, 47f, 49f
  nonretinotopic brain regions of, 5, 49–50
  posterior visual (V1) areas and, 3
  primary, 3
  processing streams of, 13, 14t, 15
  recognition and, 50, 51
  remapping, scotoma, texture filling-in and, 96–97
  reorganization after damage of, 188–89
  retinotopical areas of, 3–4, 44–45, 45f, 46, 47f, 49–50, 53, 85, 86, 92
  single-neuron properties in macaque cortex and, 40–43, 51–53
  surface, shape and, 47–50, 49f
  symmetry, elemental Gestalt grouping and, 45–47, 47f
  weak lateral activation in, 195
Visual cortical cells, xiv
Visual illusions. *See* Illusory contour
Visual motion, 163–64
Visual neurons, 87
  boundary finding, completion and, 154–55
  coding principle, boundary and surface processing and, 152, 153f, 154
  color filling-in, behavioral responses and signals of, 120–23, 122f, 123–25
  color filling-in, perception v. representation of, 107–8, 108f–109f
  context sensitivity of, 5
  higher center and, 107
  neural representation v. perception and, 107–8, 108f–109f
  reactivation of deprived, 190
  single, 5, 40–43, 51–52
  synchrony, 52
Visual system
  blind spot filling-in as early stage of, xv
  GABAergic circuitry, spatial limits of neural interpolation and, 299, 300f, 301–2
  remapping, 299–301, 304, 306, 307
Visual-search tasks
  modal and amodal completion and, 135, 136f, 137–39, 138f, 140f, 141–44, 142f, 148
Volchan, E., 181
Von der Heydt, R., 41, 126, 181

Walker, R., 213f, 219
Wall, J., 281
Wang, X., 282
Warrington, E.K., 211, 212f, 219
Watanabe, T., 134
Webster, M.A., 66
Weighting functions, 154–55, 163
Weinberger, G., 232
Weiskrantz, L., 212f
Weisstein effect, 34
Welchman, A.E., 91
West Havaen-Yale Multidimensional Pain Inventory, 237
Westheimer, G., 97, 182, 183
Wiesel, T.N., xii, 40, 97, 183, 189, 190, 299, 301
Williams, D., 211, 212f, 214
Williamson, J.R., 30
Williamson, S.J., 247n1
Wilson, F., 282, 284
Wise, S.P., 255, 257f, 258, 273
Wissel, J., 262
Wouters, G., 306
Wu, Y.L., 304

Yan, J., 296
Yin, C., 167, 168
Young, A.., 213f, 219

Zhang, X., 112
Zhang, Y., 183
Zhou, H., 112
Ziemann, U., 262
Zipser, K., 96